Nicotine:
The Drug That Never Was

Volume I:

The Biggest Medical Mistake of the 20th Century

by
Chris Holmes

Copyright © 2007 by Chris Holmes

All Rights Reserved

ISBN: 978-0-9556829-0-2

A Surfeit of Evidence

Some readers may consider, by the time they reach the end of Volume I, that I have not only proved that Nicotine Replacement Therapy (NRT) is useless and based upon a myth - and therefore a scandalous waste of taxpayers' money in the UK - but made the case over and over and over again, in a way that could easily be regarded as overkill.

I had to. For if I had not made this book into an absolutely cast-iron case that nobody with half a brain could possibly refute, the backlash from the medical authorities would have been very aggressive, possibly even threatening my profession as a whole. However, as I have spent several years making this case so solid that a hefty meteorite would bounce off it, they can only read it, weep, scrap NRT and start re-writing the medical textbooks.

As for General Medical Practitioners, I am confident that all but a few will breathe a sigh of relief that they will no longer be obliged to write out prescriptions for something which doesn't work in the vast majority of cases and is obviously not medicinal.

So if I go on a bit, and repeat myself rather more than is necessary for an intelligent reader, please forgive me but it is armour-plating, I anticipate rather a lot of flak, you see. As Boo-Boo correctly observed, "The Ranger's not gonna like this, Yogi."

Dedication

This book is dedicated to the memory of Dr John Elliotson (1791-1868), who was once the President of the Royal Medical and Surgical Society and one of the Founders of University College Hospital, London, where he became its first Professor of Medicine. When I learned of what happened to him, and others like him, I became so angry at the injustice and stupidity of it that I knew I had to do something to win proper public recognition for the work of those pioneering surgeons and the role of hypnosis – which was then known as mesmerism or animal magnetism – in the dramatic success they won briefly, before prejudice and jealousy thwarted the proper development of those methods.

John Elliotson was undoubtedly one of the most talented and enthusiastic medical minds of his generation. His career was in dramatic ascendancy at the same time that the medical world stood at the threshold of exciting new discoveries about ways in which the mind of the patient can be trained to help enormously in the process of the medical treatment of disease or injury, and recovery from it. His name should be as familiar to the public as Alexander Fleming or Louis Pasteur, but he was the victim of a conspiracy of lesser men, who robbed him of the success and historic recognition that would certainly have been his, if there had not been a ruthless and idiotic campaign to stamp out mesmerism within the medical profession, exiling all those who would not conform. The result was that mind-body medicine was set back two centuries, and the mind was then knocked out of the equation completely, with ether.

Ether. Chloroform. Opium. Morphine. Heroin. Cocaine. Barbiturates. Valium. Amphetamines. Ecstasy. Prozac. Zyban. Never did anyone any harm, did they? Not much, they didn't – and all were developed and prescribed at one time or another by the medical profession, many hailed as wonder drugs. Oh, and let's not forget the most poisonous and useless one of the lot: nicotine. The only difference is, nicotine has never been a medicine because it's not a drug at all. The nicotine myth dies right here.

Mind-Body medicine is back. With a vengeance.

Table of Contents

Nicotine: The Drug That Never Was
Volume I: The Biggest Medical Mistake of the 20th Century

Acknowledgements..i
Anecdote...iii
Are You Trying to Tell Me How to Read?.................................v

Section One...1
The Emperor's New Clothes
The Biggest Medical Mistake of the 20th Century
Welcome, Skeptics!

Section Two..17
Stage Hypnosis (The Shorter Explanation)
A note on Paul McKenna
Case Mysteries No.1

Section Three...57
Cravings are Not Withdrawal Symptoms
Case Mysteries No.2

Section Four..73
Introducing: The Subconscious Mind
Case Mysteries No.3

Section Five...129
Why the Nicotine Addiction Theory is Wrong
Case Mysteries No.4

Section Six..185
Trance and Suggestion:
a). What Really Happens in a Hypnotherapy Session
b). The Role of Suggestion: How and Why We Respond

Section Seven..231
Why Nicotine is not even a Drug
also The Inhalation of Smoke
& Rattus Humanus

Section Eight..261
How we Shut Down Cravings in Therapy
Case Mysteries No.5

Section Nine..295
The Stupidity of Nicotine Replacement 'Therapy'
also, Marketing, Slander and Excuses:
i). The Promotion of a Poison
ii). Peddling Doubt
iii). Beggaring Belief

Section Ten..349
The Compulsive Habit Structure
Case Mysteries No.6
A Pause for Breath

The second volume follows directly on from the first, and the contents of that volume will be as follows:

Nicotine: The Drug That Never Was
Volume II: A Change of Mind

Section 11 <u>The Beliefs & Suggestions that Support the Habit</u>
also Smoking and Self-Harm: A Parallel

Section 12 <u>The Willpower Myth</u>
Case Mysteries No.7

Section 13 <u>Why Doctors Do Not Provide Hypnotherapy</u>
Case Mysteries No.8

Section 14 <u>Those Two Imposters: 'Success' and 'Failure'</u>
- Success Rates
- Relapse is Not Failure
- Removing the Fear of Failure

Section 15 <u>The Art of Hypnotherapy in Practice</u>
- Waking suggestion
- Some Useful Laws of Hypnotherapy
- How to Choose a Good Hypnotherapist
- How to Accept Suggestions Successfully

Section 16 <u>Stage Hypnosis (part 2)</u>
Case Mysteries No.9

Section 17 <u>Hypnotherapy v Science:</u>
The Myopia of the conscious mind (A Historical Perspective)
Case Mysteries No.10

This volume will be available in 2008.

Acknowledgements

First of all I would like to thank those clients who never turned up for their hypnotherapy appointments with me over the last few years, thus allowing me the time to write this book - and these acknowledgements, come to that. Yes, thank you, Gina Potts! (She evidently decided at the last minute to continue inhaling toxic gases for a while, and this page is the happy indirect result.) God knows I could never have written any of this at home. So if everyone who booked a hypnotherapy session with me had actually turned up there would be no book. This means that every one of you no-shows has played a part, however negatively, in the creation of a literary landmark. In fact I can truly say that I could never have completed this work without your laziness, unreliability, fecklessness, cowardice, faithlessness and procrastination! So well done.

I would also like to thank all the hypnotherapists from whom I have learned many amazing things over the years. There are too many to mention them all but I would especially like to thank Gerry Kein of Omni Hypnosis in DeLand, Florida whom I have never met but whose training videos line the bookshelves in my office, eclipsing all other contributors to the sum of my professional learnings. I think I've got about forty recordings of his teaching seminars altogether, and I still want more. Production quality endearingly poor, teaching quality pure gold. Why not go to www.omnihypnosis.com and order yourself something wonderful.

Most of all I would like to thank my family for their love and patience, especially my wife, Beverley, who has helped me enormously with the editing and proof-reading of this book, kindly explaining which bits were rubbish and pointing out when I should particularly avoid trying to be funny. I need that kind of advice because this is a very, very serious book. Please try never to forget that even if you do find yourself chuckling from time to time. Everyone likes a laugh but I would remind you that we are changing medical history here, so please, no snickering during the momentous bits. We don't want to chortle our way right out of that Nobel Prize Nomination.

Anecdote

When I was first setting up my hypnotherapy practice, I spent a good deal of time delivering little business cards to thousands of houses in the South Manchester area, because when you launch a new hypnotherapy practice there is quite a long phase at the beginning when nobody calls you at all, so you have to do something about it. One day I was approaching a house when a woman walked out of the front door and we met on the drive, whereupon I handed over my card with some polite utterance I was soon to regret.

"What's this?" she asked, with a voice like icy effluent.

"Ah, it's hypnotherapy actually. To stop smoking, that sort of thing."

"Don't smoke!" She tried to hand it back, but I was already walking away. She followed me, and caught me up on her neighbour's drive. She held the card up and announced: "This... is not... with God."

"I beg your pardon?" I felt I was owed a better sentence than that.

She glanced at the card again. "Are you... involved with this?"

"Yes." She had me there. I certainly was.

"Then you need God in your life! This is not... this is without God..."

"You mean hypnosis?"

"Yes! This... opens up the mind, and *other things* can come through!" She was the most inarticulate ranter I had ever heard, and she was boring me now so I took back my little Stop Smoking card.

"Lady," I said, "you have a very strange notion of what hypnosis is. I'm sure God would have no problem with what I do." I was tempted to add that she had a face like a melted welly but I rose above it, thanks to God.

Are You Trying to Tell Me How To Read?

Just before we begin to change medical history, I'd like to draw your attention to a couple of things. First, I would like you to notice *how* you've decided to read this book. Consider the options below for some basic guidance, then feel free to make any adjustments to suit your own position:

1. "I'm intending to read the unsubstantiated, rambling assertions of Mr Holmes with frank disbelief."

2. "I normally sit at the feet of Mr Holmes and already believe every word he utters even before he utters it."

Most people find themselves somewhere between position one and two, perhaps leaning more toward one extreme than the other. Now, human beings possess an extraordinary capacity for *learning new things,* which is one of the abilities that has enabled our species to thrive to such a ridiculous and harmful extent. However, our individual ability to learn is seriously impaired if we have *no bloody intention* of learning anything new just now, on account of the fact that we already know everything worth knowing and life is short.

Is your Learning Capacity switched on, or off? As you prepare to delve further into this, are you just going to skim through it looking out for anything you can immediately disagree with, or are you looking forward to rich new understandings and fresh knowledge? Might you be - even now perhaps - preparing a critique? Or are you setting off on a journey of discovery... maybe self-discovery... and excited about the promise of this bold exploration?

It is probably not an either/or for most people, but a bit of both. I just wanted you to recognise right at the beginning what your starting-point was: which end of the scale you were leaning towards. Then maybe at the end it will be easier to see how much the book has 'moved' you, so to speak.

The second thing I'd like to draw to your attention is the fact that *both of you* may be reading this. Of course you already knew that one of you was reading this because you are conscious of that. In other words, your conscious mind knew it was reading this.

What your conscious mind probably did not know – and might not believe, unless you already know a lot about these things – is that your Subconscious mind could well be reading it too. In fact your Subconscious mind is apt to be even more interested in this book than your conscious mind right from the start, because it will quickly pick up on the fact that this book is mainly *about* the Subconscious mind. Consequently your Subconscious is likely to get quite excited about it - so few books are!

But there's a lot in here about the conscious mind too, of course. It isn't going to feel left out. In fact this book is going to explain a lot of things that the conscious mind has often wondered about, and probably worried about too, for years. And that can't be a bad thing, can it?

Section One

The Emperor's New Clothes

Many of you will be familiar with the story of the Emperor's New Clothes, a lovely little tale of deception in which a whole country, starting with its Emperor and all his most trusted advisors and then everybody else in the land were hoodwinked - purely by suggestion - into believing that the Emperor had a magnificent new set of clothes, but that the clothes were completely invisible to a fool. This brilliant lie was devised by two unscrupulous 'tailors', who correctly guessed that most people will fall into line with an idea provided other people apparently believe it, and especially if they regard those people as superior to themselves.

So the tailors began by convincing the Emperor that the fabrics they would be bringing to show him were so fine, so magnificent, that only wise and intelligent people were able to appreciate them - indeed a complete fool would not even be able to see them at all. Naturally the Emperor couldn't wait to see them, but imagine his horror to find that he, the Emperor himself, could not see the fabrics! Now of course there were no fabrics in reality, it was all a confidence trick, but the Emperor's *fear* that this must mean he was a fool himself - and that other people would find out that he was a fool - completely overrode his critical judgement and his instinct was to protect himself by dissembling. So he pretended he could see the fabrics, and after admiring them for a while and perusing various possible choices, he began to feel comfortable with the whole pantomime and really settle into his new acting role.

Later, when his closest advisers were entrusted with an opportunity for a preview of the new outfit, they too had already been primed with the suggestion that fools could not see the clothes at all. So when they each found to their shock that they were unable to perceive them but the Emperor apparently could, their first thought was also to protect themselves by hiding their 'foolishness' from the Emperor or they would quickly lose their advisory positions. And once you have the Emperor and all his most trusted advisers singing from the same hymnsheet, who then is going to sound a wrong note? Everybody else fell into line, assuming others could see the clothes and that they were wonderful, so the safest thing to do was act as if they could see them too. Pretty soon everyone was settled into their acting role, until indeed it seemed to everyone as though the New Clothes were truly marvelous.

And then one small child, who knew nothing about the difference between wisdom and foolishness, simply stated the obvious:

"Look! The Emperor has got no clothes on!"

What has all that to do with this book? Simply this: there are certain established 'facts' that many people genuinely believe to be true, but which they originally came to believe mainly because they were told to believe that by other people, and because it seemed plausible on the face of it. This is subsequently made to seem more convincing by the fact that the majority of other people apparently believe that too. As you read what follows, there may be things that do not sound true to you at first *just because* they directly contradict 'facts' that are likely to be well-established in your mind already. Here's one now:

"I can't stop smoking because I'm addicted to nicotine!"

Sounds convincing enough, doesn't it? I mean if it wasn't true, then why would so many people say it?

Well everybody used to say the Earth was flat, and if you had been there at the time that would have been very convincing too, would it not? I mean look at it - it's flat, obviously! And yet we now know it is not, so 'common knowledge' can actually be dead wrong whilst appearing to be true: the Earth did generally seem, upon immediate observation, flat. Everyone was accustomed to that idea, and comfortable with it. That was the way it was. So of course the first person to contradict that and try to explain that in reality, the Earth is like a huge ball spinning through space... well, that person will have encountered some serious skepticism. Very probably people even scoffed, and that's never pleasant, is it? Possibly tears were shed at the time. Perhaps there were even fisticuffs.

Nowadays though, we all know that the Earth is round and we smile at the idea that people used to think otherwise. Yet the only reason we know that now is because somebody, somewhere, at some point in history had the nerve to stand up and say so *first*.

That person – who crops up, occasionally, in history – is taking a big risk, stepping out of line like that. Not singing in tune with the rest. Daring to contradict the Emperor and all his most trusted advisers. He may, like the small child in the story, manage to get everybody to suddenly see the truth, especially if it is as simple as it was in that story.

But what if – and this is me facing my fear, now - it is nowhere near that simple? What if there is some interesting complexity to it... maybe nobody will listen! The lone voice may be shouted down, hounded, persecuted even. Not because they are wrong but because it can be a little alarming, in a way, to be told that something you have always assumed was true is in fact false. That the truth is something rather different, changing the meaning of a thing you thought you already understood. This can be especially disconcerting if you have never heard any of this said before. It can be disorientating and most people don't like that, they prefer stability, familiarity and faith. How can we have faith in the stability of our world if one new voice completely contradicts 'common knowledge' and turns out to be right? That would mean that all the people who told us otherwise are wrong - and if they are wrong about that, what about all the other things they told us? Might they be wrong about those things too?

Far easier – far more comfortable, perhaps – to just assume that this new voice is the 'wrong' part and all the things we were told were right after all... and everything is okay... and we don't have to worry, or think, or change anything... we can leave everything as it is, and just go back to sleep...

But it is not really disturbing, is it, once you have got used to the idea, that the Sun does not go around the Earth, but that our planet orbits the Sun? And surely it is more interesting to learn that the Earth is not flat but a globe, spinning majestically through the Solar System? And although what I have to tell you here, in this book, is not as dramatic as any of that, it is perhaps even more interesting from a human perspective, because it is all about human behaviour and the actual workings of the human mind. And whether you are a smoker or not, we are all affected by how well, or how badly, the human mind is being understood. So here we go!

N.B. If you really want to understand everything in this book completely, it is quite a good idea to read the whole thing, preferably in the right order. I mention this because I hardly ever do that. I start books in the middle, then read a bit somewhere near the beginning, glance at the ending and then wonder why the writer doesn't seem to have explained things very well. Actually I wrote this book pretty much in that way but then I spent absolutely ages reorganising it, so it should make more sense to normal people. So please, don't go reading it the way I would.

Ah! I've just realised I should probably have put this warning somewhere in the middle, shouldn't I? Oh, sod it – I should just be grateful if you are reading any of it really.

The Biggest Medical Mistake of the Twentieth Century

This book will clearly explain three things: firstly, that stopping smoking need not be a struggle at all, in fact for most people it is really quick and easy if you find a talented, well-trained and experienced hypnotherapist who knows how to help you do that. (Not all hypnotherapists are, but then it is the same with every other profession.) Secondly, I need to explain why hypnotherapy is quite different from what most people think it is: not mysterious in any way, effortless for the client and totally safe. Thirdly – and this is the bit that is going to confuse many people all over the world - that nicotine is not a drug at all but simply a poison, and that the theory of 'physical addiction to nicotine' has always been completely wrong.

Cravings are real of course, but they have nothing to do with the contents of the smoke at all and can be easily shut down using hypnotherapy because they are not nicotine withdrawal symptoms. The truth is that cravings have nothing to do with nicotine. They are signals (compulsions, urges, impulses) controlled by the brain. Tobacco smoking is not a drug addiction but a compulsive habit, and I will explain the differences precisely and conclusively in this book.

I will further show that habitual tobacco smoking is not the act of taking a drug, and indeed never was. It is just a compulsive habit of lighting up cigarettes and smoking them, and the 'compulsive' part has nothing whatever to do with any of the chemicals in the smoke. The impulse to pick up a cigarette and light it can be permanently removed with hypnotherapy, usually in one session. Sometimes it takes two, and in just a few cases it may take several sessions, as smokers vary a bit in terms of their outlook and attitudes, and therefore how readily they respond to the change process. This process will work for the majority of people right away and does not involve any effort on their part, just a genuine preference to be a non-smoker, on balance.

Even if the smoker is in two minds about stopping – which many are - this is something we take care of during the ordinary course of the therapy. I have personally conducted these sessions with thousands of smokers and find success really quite easy to achieve the majority of the time now that I have plenty of practical experience. It's a complex subject but it isn't difficult for a good hypnotherapist who specialises in this area, and for the smoker it is effortless.

None of this can be done against the smoker's will of course, but it is easy enough to achieve provided the person wishes they had never started smoking and is content for the change to take place on that occasion. Nevertheless it is worth noting that smoking clients usually do not expect the hypnotherapy to be successful - in fact they are often astonished that it removes the problem so easily, with no apparent effort on their part. These low expectations of success are usually the result of previous attempts to stop smoking using other methods, which involved lots of effort and yet were unsuccessful. The fact that many people are of the general opinion that it is terribly hard to stop smoking and that there is 'no magic cure' compounds these low expectations. Of course the people who voice these opinions are genuinely unaware it is not true. Not that hypnotherapy is magic of course, as I will explain here.

The Unique Aspect of this Book

This is not the first published work to challenge the idea that tobacco smoking is a drug addiction. Others have found fault with that idea, yet have been unable to account for the apparent difficulty many smokers have in quitting permanently, because they did not understand the nature of the compulsive element of the habit, nor did they know of an easy therapeutic solution. This is the first book – to my knowledge – which explains the compulsive element in the context of the real phenomenon, the Compulsive Habit. Section Ten defines the various common types and features of that organised behavioural phenomenon. As a crucial part of these explanations, compulsive habits are properly identified as distinct from addictions, and as a result, the rather woolly current notion of addiction is superceded by a more accurate and useful model. During the course of Volumes I and II, all aspects of the smoking problem will be explained in full and the appropriate corrective therapy identified and explained, with the added benefit that this therapy can be used to solve many similar problems previously regarded as resistant to therapeutic intervention. (Those would be interventions that did not involve talking to the Subconscious, or else approached that in some inadequate fashion.)

Not everyone believes in the notion of nicotine addiction, but so many currently do that it is necessary to devote most of Volume I to destroying that idea completely. I am well aware that the systematic destruction of the nicotine hypothesis in Volume I builds up to a degree that could certainly be described as relentless, possibly even obsessive at times. If it gets repetitious I make no apology, since it is my outright intention to build up a case so undeniably strong, within this single volume, that it forces the medical authorities in the end to abandon the use of all nicotine products because they are entirely based upon a myth, and they are a risk to health.

This is also the first book to reassure smokers that their difficulty in quitting or frequent relapses are entirely understandable if they have not had effective hypnotherapy to eliminate the compulsive habit of smoking. These difficulties should not be regarded as 'failure', and as I shall explain, willpower is almost irrelevant in reality. Lack of success is predictable when the wrong methods are being incessantly promoted.

Once I have established that the theory of physical addiction to nicotine is a fundamental mistake, it follows that Nicotine Replacement Therapy is not needed by anyone because the compulsive urge to light up is actually a signal generated by the brain - not connected to nicotine levels in any way - a fact which will be proven in this book simply by logical argument. Nicotine is not the reason anyone starts smoking nor is it the reason they continue, even if they are currently under the impression that it is. Neither is nicotine the real reason they find it difficult to stop smoking - cravings are - and effective hypnotherapy can shut those impulses down without bothering about nicotine at all. And if you find yourself doubting any of that at this stage, it is just because you have not yet read the details.

Once all the details are properly explained, anyone can see the naked truth - very much like the Emperor's New Clothes, in fact.

This is also the first book – to my knowledge – to throw down a direct challenge to the drug companies that manufacture Nicotine Replacement products: why do these items exist at all? These products are based on a myth and their actual success rates are virtually no higher than willpower, as I will prove using figures from the Department of Health, and other similar official sources. The whole idea of nicotine replacement is a dangerous mistake, since nicotine is highly poisonous, and in reality it is of no greater significance in the daily operation of a smoking habit than carbon monoxide.

It will become evident through all of this that no-one has ever needed nicotine at all, although smokers may well feel that they 'need' to smoke. They certainly don't need nicotine 'replacing', in truth it is dangerous, which is exactly why the British government should not be wasting vast sums of taxpayers' money every year on nicotine replacement products or the services that promote and supply these products, especially when there is a much safer and far more successful method in hypnotherapy. That money would be better spent on providing good quality hypnotherapy services for the public and training thousands more people to become expert hypnotherapists, for we can help with lots of other problems too.

No-one should be using nicotine products even if the drug companies were giving them away free. Nicotine in any form – including patches and lozenges - can cause heart attacks, strokes, thrombosis, damage to blood circulation and can also cause cancer. Ask any doctor. And the huge failure-rate of those methods means it isn't worth the risk, especially since hypnotherapy causes none of those things, and neither does acupuncture, which also has a higher success rate than nicotine products, as I will show. In fact these methods are entirely safe, and hypnotherapy was officially recognised as a valid therapeutic method by the British Medical Association as long ago as 1955. And yet, over half a century later, hypnotherapy is still not generally available on the NHS.

To be fair to the Government it is highly unlikely they will have received any accurate information about the effectiveness of hypnotherapy when they made their decision to make Nicotine Replacement products available on prescription early in 2001. From the advice they will probably have received from medical advisers, scientists and the drug companies that manufacture nicotine products it is quite possible that the politicians may genuinely have been unaware there was any better method, *but there is,* and it is a far more suitable method in every respect so it is time to sweep away that ignorance now.

Part of the problem is, if anyone even mentions hypnotherapy to medical authorities, doctors and the scientific community many of those people – not *all* of them, I hasten to add, but it is fair to say the majority - will immediately feel inclined to cast doubt, almost as a knee-jerk reaction, saying: "There isn't the evidence", or "Hypnotherapy is not proven" etc. Not because that is true, but just because that is what they have heard other medical people say, or were led to believe during their medical training. Also, because they do not already understand how it works they assume it probably doesn't, which makes them no different from the general public in their intellectual blankness on the subject of hypnotherapy. Their opinion on that particular subject then carries no weight, but very often a good deal of prejudice. This is very misleading, because:

a) There has been scientific evidence supporting the effectiveness of hypnotherapy for decades, as I will show in both Volumes.

b) There would be far more scientific evidence anyway if medical authorities had not been largely ignoring hypnotherapy for 150 years.

c) As well as all the evidence presented in this book, I can prove the truth of what I'm saying by demonstration. Not in the form of some stage trick or parlour game, but through proper extensive trials involving many smokers.

People are dying from tobacco at the rate of 120,000 each year in this country. This equates to six million deaths every 50 years, which means that tobacco is not merely a health-risk but a holocaust. Since that is just the figure for the UK, and the global figures almost amount to a holocaust *every year,* clearly we need the best solution being offered to every smoker as a matter of urgency. Nicotine Replacement turns out to be a gigantic failure, which is hardly surprising since it is misconceived to begin with.

As I will explain in detail, what smokers refer to as a 'craving' is in fact a compelling signal produced by the brain but experienced in the body, like a pang, which has nothing to do with falling nicotine levels at all so it is not a 'withdrawal symptom'. In fact a craving has no chemical *cause,* although of course brain chemicals are bound to be involved in the transmission of the signals. Cravings are experienced in the body because the Subconscious mind is using the body as a signalling system to get an idea across to the conscious mind. The conscious mind is apt to interpret the signal as a 'bodily need', in fact it usually does. In truth cravings are not real needs at all but 'prompts' from the Subconscious mind. They are easily shut down by hypnotherapy provided the hypnotherapist is a competent one who knows how to do that, and the smoker is content to become a non-smoker on that day. If that change does not take place right away, the reason will probably be a conflict in the smoker's Subconscious about quitting: I will use case histories to demonstrate typical examples of this sort of delay and how it can sometimes be corrected, as well as explanations of why it sometimes cannot.

Now Consider the Wider Implications

All of this applies not only to tobacco cravings but also: food cravings, chocolate cravings, alcohol cravings, the compulsive impulse to gamble... even 'love' cravings like longing, infatuation or jealousy. You see we get lots of cravings, they are not all about tobacco. People assume they are just stuck with those feelings but that is only because they do not know anything about hypnotherapy. Eliminating these annoying pangs and impulses is a normal part of my everyday work, and of course clients are astonished by the change because they really were not expecting it to be that easy.

I am not a scientist or a doctor of any kind, neither do I pretend, nor wish to be. They know nothing about these matters, no more than the man in the street because their training and expertise is in other areas. I am a qualified and registered full-time private practitioner of hypnotherapy, and spend most of my professional time helping people to get rid of their smoking habits, often in one session. Of course I deal with many other issues too but the greatest demand is still the smoking problem, with weight-loss a close second. Both issues involve compulsive habitual behaviour which is outside our conscious control. The Subconscious is controlling it fine though, and is simply unaware of any conscious decision to change it, or any of the reasons for the decision.

Hypnotherapy makes the Subconscious mind aware that the behaviour is under review, and the reasons for that. The Subconscious may act upon that information but it does not have to. The hypnotherapist changes nothing, but is arguing a case as if before an independent judge. To win a Subconscious ruling in favour of the change, it is up to the hypnotherapist to argue a good case and up to the client to be generally accepting of the change. Get those elements right and change is effortless, which of course is astonishing to the client's conscious mind because it did not do a thing, and frankly (in most cases) wasn't expecting it to work.

Stopping smoking is commonly thought to be difficult - which it is, if hypnotherapy is *not* involved - just like changing any other habit. That is why we recognise the general validity of the expression "Old habits die hard". Yet with hypnotherapy change is quick, easy and permanent for the majority of smokers. This amazes the person experiencing the change because both smoking and hypnotherapy are greatly misunderstood by the population at large. This book aims to correct that, and although it may seem an ambitious aim it is actually long overdue. Millions of people all over the world have suffered and died quite unnecessarily partly because of these misunderstandings, and not just from smoking but many other damaging habits too.

Everything I am explaining here can be demonstrated - under the proper conditions - many times over, if that is what is necessary to convince the world that what I am explaining is true. In fact I welcome any independently-assessed opportunities to prove my case by repeated demonstrations, as this is obviously an urgent health issue. The nicotine myth is surely the biggest medical mistake of the twentieth century, with implications and enormous costs that threaten to spill over for decades into this century also, if it is not corrected. The consequences for ordinary people the world over are dire: continued belief in 'nicotine addiction' perpetuates the notion that stopping smoking is necessarily difficult, which prevents millions of people from even trying to quit. As does the fear of weight-gain, which the hypnotherapist can also prevent in most cases, as part of the normal stop-smoking session.

The poor success rates for nicotine replacement products also perpetuates the myth that quitting is difficult, whereas the public (in the U.K. at least) have actually been *steered away* from complementary therapies in general by the main agencies involved in the official 'Quitting' organisations, which always guide smokers towards the quit products made by drug companies. In the past these agencies have consistently misled the public by wrongly stating that there is "no scientific evidence" to support the success of complementary therapies like hypnotherapy. This is not true at all, as I will show here.

Whether the public were being *deliberately* misled is an open question. In human affairs I tend to assume (at first) that ignorance is a more likely explanation than conspiracy because ignorance is so much more common. Recently the quitting organisations have been a bit less discouraging about hypnotherapy particularly but they still advise the use of nicotine products first and certainly will not mention complimentary therapies of any kind unless asked directly about them. Are these quitting 'charities' as independent as they are supposed to be? We shall see.

I am fully aware that some of the information I am presenting here will be far-reaching in implications - global, in fact - and could well be politically and commercially explosive. Nicotine Replacement products alone for example represent a global market reckoned to be worth more than 1.2 billion dollars a year already. That is why presenting my direct refutation of the established myth of 'nicotine addiction' here fills me with trepidation. I feel as if I am walking alone into a den of lions. I may be ruthlessly attacked by all the vested interests involved, I may be ignored or the message may hit home the world over - which could precipitate a revolution in the treatment of many conditions, not just smoking. Only if I were ignored would I be able to continue with my happy, quiet life and that's why I'm somewhat uneasy about what might happen next.

Why publish this book at all, then? Because I know for sure that everything you read here is true and it would be wrong to allow the mistakes, the ignorance, the waste of resources and especially the exploitation of millions of smokers to continue by not even attempting to explain to the world the facts I explain to individual smokers in my office every day. This knowledge helps them to get free and it is now my determination to present it to the world. But I may have my work cut out to begin with, to convince the world at large. For as a wise man once said:

"It is easier to go on believing what you've always been told, than to recognise the truth you've never heard before."

Having said all that, this book is not going to be like all those boring self-help books which just tell you what you know already, and offer you advice you could easily give yourself. That's not my style, we can have some fun along the way. But I really must not go any further without saying:

Welcome, Skeptics!

You certainly do not need to be skeptical about hypnosis to benefit from reading this book. Yet it is not really a book aimed at the experts and devotees of hypnotism. Rather this has been written for any ordinary person who has ever wondered what the truth about hypnotism is. Since this curiosity is almost universal, I suppose the book is for everyone because we are all naturally interested in how our minds really work and what the mind is capable of. That includes skeptics, and I welcome skeptics particularly because I suppose I am one myself. When I was first learning about hypnosis I was not interested in showmanship or possessing 'secret' knowledge, but in finding out what was genuine and what could actually be achieved with the use of this knowledge. Then as a therapist, putting it to some practical use as often as possible.

I don't like mysteries. Well, that's not true actually - I do like mysteries, but only because they present a challenge. Mysteries are fascinating because they mark out the 'beyond' of our current understanding and inspire us to seek to understand more. Clients who come to me for hypnotherapy often tell me right away that they are skeptical. So I immediately ask them: "On what detailed knowledge and experience of hypnosis is that skepticism based?" They then have to admit that they don't actually have any detailed knowledge or experience of hypnosis - which I already knew because if they did, they would not be skeptical at all. Just interested.

Skepticism is simply an intelligent conscious attitude to all things unfamiliar. It is quite different from cynicism in this respect. Skeptics are quite prepared to suspend their skepticism in due course, if things are proved or adequately demonstrated to be genuine. This is because skepticism does not interfere with our learning capacity. Cynicism on the other hand - usually born of hurt, disappointment and general disaffection with life - seriously impairs learning faculties and is really a bitter state of mind that amounts to an intellectual disability. If a client tells me they are a cynic, I point out the difference and reassure them: "If you were truly a cynic, you would not be here!"

So if you, gentle reader, have ever thought of yourself as a cynic where hypnosis is concerned, I suggest that since you have got this far you may have been a little hard on yourself. And since cynicism is only ever regarded as a good thing by cynics - and by the rest of us as a bad attitude or even a disability - you should hesitate to put yourself down in that way regarding anything in which you are simply not yet an expert.

What do ordinary people know about hypnosis? What have they been told, what have they seen or *think* they have seen? What have they personally experienced? What have they read, and in what kind of publication did they read it? What might they have heard somebody say, once, which stuck in their mind?

In truth, the general impressions most people have in their minds regarding hypnosis are very vague, and even when they are more particular it is rare to find someone with an accurate understanding of hypnosis who is not an experienced professional hypnotist. So to begin our journey of enlightenment we must start with what everyone *has* seen - the aspect of hypnosis upon which all general impressions and misunderstandings of the subject are actually based - which is not hypnotherapy at all, but:

Section Two

Stage Hypnosis (The Shorter Explanation)

There are two types of hypnotist: stage hypnotists and hypnotherapists. Stage hypnotists are part of the world of entertainment and they work with crowds, whereas hypnotherapists usually work with single individuals to help them resolve some problem or other. The aim of stage hypnosis is to astonish and entertain the audience without explaining anything at all, so that the overall effect is puzzling and hopefully amusing. The sole aim of hypnotherapy is to help people with problems they do not seem to be able to overcome simply through their own efforts. In my practice, I also educate clients throughout the process itself, so that there is no mystery to it. Not all hypnotherapists adopt that approach, for there are many different ways of conducting hypnotherapy sessions.

N.B. In the U.K. there are *very* few hypnotists who do both stage performances and expert hypnotherapy, as the talents required for each are so completely different.

First, a few Frequently Asked Questions:

Is stage hypnosis a fraud? No.

Is stage hypnosis what it appears to be? No.

Is it true that the stage hypnotist is controlling people's minds? No.

Is it true that some people cannot be hypnotised? No, that is a misunderstanding caused by the fact that some people do not go into trance upon cue.

Do some people simply <u>choose</u> not to respond at the time? Absolutely, and they may have various reasons for exercising that preference.

Can hypnotists <u>make</u> you go into trance? A stage hypnotist cannot make anyone do anything. But he can certainly make it look as if he can.

Do people respond to suggestions <u>because</u> they are in a trance? No.

Does being in a trance make a person more suggestible? Actually, no! This is a very common notion, but it is really a misunderstanding. A suggestion either appeals to an individual or it does not, but the key to understanding 'surprising' responses is to recognise that a suggestion which might have no appeal for the Subconscious may yet appeal to the conscious mind, and vice versa. These two mental departments do not always hold the same view, which is often the situation when someone comments that they are "in two minds" about something.

The only real difference that trance makes is this: when a person is not in trance, the Subconscious is generally inattentive to social interaction, so it never actively considers the suggestion at all because it isn't really paying attention anyway. Therefore if the conscious mind finds the suggestion unappealing for any reason, there will be no response.

When that person is in trance, the conscious mind would still have the same lack of motivation regarding that suggestion, but the idea would then also be actively considered by the Subconscious, which might have its own reasons for looking at it differently. But equally it might not, so it is inaccurate to regard the trance state itself as a 'state of heightened suggestibility'. It would be more true to say that being in trance increases overall mental attentiveness, and therefore increases the overall *potential* motivation to respond. But the suggestion itself still has to have some appeal to that individual at some level, or trance makes no difference at all.

Do people tend to be more imaginative when in trance? Absolutely, and it is observable that some individuals are blessed with considerably more imaginative powers than others. Like any other mental or physical ability, creative imagination is unevenly distributed. This is undoubtedly one of the key factors that has led to the ignorant notion that some people are 'better hypnotic subjects' than others. Likewise, the perjorative comments that some people are "more suggestible" or "more susceptible" than others – comments usually made by persons whose imaginative powers are feeble – are an ignorant assumption in reality. A feeble imagination would certainly make a person a poor candidate for stage hypnosis, but it wouldn't stop them from being perfectly successful in hypnotherapy provided the session was presented in the right way. As the great Milton Erickson observed, there are no poor subjects, only inflexible hypnotherapists.

When hypnotists use the word "sleep" do they really mean sleep? No.

Are people in deep trance asleep? No.

What is sleep? A state of restricted activity for the purpose of resting and repairing mind and body, during which conscious thinking is suspended.

Does that happen in hypnosis? No, but in all trance states the Subconscious is making the decisions. Whilst the state maintains, the conscious mind is really in the position of an onlooker. It may also become dozy and inattentive, or wander off altogether for a while. What people who are new to hypnosis fail to realise at first is that this is actually a normal state of affairs that occurs regularly in everyday life.

Why do stage hypnotists use the word "sleep"? To mislead the audience. A stage hypnotist would get zero response from a person who was actually asleep, and it is the same for hypnotherapists.

Can a person come out of trance whenever they like? Yes, and sometimes they do, both on stage and in the hypnotherapist's office. It is not surprising that most choose not to, though, as trance is a more comfortable mental state than non-trance.

Is a person in trance aware of what is going on? Yes, although they may not always be paying much attention to what is going on. This can look like unawareness, but is really ordinary conscious inattention, similar to a schoolkid gazing out the window in class. Eyes open or eyes closed, same mental state.

Does being in trance make people generally less self-conscious? Yes, and this increases as trance 'deepens'. Some minor social inhibitions may temporarily disappear as a result, and this may be even more obvious in those who are exhibitionists and attention-seekers anyway.

This factor is manipulated by stage hypnotists to make it appear to the audience that a person in trance will do things at the hypnotist's bidding which they would not normally do, and of course the imagination is then left to expand on that loaded suggestion in all sorts of ways that are well outside the true scope of performance reactions. It is worth pointing out that simply being in the spotlight can elicit behaviour that is surprisingly uninhibited, but in the hypnosis show the suggestion to the audience is that it is all down to the influence of the hypnotist!

Some people watching these antics will see through that aspect of the show, and recognise that exhibitionism and attention-seeking are key factors in play, and that 'hypnosis' is an acceptable mask for that, so that the behaviour is not simply seen as showing off, which does not always win approval. However, individual responses vary, and the more imaginative the performer, the more they may 'lose themselves' in the performance. Some people are quite keen to lose their ordinary self and borrow a different persona for a while. Especially if you shine a spotlight upon them, because their emotional connection to reality is temporarily diminished as the 'real world' fades to black. For some people this is liberating.

Since a few performers can get rather too swept away by waves of applause and gales of laughter, it is the responsibility of all stage hypnotists to be mindful of the overall wellbeing and dignity of their performers, because they are doing all this in front of an audience: this is a public event. It might not occur to the performer at the time, but later they may start to wonder what other people thought of their more ridiculous antics. Such thoughts are not likely to bother them as long as the hypnotist has guided them in such a way that their role remains within the realms of good sport and entertainer, not spectacle.

In therapy, feeling less self-conscious just makes the client feel comfortable, so they respond better. Self-consciousness is an awkward state of mind in which we tend to be hesitant, uncertain and defensive. Trance does not leave you 'unguarded' in some way – as is popularly imagined by some – but simply calm, clear-minded and comfortable.

Do people in trance always speak the truth? No, that is a myth.

Will people reveal secrets because they are in hypnosis? Another myth!

Will a person in hypnosis feel compelled to answer questions? No.

If they do answer, will they feel compelled to answer truthfully? No, they are free to say what they like, which might be the biggest pile of horseshit you ever heard. Or it might be absolutely factual, or a random mixture of the two. The idea that hypnosis helps you get at the gospel truth is a dangerous myth. It must be remembered that Subconscious mental processing does not draw any clear distinction between real and imaginary in the way that the conscious mind normally tries to do. All Subconscious thinking is formulated within the Imaginary, and the notion of 'The Real' holds no special status. Similarly, the concept of 'Truth' partly unravels here: the idea that there is empirical truth is really a conscious notion, an attempt to impose order upon a chaotic world. Factually speaking, the Subconscious is more in tune with the chaotic world, where meaning isn't fixed, it is forever in play.

If a stage hypnotist commands, must the hypnotised obey? No.

If a person goes into trance, do they surrender any control at all? No.

Do stage hypnotists really <u>make</u> people do silly things? No. Invite, sure. Encourage, yes. That is as far as their influence goes.

Is the stage hypnotist just <u>acting</u> as if he is controlling people? **YES!**

If not the hypnotist, then what is truly governing their behaviour? It is their own Subconscious mind - which often controls their behaviour anyway, it is just that most people do not realise that because it has never been properly explained to them. This book will explain it all and reveal the truth about stage hypnosis and hypnotherapy. And if that ruins the illusion of stage hypnosis and causes it to become just an old-fashioned piece of theatre history, well... I think the human race will get over it.

Do hypnotists of any sort control other people's minds in any way? No, but it is possible to make it seem as if they do, and that is what stage hypnotism is all about. That is also why some people are rather afraid of it, and perhaps apprehensive about hypnotherapy too. Proper, detailed explanations dispel the imaginary fears.

<u>The Illusion of Power</u>

Stage hypnotists *apparently* control the behaviour of other people in a way nobody else seems to be able to do - this is the immediate perception of the audience, or most of them. So it should not be surprising that some people are scared of hypnotists and what they might be able to do, as if they are some sort of modern witchdoctor who may be able to put a spell on you and perhaps take possession of your very soul, or make you do things you otherwise wouldn't do. And because we therapists are hypnotists too – you know, 'hypnotising' people, like we do – then the common assumption is that we too might be able to control people, and make them do things they wouldn't otherwise do.

No hypnotist can make anybody do anything. In hypnotherapy, it is not the therapist that makes things change anyway, it is the client's Subconscious mind. The client cannot explain the situation to their own Subconscious, but the therapist can, and if the therapist has real talent in the art of communication and understands the Subconscious mind well, the combination of that skill and the power of the human Subconscious mind can help people to change all sorts of things they might not find easy to adjust simply with conscious efforts: like stop smoking, or lose weight. Gain confidence, pass a driving test, improve sporting skills, overcome fears, stop overeating, sleep better, ease pain, enjoy public speaking, get fit, resolve inner conflicts, put past turmoils to rest, recover from depression, drink less alcohol, stop gambling, come to terms with painful loss, learn to enjoy life again, overcome the fear of failure... spread their wings and fly. Metaphorically, of course.

Can stage hypnotists also help people to do all those things? No, the vast majority of them could not because they are not therapists, they have never learned to do any of those things. There is a common assumption that hypnotists influence the behaviour of a person *by hypnotising them,* as if that is all you need to do! Therefore many people are under the impression that anyone who knows how to hypnotise people would therefore also be able to help them stop smoking or achieve any of those other changes. This is not so – if someone is in trance, that merely gives the hypnotist an opportunity to present ideas or suggestions to that person's Subconscious mind. The Subconscious certainly doesn't have to accept them, or act upon them. That's entirely optional, and entirely for the Subconscious to decide. Even if a person is in the deepest trance possible, nothing changes that.

Stage hypnotists will not usually have any experience of talking to the Subconscious about grief, gambling or major emotional issues, because they are professional entertainers. Therapy is not what they do. But they can get some people - under the right circumstances of course - to react in a surprising way to the suggestion that their hands are stuck together and they cannot pull them apart, or that all the people in the audience have got no clothes on. The only reason anyone in the audience is surprised by that is because they do not know enough about the human mind to understand what is actually happening. The audience are also being invited to believe that the hypnotist has cast some sort of magical influence upon those people taking part – a notion that would indeed be disconcerting if only it were true. Of course appearances can be deceptive, as I shall explain.

A World of Difference

Stage hypnotism is to hypnotherapy what darts is to acupuncture. Darts might be more entertaining to watch but it is never going to be of much practical use, is it? Acupuncturists can do many wonderful things – especially the real experts – but because that process is not very gripping to watch it gets less exposure in the media, with the result that people in the U.K. are far more familiar with the spectacle of darts than the wonders of acupuncture. Since virtually anyone can benefit from a bit of acupuncture now and then, but the game of darts has no useful application for anyone, this is a bit of a shame. Stage hypnosis shows might raise a few laughs and give a few amateur clowns their fifteen minutes of local fame, but that is about the limit. Unfortunately, this can make the unimaginative and skeptical observer assume that hypnosis is of little practical use, or even fake. Some fall for the suggestion that the hypnotist is controlling others, and assume hypnosis is a risky business.

Is there any *real* reason to fear hypnosis? None. People do not really fear hypnosis anyway, they fear the unknown. Once hypnosis is properly explained and understood it is not possible to fear it. The 'unknown' aspect – and this is currently true for most humans on this planet - is actually the Subconscious mind. Being afraid of your Subconscious mind is like being afraid of your spine, or your liver. Being scared of your ears. Your Subconscious mind formed in the womb like every other atom of your being. Before you even developed a thinking conscious awareness, your Subconscious was already busy with the project of your survival and growth. It has ultimate control of everything from your skin inwards, and directs quite a lot of your behaviour too. Hypnotists do not control the Subconscious, the Subconscious does what it likes. But it does rather like to play games...

Now originally, I wrote a detailed explanation of stage hypnosis which set out precisely how it really works and why it is no cause for alarm, but it ended up being a bit too long because it is all very interesting and I got a bit carried away. Generally I would prefer to quickly get on with what this book is actually about - nicotine and smoking - and keep each section reasonably short and readable. That way the whole thing is enjoyable and no-one feels overwhelmed by complexity or bored by too much detail. So I decided to move the longer explanation to the end of the book (ie. the end of Volume II), for those of you who are interested in extensive detail about stage hypnosis shows. I'll keep this bit fairly introductory.

The stage hypnotist is constantly playing off the fact that his audience knows nothing about the Subconscious mind, and is using this state of affairs to help him create the impression in the minds of the audience that he is controlling the behaviour of the people on the stage. Many people do not even realise they have a Subconscious mind, they certainly do not know what it does, or how it operates. All of us were raised and educated as if the Subconscious does not exist.

The Initial Rejection of the idea of a Subconscious

By the time you first heard of this thing called "the Subconscious mind" your conscious mind had already been convinced that it (the conscious mind) is in charge of all our decisions and behaviour. From an early age we are given to understand that we ought to have conscious control in everything, *think* about what we are doing and have reasons for our choices and the direction of all activity. In early childhood we struggle with this continually, and our behaviour is often criticised by adults for being too emotional, irrational and spontaneous. We are encouraged to repress that kind of behaviour and develop more logical, rational and calculated behaviour directed by the conscious analytical mind. Gradually the conscious mind becomes convinced that it is, or should be, in control of everything – especially when we are dealing with the world around us and other people, ie. external reality.

As a result of that developmental process, the first time we ever hear mention of a *Sub*conscious mind - much later on, perhaps in our teens - the conscious mind does not like the sound of it: "How can there be *another* mind I know nothing about, doing other things? Ooh, no!" The conscious mind pushes that idea away, as if the very existence of a Subconscious mind is vaguely alarming. So if you find yourself doubting – on a conscious, rational level – that any of what I am telling you is true, that is perfectly normal and pretty much to be expected, until a deeper understanding is gained as we proceed.

Yes, initial fears and doubts on a conscious level are normal when the conscious mind is confronted with anything to do with the Subconscious, which is essentially what Stage Hypnosis does. And the aim is to do that in the most astonishing way of course, so as to make a lasting impression. But it is essential, if stage hypnosis is to have its full impact on the audience, that the people in the audience have very little conscious understanding of the existence and nature of the Subconscious, because the more you know about the Subconscious the less surprising stage hypnosis is... until you reach the point where it is entirely predictable and there is nothing astonishing or mysterious about it at all.

Since the 'Age of Enlightenment' and the rise of modern science, all the academic respect and regard has been bestowed upon the conscious, rational part of the mind, as if it is the only reliable and trustworthy aspect of mental processing, and should therefore be assumed to be supreme in every kind of task. This is a gross overestimation of the power and significance of the conscious intellect, but that phase can now be regarded historically as a necessary step in the overall development of human intelligence, because it challenged traditional belief systems to prove themselves. All well and good, but the problem now is, that having accepted the flattering idea that it is in charge of all our decisions and behaviour, the conscious mind doesn't want to surrender that notion, so it usually attempts to deny the existence or the significance of the Subconscious mind. This is not true of everybody individually of course, but it is especially noticeable in some people. In hypnotherapy, we often refer to these people as 'analytical types'.

Like most labels, the 'analytical' tag is half-nonsense because we all possess the ability to be analytical. We can also learn how to enhance our analytical abilities too, through education or reading murder mysteries, that sort of thing. The funny thing is that analytical types often pride themselves upon being analytical, which they assume is the highest level of intelligence, when in fact it is only one of our mental faculties. All of our mental faculties, operating collectively, make up human intelligence, which has outstanding potential. To rely too heavily on analytical thinking de-humanises us, as it neglects the emotional arena to a disturbing and potentially ruthless degree. The effect of this ranges from simple insensitivity and social clumsiness at best, to Auschwitz at worst. Unemotional analysis of a problem should not be assumed to be the highest level of thinking, since it can lead to a (final) solution which is in fact monstrous.

The Nazis assumed that repressing or denying emotion made them stronger, whilst expecting that their enemies' indulgence of their emotional side left them weak and vulnerable. Actually it just made the Nazis brutal and thuggish, so they were overwhelmed by the enormous fury (emotional) that rose against them on all sides, which they failed to anticipate because they had narrowed the scope of their thinking, flattering themselves that they were now superior when in reality they were not very clever at all. In their cruel contempt for their enemies, they under-estimated them – a fatal error. (It's the same with the Daleks, which seem to me to be obviously modelled on Hitler's SS troops: they bark orders in clipped and harshly-accented English, orders which must be obeyed without question or hesitation, or you will be "exterminated" - a very loaded word for the creators to have chosen.)

Occasionally some fool reminds us that the fascists did at least make the trains run on time, as if that is evidence of some social improvement. Of course that does include the cattle trucks that took millions of innocent people to extermination camps – that system was very efficient, thanks to the organizational skills of the conscious, analytical, unemotional mind.

On a less horrifying level, we can see this argument between the analytical and emotional aspects of intelligence being thrashed out in many of the original episodes of *Star Trek*. The character of Spock, who significantly is the Science Officer, is only half-human because he is also partly Vulcan, and he lacks human emotions. Captain James Kirk represents the heart and soul of humanity by contrast, which Spock finds "fascinating" but also rather incomprehensible because it often appears "illogical". The regular debates between the two characters frequently explore the relative advantages and disadvantages of these two perspectives, and although there is mutual respect because Spock is certainly not ruthless or brutal, the audience is invited to recognise how Spock's overall perspective – and therefore his understanding - is often limited by the dominance of cold logic. However useful logic may be, for social creatures it is not enough. Psychopaths also have problems understanding emotions in other people because they have little or no development in this area, which makes it very difficult for them to have any real sense of social responsibility, and they often fall back upon mimicking the emotional responses they see in the behaviour of others.

Some serious readers may raise an eyebrow about references to *Dr Who* or *Star Trek,* as if a book about the workings of the human mind can hardly be taken seriously if it refers to such things. Actually, although these popular dramas can include elements that are silly or fanciful, on a deeper level there are subtexts which address real human fears, and how we confront those fears. The people who first dreamed up the Daleks had been genuinely threatened, not long before, by the prospect of invasion by a cruel and heartless enemy bent on destruction and subjugation. And the original *Star Trek* series, however ridiculous the costumes and the aliens sometimes were, often attempted to address the problems of relating to the wider Universe from a human (albeit American) perspective, using 'alien' life forms to represent different belief and value systems. How these various discourses compete within the drama is the real meaning of the show, as humanity examines itself and questions itself, only to reaffirm itself again by the end of every episode. The tension between Spock's analytical outlook and Jim Kirk's humanist (and therefore more complex) view is very interesting, especially for the 1960s when Science was probably at its most self-confident in the West. Even at that point in history, cold analytical scientific thinking is being challenged, and the accusation is that it lacks something which is essential to our humanity.

Back to Earth

The conscious mind is not the whole of the human mind, it is only a part of it. We are taught nothing about the rest of it, which makes many people unaware that there *is* another, active part of the human mind. I recall reading once in some scientific journal that when we go to sleep (i.e. when the conscious mind is not active), electrical activity in the brain is reduced by only 12%. If true, this would indicate that only 12% of the human mind's activities are involved in the operation of consciousness. The other 88% is evidently the Subconscious and that never shuts down at all. It doesn't need to sleep, it is constantly active, although it may be fairly low-key activity much of the time. This actual balance of power, if indeed accurate, is unlikely to surprise hypnotherapists who are well aware that the Subconscious mind controls a lot of systems.

This physical observation concerning the brain's electrical activity is also likely to be the origin of the common assertion that: "We only use 10% of our brain". The suggestion that 90% of the brain is just hanging around, waiting for some quantum leap in human development that might at last give it something to do, is one which tempts me to retort: "You could begin by using some of your 90% spare mental capacity to question just how dumb was that statement from the allegedly-active 10%. Who knows, you could maybe get a debate going."

Of course the human mind is not 90% like the *Marie Celeste,* just drifting aimlessly with no-one aboard. Although I have met the odd person who was 20-30% that way, they stood out. Most of us are using the whole of the brain, of course – witness the fact that if any part of the brain is damaged, things go wrong, at least temporarily. You never hear of someone being shot in the head, but back in work the next day saying: "No really, I'm fine, luckily the bullet only tore through the empty, inactive part of my brain I never used anyway. I won't miss the back of my head at all - we only use 10% of our brains of course, and for me that's this itty-bit at the front here, so they've just boarded it up at the back... see? Painted it like my hair. It's a bit flat I guess, but I won't see it anyhow. And it does give me extra stability whenever I lay down."

Once somebody noticed that electrical activity in the brain only dropped by about 12% when we fall asleep, their bright little conscious mind – which assumed that its own mental activities represented the whole of the useful activity of the mind, bless it – leapt to the conclusion that only 12% of the mind was being used, when the truth is that only 12% is used by the conscious mind. The notion that the other 88% is spare mental capacity which the conscious mind could theoretically expand into, is one the Subconscious would find most amusing, I'm sure. In any case, whatever the real percentages may be, there is no doubt that although we are taught to put so much faith in the conscious analytical mind, the Subconscious is vastly more powerful and influencial.

Influencial, certainly – but is the Subconscious mind also *easily influenced?* This is the crux of the matter, the real source of fears and misconceptions about hypnosis, especially amongst analytical people. Stage hypnosis deliberately *makes it look* as though the Subconscious is influenced ridiculously easily - that people can be 'made' to act foolishly, and apparently cannot help repeating foolish behaviour on command, as it were. But if that were actually true, hypnotists would be the High Priests of the entire world and have everybody dancing to all sorts of amusing tunes. That kind of power would certainly corrupt, there is no doubt. So why isn't it happening?

Well if you are by inclination a conspiracy theorist I suppose you could argue that it *is* happening, but I would immediately point out that if it were that simple, there would be many more examples of it going on all over the place, not just on the stage. A popular comedy sketch show on British television called *Little Britain* features a spoof stage hypnotist who goes around changing the beliefs and behaviour of everyone around him for his own petty convenience, and very funny it is too. That is exactly the sort of thing some people would do with hypnosis if it were possible. The fact that it only appears in stage performances makes it obvious that hypnotists cannot control the behaviour of others in reality, because there would be endless unworthy opportunities for hypnotists to benefit from that if it could be done. And indeed, part of the fascination with stage hypnotism over the last century or so has been in imagining such unfair advantages and what might be gained by being able to 'control' people.

The truth is, however – and I'm sorry to have to break this to you, those of you who were just having fun fantasising about that notion - what happens on the stage only happens under those circumstances because everyone involved understands that it is *not real life* but a piece of theatre - a performance for the sake of entertainment – and they respond imaginatively within the context of that. They are only responding in that way because their Subconscious mind is aware they are engaged in a performance. It is not the hypnotist that is controlling their responses, although he wants the audience to think it is. It is really their own Subconscious mind directing their behaviour, as it often does anyway in much more ordinary situations. So if that person's Subconscious mind decides, upon this lively occasion, that it might be fun to play this game - however silly it might seem to the conscious mind - then *under those circumstances* it may go ahead and do that. But the participant is not behaving in that way because the hypnotist says so, nor is it simply because they are in trance. It is simply because they feel more inclined to join in with the game at that moment than not to, for whatever reasons of their own. If you wish to understand their true motivations at every stage of the procedure read the detailed account at the end of Volume II, which examines everything that goes on at every level of the mind during each key moment of a typical hypnotic stage performance, as well as explaining the hypnotist's actions and timing, and why it works the way it does.

If the stage hypnotist has selected his candidates for this game correctly, and behaved in an appropriate way himself by making sure the fun is genuinely amusing - and not humiliating, demeaning, disturbing or cruel - then the performance should be entertaining and the participants will not be upset afterwards, on a conscious level, by their behaviour in trance. Merely bemused.

Many hypnotherapists foam at the mouth when they speak of stage hypnosis and a few even argue that it should be banned. Personally I think that is an over-reaction, although it would be a good idea to licence stage performers and make sure they have had proper training, particularly with regard to treating the public with respect and to avoid upsetting people, which can occasionally happen at present. We therapists have to prove we have had formal training before we can get practice insurance but a stage hypnotist needs no formal qualifications whatsoever, and indeed some of them have none. A handful of well-publicised legal actions against stage hypnotists in recent years has made it more difficult for them to get affordable insurance in the U.K. for the time being, despite the fact that nearly all those cases ruled in favour of the hypnotist in the end.

That is one reason why stage hypnotism is rarely seen in large venues these days in the UK, you are more likely to see it in foreign holiday resorts, corporate functions or in a smaller venue like a pub or club, where it is not so easy for the stage hypnotist to get a decent atmosphere going, an important aspect of a good stage hypnosis performance. Hilarity and hysteria, that is really the kind of atmosphere the stage hypnotist aims to create. The bigger the crowd, the bigger the reaction. The louder the laughter and the applause, the more encouragement there is for the volunteers taking part to get even wilder and more carried away.

But the real problem for *therapists* is that stage hypnosis deliberately creates a false impression of hypnosis in the minds of the audience. Just because of this many people would hesitate before consulting a hypnotherapist. Even those that do opt for therapy usually have completely the wrong impression of what hypnotherapy is. In every session with a client who is new to hypnotherapy – which for me is about seven hundred sessions a year - I have to spend at least twenty minutes each time explaining what hypnosis *isn't*. There cannot be many professions in which that is necessary.

The truth is the vast majority of people in this country have never even seen any hypnotherapy let alone experienced the benefits of it - but they have certainly seen stage hypnosis, even if it was only on the TV. They do not know what the stage hypnotist was actually doing, they only know that it *seemed* as if he was controlling the behaviour of other people via some mysterious 'power' called hypnosis. So that is what most people imagine we hypnotherapists do - influence other people's behaviour using the mysterious power of hypnosis. Consequently it is not unusual to hear somebody remark: "Oh, I wouldn't go to see a hypnotist! I wouldn't want anyone messing with my mind!"

But if you are a smoker, your mind has already been thoroughly 'messed with'. You were born a non-smoker, with no interest in tobacco at all. Then a lot of outside influences came along and changed that. Some of them deliberately, hoping to make a fortune out of you regardless of the harm you suffered in the process. All I do as a hypnotherapist is help you to return to normal, to become an air-breathing, non-smoking person once again with no interest in tobacco, just as you were to start with. It is de-hypnosis, really.

So what about those people who have sued Stage Hypnotists?

Occasionally there have been well-publicised cases of people being upset or even devastated following participation in stage hypnosis and have pursued legal claims but these cases are thankfully very rare. Although it is natural for the layman to assume that 'hypnosis' did the harm, this is actually a misunderstanding. In every case it could have been easily avoided had the minimum of proper care been taken. Stage hypnosis itself is totally harmless and not remotely upsetting, but rather fun, for the kind of people who normally choose to get involved. Anyone can participate in a stage hypnosis show if they want to, but most people do not want to. Even a few of the ones that try to join in don't respond, or don't respond much and this is really because they are really only testing the hypnotist to see if he can 'make' them do things. Stage hypnosis requires a performance, and most people have no inclination to perform no matter what the circumstances, whether they are in trance or not.

However, some people do. There are quite a lot of people around who have some general inclination to perform, even if they are not talented in any way. This is the reason for the popularity of things like line-dancing and karaoke. Many of the people doing that know that they are not especially talented but they want to do it anyway, because performing is fun. At least, it is if you are a performer by nature, or can find the performer within you. Not everyone appreciates an audience when they are doing things like that, but some enjoy it more when there is one. And for certain types of natural performer, the bigger the audience, the more exciting performing becomes.

All kinds of people can find the performer within them during a stage hypnosis show, because the imagination plays such a key role in the whole thing. So some of the people who surprise themselves – and their friends – by acting it up on the stage may normally be quiet socially, or even shy. It might not be obvious that they have a powerful imagination and the soul of a performer somewhere deep inside. Nevertheless, the majority of people that volunteer themselves for stage hypnosis are not shy at all, but outgoing, attention-seeking livewires who don't give a damn about making a fool of themselves and often clown around anyway just for a laugh.

People who do not really approve of that sort of carry-on usually prefer to avoid the stage altogether if they can, at any sort of public entertainment. They are more serious, and don't want to be the centre of attention in that way because they *are* afraid of making a fool of themselves. Very occasionally one of these people is persuaded - despite their obvious reluctance - to get up on the stage and join in the performance. Sometimes the stage hypnotist will find this type of person difficult to work with for obvious reasons and send them back to their seat anyway, so there is no harm done.

But not always. There is a difference, you see, between what your conscious mind thinks is fun and what the Subconscious mind finds amusing. The conscious mind is responsible for dealing with the World Around You and Other People and consequently may come to care about things like what other people think of you, or your reputation and dignity. The conscious mind of certain individuals may regard their reputation, dignity or standing in the community as highly important and may therefore prefer, usually, to inhibit any behaviour which is unbecoming or undignified, or not in keeping with their projected self-image. I don't mean to be denigrating - different people value different things, and each person's values should be treated with respect. It's just that their Subconscious mind has never needed to concern itself with any of that because the conscious mind takes care of that sort of thing. So if the Subconscious (which is making all the decisions whenever we are in trance) spontaneously accepts the suggestion that, under these theatrical circumstances and just to give everyone a laugh, it might be fun to play some silly games for a bit, the Subconscious would be completely unaware of the very different concerns of the conscious mind.

This would actually be the case for the majority of people watching, but it presents no problem because they are allowed to exercise their preference to sit it out. This is just as it should be, because the majority of the audience would find the antics of stage hypnosis unappealing personally, and although they might be undisturbed by watching some other clown do it, they may feel that they would sooner die than *be seen doing that* themselves.

Now, it is important to emphasize that this is only the view held by the *conscious* mind. The tiny number of people who report suffering depression, anxiety or distress after being involved with stage hypnosis are almost exclusively people who actually would have preferred *not* to participate themselves but were persuaded or felt obliged to change their decision. After the performance was over, it was really their conscious mind's dismay at thoughts of what other people now thought of them after they were seen participating in that ridiculous performance, coupled with an inability to understand *why* they didn't inhibit that behaviour – a feeling of conscious powerlessness – which led to mental strain or breakdown in the conscious mind.

It is this lack of understanding of their own behaviour – only because they do not even realise they *have* a Subconscious mind, let alone that it controls a good deal of their behaviour - which causes these people to conclude that the hypnotist must have had them 'in his power'. This is certainly what the stage hypnotist wants the audience to conclude, so he behaves as if that were the case. The truth is, he doesn't have any power. The hypnotist is simply suggesting a game and their Subconscious mind is responding because *it* has no objection. It is the conscious mind that may have a serious objection in these rare cases, and because the conscious mind has always believed it is the Centre of All Operations in the mind – the decision-maker - it cannot understand why it was allowing that behaviour to continue, or becomes distressed because it apparently could not prevent it. But actually, we're all very familiar with *that* phenomenon:

Conscious Resolutions v. Actual Behaviour
===

Ever been on a diet? Have you ever consciously decided, firmly and determinedly that you are *not* going to eat any more chocolate biscuits, and then been dismayed to find that you're doing it anyway? As you munch away, a little disheartened voice inside your head is saying: "You *know* you shouldn't be doing this, why are you doing this again? You decided!" This is your conscious mind talking to itself, not able to inhibit that behaviour because the Subconscious is dominant when it comes to eating habits, and not understanding that the recent conscious decision to stop eating fattening rubbish is something of which your Subconscious mind is totally unaware. (The Subconscious is also unaware that fat is an issue, or that biscuits are fattening.) So the compulsive urge (craving) to eat those things again is triggered as per the usual behavioural pattern. All eating behaviour is habitual so the conscious mind doesn't control it in the first place. You are consciously aware that you're doing it, but it is not the conscious mind that is driving the behaviour, nor can it easily oppose it.

This kind of experience results in the expression 'old habits die hard', and other common expressions like "Everybody knows it's really difficult to stop smoking". Sure it is, if you don't consult the part of the mind that operates the behaviour. Otherwise you have nothing but willpower with which to oppose the Subconscious drive, and we all know from long experience that willpower alone is not going to bring about permanent change the vast majority of the time where habits are concerned.

I'm not suggesting that willpower is useless, by the way. Far from it, we use it regularly to considerable effect, but it isn't much use when it comes to altering established habitual behaviour. Yet many people end up believing that they 'lack willpower', and both smokers and dieters are especially prone to accepting this suggestion. Not because it's true, but because they don't know why it *isn't* true, and because they find that they cannot change certain behaviours with a conscious effort alone. If you have ever been accused of lacking willpower – or have accused yourself - to find out why that is an unfair and ignorant accusation, discover the true nature of willpower in Section 12 (Volume II) *The Willpower Myth*. It explains a lot.

First Principles
=

There will be plenty more useful information about the conscious mind and the Subconscious later, but for the time being it is enough to know that the conscious mind roughly equates to the thinking you know you are doing, and everything else that goes on in the mind is part of the Subconscious. So let us just get that firmly established:

conscious mind = the thinking you are aware of doing

Subconscious = everything else that is going on in the mind

If this seems simplistic, that is because it is a first principle for practical purposes. Learning must always begin with basics we can quickly grasp and upon which we may safely build, because they are true enough to function as true the vast majority of the time. Complications and subtle contradictions are fascinating to consider later, when we have real confidence and those questions can lead to deeper understanding of complexity, not just confuse us.

It is also useful to know, at this stage, that there is a basic division of labour between the two, best summed up thus:

The conscious mind is generally responsible for working out how to deal with external reality and other people in an everyday sense, using logic and reason to do that, and generally regards 'real' as more significant than 'imaginary'.

The Subconscious mind orchestrates all bodily functions, instant reactions (reflexes), habitual behaviour, sexual behaviour, and also all emotional reactions and emotionally-motivated behaviour. The Subconscious is also the locus of the creative imagination, and does not regard rationality as having any special status amongst various useful modes of mental activity. It uses emotions (feelings) to motivate us generally and impulses (urges) to prompt us to do or repeat something in particular.

Occasionally when I am explaining these things for practical purposes, a client might ask me what 'the unconscious' is, or how any of this relates to Freud's notions of the ego and the id. And indeed there may be other models of the mind's workings with which psychologists, psychoanalysts and various other 'mind scientists' may be familiar, some of which I'm sure are complicated enough to prove just how unusually clever those people must be, even if they don't actually end up helping you very much. For the straightforward purpose of understanding this book though, I would say quite simply: forget all that. The conscious mind is the thinking you know you are doing, everything else is part of the Subconscious. Let's keep things simple and useful because hypnotherapy should always be 100% practical. It is all about *changing things,* preferably now. This is the essential difference between endlessly analysing and labelling things because you don't know how to change them quickly, and the dynamic, rapid results of hypnotherapy and NLP. (If you don't know what NLP is, that doesn't matter but it has some things in common with hypnotherapy, particularly in the sense that the aim of NLP is to correct a problem with a swift and practical method which simply removes the problem, no messing about. I explain a little about it in Case Mysteries No.8 in Section 13, Volume II.)

It is also helpful to recognise at this early stage that the conscious mind does not believe in the Subconscious, except perhaps in theory. In fact, many people do not even realise they *have* a Subconscious mind, let alone understand what it is for and how it operates. So when I go on to explain that the Subconscious is usually dominant – that is, more influencial than the conscious mind – some folks may not like the sound of that and a common reaction on a conscious level is to disbelieve it initially. The conscious mind has been encouraged to assume it is in charge of all decisions and behaviour from an early age. But if culture and education convince a person that their conscious mind is supposed to be in charge of all actions and choices, they keep bumping up against the fact that it is not true, and this is why people end up fighting battles with themselves over all sorts of things, and sometimes getting very wound up about it too, which can often cause rows with family and loved ones.

All stage hypnosis actually does is demonstrate this simple fact: that the conscious mind does not control everything, even though it thinks it does. The trouble is, it also confuses the picture by suggesting that the hypnotist is controlling their behaviour, which is actually an impossibility unless you believe in the existence of some sort of magic power. In truth, the stage antics are Subconscious responses not conscious choices. The Subconscious is clearly shown to be dominant - the Subconscious 'will' can override the conscious 'won't' – but only in people who are essentially happy to play the game. The hypnotist has no power over anyone, because if there is no desire (Subconscious will or motivation) to play the game, there is no response anyway. But the preference there - to play or not play - is actually a Subconscious decision too, because the Subconscious can sometimes choose to respond to all sorts of things the conscious mind would not tend to bother with, so people can end up surprising themselves in the anarchic atmosphere of a lively stage hypnosis routine.

<u>In summary:</u> The stage hypnosis performance entirely depends upon the circumstances being right, and having willing participants available. If any reluctant participants get involved and end up playing games, there is a slight possibility that they might later struggle with feelings of embarrassment or humiliation, and may even feel as if their dignity has been destroyed. This is rare, even amongst reluctant

participants but it can have serious consequences in a tiny number of cases – and of course, even one case is one too many. Since this can be avoided entirely there is no need to ban stage hypnosis, but it would be a good idea to train and license stage hypnotists properly to make sure they treat their volunteers with care and consideration – as indeed it is fair to say most of them do already.

The only other cases of harm I am aware of either involved accidental physical injuries due to reckless suggestions from the stage hypnotist, which are easily avoided with a bit of common sense, or the use of age-regression bringing up painful childhood memories, which is now outlawed stage practice anyway. The actual harm in those latter cases really happened in childhood, so the hypnotist didn't cause it, but no entertainer should be doing anything with regression in a public arena. Not because it's dangerous, but because it is personal. Since it is not immediately obvious what previous experiences people may have had, nothing can be assumed and of course a stage is no place for handling real emotional issues from the past. Such risks can easily be avoided.

It would also be a good idea for the entertainer conducting shows like that to make sure the audience understand from the beginning that everybody should respect each other's wishes, and no member of the audience should 'volunteer' their friend or loved one for anything that the person wouldn't have chosen to do if left to themselves. There are always enough real volunteers available. Or even if there are not, let that be the stage hypnotist's problem. He is after all the only one getting paid for his role in all this.

A note on Paul McKenna

I wanted to include a brief note on Paul McKenna because he is probably the only hypnotist of any sort who is already a household name in the UK, with the possible exception of Sooty. (Did you not know Sooty was a hypnotist? Oh yes. And a real Magician.) I am often asked by clients what I think of him (McKenna I mean, not Sooty. Nobody ever asks me about Sooty. Though I live in hope.) When they ask about him, I think some of my clients are expecting my face to contort with rage at the mere mention of the name (Paul McKenna, not Sooty) but in truth I really do not have a problem with the guy at all. (Either of them. Especially Sooty.)

McKenna is an interesting figure in the field of hypnosis generally, as he has almost come to personify hypnosis in the minds of the British public and is also well-known in the USA. Originally he worked in broadcasting, and he learned the stage act from another adept performer called Andrew Newton. McKenna's media savvy helped him to develop his performances beyond live stage work and into television, and he became a very popular performer with tremendous experience, eventually becoming a household name. Largely thanks to the influence of people he met in the USA – especially Richard Bandler and John Grinder - he followed his interest in hypnosis further into the field of hypnotherapy and NLP (Neuro-Linguistic Programming: a rapid form of mental training originally developed in the USA by Bandler and Grinder).

McKenna has lately been a prolific and dynamic ambassador for hypnosis generally, and despite the fact that he has never been a professional hypnotherapist – in the sense that there has never been a Paul McKenna Hypnotherapy Clinic where ordinary people can pop in and get rid of their problems – he has routinely appeared on television shows eliminating phobias, curing shyness and demonstrating lots of things hypnosis can be useful for. There is no doubt that some people who come along to private practitioners such as myself for hypnotherapy were partly inspired to do so by seeing one of these demonstrations on television.

As stage hypnosis has always been - up to now - presented as if it is all about the 'amazing powers' of the hypnotist, what would have originally been billed as "The Amazing World of Paul McKenna" has developed over time to become much more about what the human mind is capable of, and McKenna's many CDs, books and DVDs have become more informative generally about the power of the mind. In my view, books and recordings are by no means an adequate substitute for therapy but I'm sure Paul McKenna would not disagree with that anyway. The fact is, he has never earned his living as a practising hypnotherapist. He has always been a performer, and more recently a celebrity demonstrating hypnosis to a mass audience through one broadcast or publishing medium or another. So if an ordinary person who is not a celebrity and is not appearing with him on a TV show wishes to be helped by Paul McKenna, their only option is to buy one of his books or recordings, and they sell very well.

In the professional field of hypnotherapy it is common to hear criticism of stage hypnosis and negative comments about performers like McKenna, although not everyone is negative about them. Whilst it is certainly true that the existence of stage hypnosis - as it has been presented up until this point in history - has been a tiresome problem for hypnotherapists in that many people are frightened by it and others deeply skeptical, nevertheless stage presentations can be inspirational to some people too. Many established techniques in hypnotherapy and NLP originated in stage demonstrations, and in the earliest prehistory of hypnotherapy these kind of performances kept the knowledge and techniques alive when they might otherwise have disappeared altogether. This is because for most of the last century and a half, the useful application of any sort of mesmerism or hypnosis was being ruthlessly eliminated from the medical mainstream by the prejudiced hostility of the medical authorities. (For more about this aspect of our professional history see Section 17 in Volume II: *Hypnotherapy v. Science.*)

So we must be even-handed about stage hypnosis and those people who have developed their success coming from that direction, and I wonder how much envy there is amongst the hypnotherapists who feel inclined to sneer at people like Paul McKenna, since he has made a vast amount of money compared to what the average hypnotherapist is ever going to earn and enjoys considerable international fame and recognition too. But then he has earned it, nobody handed it to him on a plate. Just like the rest of us he started with nothing but curiosity and went on a personal journey that has taken him a long way. I have never met him, but good luck to him, say I.

One amusing aspect of this though, is that however much Paul McKenna has switched to the therapeutic applications of hypnosis with his recent books and CDs, in the dumbed-down world of the media he remains a symbol of 'Amazing Powers' rather than hypnotherapy. One recent newspaper story reported how he cured a needle phobia in a female doctor who had previously won half a million pounds in compensation from the NHS, because the needle phobia prevented her continuing in her job! It says a lot about the general ignorance of hypnotherapy within the NHS that they would first let a fully-trained doctor go, and then approve a massive compensation payout for something as ordinary as a needle phobia – a little matter any decent hypnotherapist could eliminate in a single session in most cases. She could have been back at work the same week for the cost of one hypnotherapy session if they had only known that basic fact, without troubling Paul McKenna at all. But of course, the newspaper made it sound like something miraculous. The headline:

Doctor who won £1/2m for needle phobia cured

...by Paul McKenna

The Mail On Sunday, 03/07/2005, p47

Now, what that headline should read is:

Doctor who won £1/2m for needle phobia cured

...by hypnotherapy

because that is what actually happened there. But the Mail's headline makes it sound like Paul pulled off some minor miracle - using his Superhuman Powers for Good, and not Evil - as if no-one else could possibly have achieved that. Of course this says far more about media cluelessness than it does about Paul McKenna, but then again we shouldn't be surprised: if the Health Authority had no idea that any good hypnotherapist could wipe out that phobic reaction in next to no time, we shouldn't expect some *Mail On Sunday* hack to be more knowledgable about it.

Being a hypnotherapist is sometimes like being invisible. The rest of the world carries on as if we don't exist, and this has been caused largely by traditional attitudes within the medical establishment, plus the fact that rowdy stage shows make hypnosis look like nothing more than some disreputable charade.

Professional life for hypnotherapists is a bit like being a member of one of JK Rowling's wizarding families. The wizards are fully aware of the reality of the magic, indeed they learn it in school just like any other knowledge. Yet in the real world they are surrounded by 'muggles', non-wizarding folk who not only fail to see the reality of the magic, but also fail to understand that it is all quite normal to wizards and very much an everyday thing. The only difference is, the wizards in the Harry Potter books are trying to keep their magic world hidden anyway, whereas hypnotherapists often try to draw attention to the wonders of hypnotherapy, but people have been turning away muttering: "No, no, it cannot possibly be!" for the last 150 years, and not just in the UK either but all over the Western World. What it comes down to is that ordinary people are more prepared to believe in Paul McKenna's Amazing Powers than their own. I think that is a real shame, and I do hope this book changes that for everyone who reads it. However, it is important to understand that this is a guidebook to:

Self-Knowledge, not Self-Help

A Note on Paul McKenna

This is not your run-of-the-mill self-help book. I am not saying to you: "Read my marvellous book and by the end of it you'll be a happy non-smoker!" No, because I am a therapist with considerable experience in this area, and I know there is a lot more to it than that. I am not simply selling you a product here. Some people might stop smoking after reading this book without doing anything else about it, but most smokers will only find that easy with the professional assistance of a good therapist. People differ, you see - not only in their habits but also in the way their minds work.

Most people who buy self-help books find that even if they read them, and judge the message appropriate and useful, still their habitual or emotional behaviour does not change. This is because the process of reading a book like that is bound to be analytical. Within the text they are reading, typical behaviour is being analysed and the reader is invited to reconsider and think about their actions and reactions in particular situations. Guess which part of the mind does that kind of thinking? That's right, the conscious mind. Guess which part of your mind controls emotional or habitual behaviour? The Subconscious, which is precisely why new conscious decisions to change those things rarely achieve easy or permanent success. Because of the very nature of the book, your conscious mind is reading it alone. If it were Harry Potter or The Lord of the Rings, then the imaginative Subconscious would probably be right there with it, but not this boring crap about calories or tobacco. The Subconscious is picking up nothing from any reading process unless the subject fires the imagination, you see.

This doesn't make self-help books completely worthless, of course. It just makes them almost completely worthless, and no substitute for a bit of decent hypnotherapy.

<u>So Why Bother Reading This Book, Then?</u>

Well, you don't have to. Millions aren't going to, however many do - and as a result of not bothering to read this, those unfortunate people will continue to be nonplussed about their failure to change their habitual behaviour even when they want to really. But if you read this book and *then* have hypnotherapy to stop smoking, or whatever, you are more likely to succeed immediately than if you just go to see a hypnotherapist without knowing what it is all about beforehand. This is due to the fact that many hypnotherapists do not explain things in enough detail, because they were never told how important it is to do that.

So I am going to explain to you exactly what is really going on with the smoking habit - why it is very hard to stop smoking any other way, why it is not a drug addiction and what cravings really are - and then, crucially, how we shut the cravings down forever and why willpower is not required at all. And lots of other vital information, including *how to respond successfully to hypnotherapy* – something which, astonishingly, some hypnotherapists do not bother to tell their clients. Then there are all the other issues that can be resolved with hypnotherapy, about which you may not previously have heard.

I hope you will find it all very enlightening and entertaining, but most of all, this book will make you wiser; and if you also find that after reading this you seem to be more popular and better-looking, you should not be surprised. You may further notice that people who do not read this book seem to age more rapidly, smell a bit funny and become disaffected with life. They will prove more likely to get parking or speeding tickets than you are too, so you see it really is well worth reading the book, and recommending it to everyone you care about. You might also relish deliberately not telling certain people about it. Enjoy.

Interlude: Case Mysteries No.1

Now let's forget all that for a while and have some fun. Years ago, before I got into hypnotherapy I used to dread being asked what I did for a living because I had quite a boring job and I certainly didn't want to talk about it. So if I was at a party and somebody asked me "What line are you in?" I would always say something vague and dismissive like "I'm in sales" or "I'm a systems analyst", something of that sort. Which was fine unless the other person also happened to be a systems analyst and wanted to talk shop, in which case I was on a bit of a sticky wicket. I don't really know what a systems analyst does. I have trouble analysing a one-way system.

So I am happy to acknowledge after years of dreading these conversations and therefore nearly all social events, that the prospect of being able to say: "Actually, I'm a hypnotist!" appealed to me enormously. I knew how interested I would be if I heard someone say that and assumed many other people would be similarly intrigued. And I was right.

Once I had finished my initial training, no sooner was the ink on my first graduation certificate dry than I was eagerly on the lookout for an ideal opportunity to casually drop into the conversation at some social event the fascinating fact that there was a hypnotist present. I didn't have to wait long and indeed the reaction was every bit as satisfying as I had hoped. Those of you who have never been embarrassed (for years!) by the dullness of your occupation can only guess at the piquancy of that moment, as everyone within earshot suddenly turned around because someone exclaimed: "Really? You're a *hypnotist?* Ooh Dave, come over here a minute: this chap's a hypnotist! Oh you must tell us all about it, that sounds really interesting - we love anything like that don't we Dave, anything to do with the mind! How long have you been doing that?"

You have to understand this was the first time anyone had ever been excited about my work and they actually *wanted* me to talk about it! Unlike before, their eyes did not glaze over. They did not wander away muttering "I must just ask Jeff something..." No, they listened and they asked me questions. They positively encouraged me to continue indefinitely. So I did. In fact you could not shut me up, and for the first year or two I relished any opportunity to bask in my new-found status as a Person with an Interesting Job. But of course I soon realised I was having the same conversations over and over again, and the novelty wore off. Then it became dull. Then it became positively irritating, until finally the day came when I took my wife aside just before some wedding reception, and said: "For God's sake don't mention hypnosis to anyone if you can possibly avoid it."

I haven't quite gone full circle yet and actually lied about my occupation, and I wouldn't want you to think for a moment that I am ashamed of being a hypnotherapist – quite the contrary. It's just that there are only so many hypnosis conversations you can have with people who don't really have a clue what you do. And to make matters worse, everyone thinks they *do* have a general idea about what hypnotherapists do but they are quite wrong about nearly all of it, which means that most of those conversations are really about what hypnosis is not.

The other problem with all that is: at first, when I really wanted to talk about it socially I was no expert really - rather a beginner in fact, with a beginner's natural enthusiasm and ebullience. The more experienced I became and the deeper my understanding of what I was doing, the less I felt like having ABC conversations about hypnosis because people will sometimes make the stupidest comments and ask such dumb questions that you can no longer bear it after a while. For example:

"Really? You're a hypnotherapist? Now tell me, because I've always wanted to know: Does it *really work*?"

To which I am nowadays tempted to answer: "No, actually, hypnotherapy doesn't work at all - in fact I am a complete fraud! I spend all my professional time conning money out of credulous fools who benefit not one bit from my mumbo-jumbo, just as you always assumed without really knowing anything about it. Clever you!"

I mean to say it is such a rude question, isn't it? Can you imagine asking a police officer: "Now tell me, because I've often wondered – do you ever catch anyone?" Or a surgeon: "Does anyone survive, at all?" Yet this is a question hypnotherapists are often asked. And even if we manage to answer that one politely, all too often it is followed up by dumb question No.2:

"It doesn't work for everyone, though, does it?"

This is particularly irritating because there can be only one answer to that question, since there isn't a therapy in the world that works for everyone. Even aspirin doesn't work for everyone. Pretty good remedy though, isn't it? Penicillin doesn't work for everyone, some people are actually allegic to it. Nevertheless it has saved millions of lives and alleviated untold suffering since it was discovered. Can you imagine anyone saying to themselves: "Whoops! Picked up a dose of the clap, better get some penicillin – no wait: it doesn't work for everyone, I think I'll just see how it goes"?

How many people out there are still smoking simply because when they mentioned - in the pub perhaps - that they were thinking of trying hypnotherapy, some negative know-all who actually knows nothing about hypnosis at all poured cold water on the idea by saying: "Ah, but it doesn't work for everyone, does it?" Quite right, Einstein. That factor is not peculiar to hypnotherapy. A triple heart by-pass doesn't succeed in every case but I don't think I'll let that put me off should it be recommended at some stage. The know-all in the pub would never pour scorn on the triple heart by-pass, yet the only real difference is that a negative outcome in hypnotherapy means you go out exactly the same as you went in, there are no other consequences. That's the worst case scenario: nothing happens. And that's not the usual outcome, but of course it does happen sometimes. When it does there is always a reason for it, and if the therapist can find the reason it can often be overcome anyway.

Now, sometime during the early stages of writing this book my father gave me some advice. He said: "You might as well forget it Chris, you never finish anything." Well actually he never said that, but he probably thought it. No, what he actually said was: "Why don't you put in a few case histories?" and I groaned inwardly. (Which can hurt by the way, so I don't recommend it.) I knew it was good advice in terms of the structure of the book, it's just that I'm cautious about the validity of case histories because they can oversimplify things. Also, as far as the reader is concerned the author might have just invented the whole scenario. When the case history ends with success, the reader has no idea if the therapist was really so successful with that client or even if the client truly existed at all.

Then I thought of a useful angle from which to approach this. You might expect that if someone like myself is going to write a book about hypnotherapy for the general public and include some case histories, that these would be shining examples of hypnotherapy working well. But you know, when therapy goes well - as it usually does, by the way – that is the source of most of the job satisfaction but as a therapist I don't find that case very interesting at all because I've seen that happen many times before, so I haven't learned anything new. All of the cases from which I really learned something new were the ones that didn't go well, or didn't go well at first – because there is always a reason. So I decided to write about some of those, then I can demonstrate *why* hypnotherapy doesn't work for everyone, or doesn't immediately work. I can show by example that there are reasons for the delay in response, or the relapse, which can often be overcome anyway once you know what the reasons are.

The commonest misunderstanding of hypnotherapy amongst the public is that it either 'works' (with a snap of the fingers, just like Paul McKenna!) or it doesn't work. So if a client doesn't succeed immediately they may well assume hypnotherapy has 'failed' - or perhaps more commonly that *they* have 'failed' - and some of those clients see no point in continuing with the process just because they didn't immediately respond. This is perhaps understandable but actually it is an erroneous assumption. The Subconscious mind does not change anything without a reason. And it does not *hesitate* to change anything without a reason either, which means that if we can identify the reason we can negotiate, often successfully. So when matters do not proceed smoothly it then becomes an interesting Mystery and I get my detective hat on and start searching for the clues that will lead to success. Sometimes it is simply that the timing is wrong, nothing more - I will illustrate that too by example. But there are times, I'm afraid, when the therapist was simply never going to get anywhere and I'd like to offer as the first of my "Case Mysteries", the strange story of:

The Cartoon Man

This case stands out in my mind as one of the most bizarre episodes ever to happen in my office and I sometimes wonder briefly if I dreamed it because I have never experienced a session anything like it before or since. It happened fairly early on in my career - perhaps a little over a year after I launched Central Hypnotherapy, just as I was beginning to gain some real confidence. But however confident a therapist may become, nothing prepares you for this sort of weird episode.

I don't divulge real names of course but he had one of those names where the first name and the surname sound similar: like Brian Briggs, or Digby Duggan, some sort of name like that. It was a smoking session, and of course smokers come in all shapes and sizes but this fellow had a very unusual appearance in that he was tall and thin, had black hair that seemed to rise up vertically and the thickest spectacles I had ever seen, which made his eyes appear huge. He wore a brown raincoat that had a rolled-up copy of The Racing Post sticking out of one pocket. Or maybe I just dreamed that bit. There was a newspaper anyway. In short he looked like a cartoon, and that was just the beginning of the surreality.

Only slightly thrown by the enormously-magnified eyes blinking at me, I began the process of explaining in detail how hypnotherapy works and how to respond to it, which is an important part of the procedure. Hypnotherapy is not what people think it is - not something I do to them, but a learning process. In my view it really helps the person respond properly if it is all carefully explained beforehand, but immediately I encountered a problem in this case. Cartoon Man wasn't listening. Instead he was talking over the top of my explanations, saying repeatedly: "Yeh, yeh, oh yeh, yeh, yeh....oh, yeh....aye.... yeh, oh yeh..." He was repeating this affirmation virtually non-stop, it would have been impossible for him to take in any of what I was saying. In fact I found it very difficult to continue talking, and kept stopping and starting. When I stopped, he stopped and just blinked massively at me. But as soon as I began talking again, he was off once more: "Yeh, yeh, yeh, yeh, oh yeh..."

Nowadays I would handle this rather differently but at the time I was so confused by this phenomenon that I had no idea how to adjust in any useful way, so I just ploughed on. I should have stopped the session really and I might as well have sent him on his way: there was little chance that this individual was going to experience insightful change that day. Or any day, I suspect. But in those days I was not very experienced, and not very busy either so I welcomed all comers and was very glad of the income and the experience. Usually. Alright, if I'm honest I simply needed the money so I gritted my teeth and got on with it.

And so it continued for about forty minutes, me explaining hypnotherapy to a man I knew perfectly well was not taking in a word of it, and the constant repetition of Yeh, yeh, yeh, was doing funny things to my head. A weird version of the Beatles classic "She Loves You, Yeh Yeh Yeh" was playing in my mind at one point. The only time Blinky said anything else was towards the end of my explanations, as I was racing towards the finish... when he suddenly said in a contented voice of slow, calm reflection: "Y' know though, I sometimes think... well I'm fifty five now... if I do get lung cancer.... I've had quite a good innings."

Case Mysteries 1: The Cartoon Man

There's motivation for you, I thought. There is a man determined to succeed. There is a man who is sick to death of smoking and seriously concerned about his health and survival. There is a man I can easily work with and together we will comfortably achieve success. There *is* such a man somewhere - I knew that - but Blinky obviously was not he.

What to do? Throw in the towel? Charge him double? Hit him with a blunt instrument? Laugh? Or just carry on, and get paid for my time as usual? Of course I just carried on, but never have I been more certain I was wasting my breath. One wonderful thing happened though: as soon as we got into the trance part of the session he stopped saying Yeh Yeh Yeh - and the Fab Four also packed up their instruments and split the crazy scene, so some mental peace returned. It was a bit like that feeling when next door's burglar alarm stops ringing.

The rest of the session proceeded pretty much as usual, except that halfway through the trance section - during which the client's eyes are usually closed - I glanced up and caught him peeking at me, just like a child peeking at the minister during prayers. He quickly pretended that he was deep in trance of course, but the session had really been a farce from the beginning. That was just par for the course on this one but I had never seen anyone do that before – and even now, thousands of sessions later it remains unique in my experience. It is common enough for someone to open their eyes of course, but not to peep surreptitiously and then pretend they had not! That one action said everything about what was hopelessly wrong with his attitude to the proceedings.

I resisted the urge to actually kick him out at the end, but for some time after he left I just stared at the wall wondering what the hell that was supposed to be. I did wonder sometime later if he might have been deaf, but that possibility seemed unlikely since we had a perfectly ordinary phone conversation two hours later. I say "ordinary", but actually it went like this:

Ring ring: "Hello?"

"Hello, is that th'ipnotist? It's Brian Bonkers here. I'm in the pub! It's not worked."

It was the least surprising news I had ever heard. "Are you struggling, then?"

His reply was cheerful: "No, no, I wouldn't say I was struggling. I left your place, went to the bookies, then I came in 'ere for a beer, and as soon as I sat down I thought I could just do with a ciggie. So I had one. I've had three now. Thought I'd just ring and let you know it hasn't worked."

He was enjoying himself of course. Here he was, ringing me from the pub. Who rings their therapist from the pub? You can just imagine the conversations that went on in that public house that day: "Aye, well, it doesn't work for everyone, you know." " Load of old nonsense if you ask me." "I wouldn't waste me money, mate!"

But what is it – specifically - that we can learn from this? Well for one thing it is obviously essential for the client to be listening and understanding the process throughout, not just mucking about. But also it is clear that the degree of change to be expected as a result of the session is directly proportional to *the desire to change;* and Blinky was already pretty happy with his lot, all in all – even if he did get lung cancer. And despite being a pretty bizarre character in other respects, he was certainly not on his own in having that attitude. In fact we have all probably adopted that attitude at one time or another, certainly anyone who has ever been a smoker.

It's just not the attitude to adopt when you pop along to see the hypnotherapist, or you will get precisely nowhere.

<u>Could Hypnotherapy have helped this person further?</u>

In my opinion no, not with that lack of listening ability and 'couldn't-really-care-less' attitude. However, there are many different approaches to hypnotherapy. Since my former background was in education my approach tends to be explanatory and enlightening - fine for the majority but not ideal for someone like this chap. There might be a therapist out there with an approach more suitable for him but frankly I think the devil-may-care *attitude* would be a problem anyway. When the conscious mind doesn't really care about the outcome, that can actually be an advantage in the hypnotherapy process. But when the Subconscious doesn't care – when there is no *desire* for change, on an emotional level - forget it. The Cartoon Man was a fine representative of that colourful character we rarely see in therapy, though you might find one in any pub: a man fairly content to be killed off by tobacco in the end if that turned out to be his lot.

Section Three

Cravings are Not Withdrawal Symptoms

In this section I want to draw a distinction between two quite different things: the fact that habitual smokers feel the urge to smoke again and again – which of course they do – and the assertion that a physical, bodily need for nicotine is the actual cause in reality. I am directly refuting the idea that the urge to smoke is an effect of the withdrawal of nicotine specifically, or indeed any other chemical in the smoke. This book aims to prove beyond doubt that the urge to reach for tobacco has nothing to do with nicotine whatsoever – just as the urge to place a bet is not evidence of a need to be rid of banknotes.

The whole basis for the Nicotine Replacement Therapy (NRT) approach to smoking cessation relies on the suggestion that nicotine is *needed* and not just *present*. Elsewhere in the book I will be showing that smokers are clearly not smoking for the actual effects of nicotine anyway but here I want to focus on this particular claim that the habitual smoker feels a requirement for nicotine specifically, rather than just feeling an urge to smoke again. This notion that nicotine is needed is an assumption based upon observations of what apparently results from the smoker's attempts to abstain from smoking through their own efforts, or sometimes when tobacco is not immediately available. (N.B. there are two other indicators which scientists have tried to use to prove nicotine dependence and I will deal with those also in Section Five *Why the Nicotine Addiction Theory is Wrong.*) The subjective experiences of smokers in these abstinence situations has become generally termed "nicotine withdrawal" or "tobacco withdrawal" and it has been accepted by many people for a while now that this is crucial evidence of classic drug addiction and directly a matter of the presence or absence of nicotine.

Of course a lot of people regard 'nicotine addiction' simply as an established fact and if you are one of those people you may be astonished that I am challenging such a broadly-accepted idea at all. But the key fact that led me to question this in the first place is something most people would be unaware of - including medical people and scientists, unless they stumbled upon the fact accidentally – which is that a single session of hypnotherapy, if conducted appropriately, will usually eliminate the smoking problem entirely. Not only that, but without any willpower being required, with no weight-gain, no over-eating and no urge to smoke either (i.e. no cravings). This result is very often permanent. Even in cases where there is relapse later, further hypnotherapy will usually reverse it.

Since hypnotherapy is not miraculous but a complex process, obviously that does not occur in *every* case - nor does it always happen during the first session, although it usually does. I also freely acknowledge that there will be some amateurish hypnotherapists out there who do not know how to achieve those results consistently, just as there are doubtless some detectives who do not solve as many cases as other detectives. Clearly talent and good training are required but those of us who specialise in this area know we can achieve these successes more often than not, in other words more than 50% of the time.

In reality I believe my success rate with smoking is higher than that but I do not wish to make excessive claims, I would rather underestimate the true figure if anything so we can be certain of dealing in realities here. For further comments upon that subject see *Success Rates* in Section 14, Volume II. But it is obvious to anyone working in the field of smoking cessation that success rates upwards of 50% - without effort, and without unwanted side-effects - is dramatically better than any other approach to stopping smoking. So it is not surprising that anyone who does not have some kind of personal experience of hypnotherapy success might be inclined to think such results sound too good to be true. If this describes you, it is important to understand that this attitude is absolutely normal for anyone unfamiliar with what I do for a living.

Hypnotherapy *always* sounds too good to be true, not least because there is no effort in it on the part of the client. Due to the historical work-ethic in this culture, we are encouraged to believe from an early age that if we want success we have to try really hard, which might be true in many aspects of life but it is certainly not true in hypnotherapy. For the client there is no effort involved in the change process, which astonishes everyone when they first encounter it for themselves. It is quite understandable that a person who has no experience of hypnotherapy might doubt that high success rates can be achieved that easily, especially since it is commonly assumed that it is necessarily *difficult* to stop smoking.

But success rates aside, if it were true that smokers were nicotine addicts - that their bodies had become dependent upon nicotine and so cravings were physical withdrawal symptoms, their body 'needing nicotine' – then how could a hypnotherapist *ever* remove that problem? I mean it doesn't make sense: if the smoker walks into the hypnotherapy session physically dependent upon a drug, surely he would walk out the same way. So if an habitual smoker who was unable to stop smoking by their own efforts has *ever* walked out of a hypnotherapy session free of any urge to smoke – if that has ever happened *once* – it begs the question: What happened to their 'nicotine addiction'? Where did their 'withdrawal symptoms' go and why do they no longer need to 'take nicotine'? Either their body had genuinely become dependent upon nicotine or it had not; so if they are evidently non-dependent at the end of the session, did they really *need nicotine* at the start? Or did they just believe they did? Is the habitual impulse to light up a cigarette anything to do with the contents of the smoke at all?

Quite possibly there is someone, somewhere who honestly does not believe that any smoker has ever walked out of a hypnotherapy session completely free of the urge to smoke. We needn't worry about that because there are also people who do not believe in evolution, do not believe women should have equal rights to men or do not believe anyone who is not pale pink should live in this country. Yes, there are some extreme minority opinions around but most people are not stupid and will have noticed by now that someone they know, or have heard of, successfully quit smoking that way. They may know somebody who didn't too, because every quitting method has its negative outcomes. No-one is surprised when the patches don't work. But again, if this was genuinely a drug addiction how could hypnotherapy *ever* work, let alone achieve consistent success? It is certainly not possible to avoid heroin withdrawal by popping in for a single session of hypnotherapy.

Unreal Addictions

Like the popular misuse of the term *addiction* - as in: "Dave is completely addicted to that new computer game!" when the truth is, Dave simply prefers to continue playing rather than do anything else - the popular notion of *withdrawal* has also become rather vague. Nowadays we hear people say things like: "Now that *Sex and the City* has finished, I'm getting withdrawal!" meaning that they don't quite know what to do with themselves now during the time they would usually watch that TV show, or simply that they miss it because they always enjoyed watching it. Clearly that kind of experience is very different from the distressing unpleasantness that real drug addicts, such as heroin users, find themselves experiencing if no heroin is available. But it shows how much the general concept of 'addiction' and 'withdrawal' has become firmly established in the popular imagination, to the extent that all sorts of ordinary habitual and compulsive behaviours are often talked about as if they were *addictions*, and as if the necessary adjustment to, or general unwelcomeness of their removal or deprivation were *withdrawal*.

Those who are really knowledgeable about the medical side of these issues will already be aware, however, that terms like 'addiction' and 'withdrawal' are not fixed in their meaning, and not entirely agreed upon in medical and scientific circles anyway. Certainly the scientific use and application of these terms has changed considerably even over recent decades, so there can be a lot of assumptions involved in the very use of the terms.

Yet as far as the smoker is concerned the idea is pretty straighforward. He has been told he is smoking because he is addicted to a 'drug' called nicotine, so to help him stop smoking he will be given nicotine a different way. This then replaces the nicotine he 'needs' so that his 'withdrawal symptoms', the main one of which is supposedly the impulse to reach for tobacco, will be alleviated. Put simply, Nicotine Replacement Therapy is supposed to prevent cravings because cravings are supposed to be caused by a lack of nicotine.

Now I know exactly what cravings really are, and I'll explain that clearly in Section 8. But first of all let's be very clear about what they are *not*. They are not withdrawal symptoms and they are nothing to do with nicotine whatsoever. If you are a smoker and you've always believed that cravings are about nicotine, just test what I'm about to explain against your own daily experience and see if it doesn't fit perfectly.

If cravings were nicotine withdrawal symptoms they would be caused by nicotine withdrawing from the body, ie. a low level of nicotine. This is the real meaning of a withdrawal symptom - an effect directly caused by the drug withdrawing from the system and the experience is always uncomfortable, unwanted and sometimes also distressing. It generally functions as an incentive to take some more of the drug but of course it may not be the only incentive.

It is sometimes claimed - usually by some average journalist in the adult comics that are sometimes called 'tabloid newspapers' - that nicotine is "more addictive than heroin". When the smoker reads this he or she has little defence against that negative suggestion and may well add it to their personal belief system, thinking: "Well, maybe it is, *I* certainly can't stop smoking!" The fact that the journalist's claim is total rubbish won't prevent that from happening, and now the smoker feels even more helpless than before - more wretched than a heroin addict in their own imagination, with less expectation of escaping the smoking trap than ever.

The very word *addiction* hits the imaginative Subconscious mind like a prison door slamming shut. The cultural stereotype of the drug addict is a hopeless, powerless slave who has almost descended into a sub-human form. Indeed one of the comments smokers often make is that they hate the feeling that tobacco is apparently controlling them. In reality that is only an illusion in the conscious mind - it is their Subconscious that is truly governing their behaviour, not tobacco.

Real drug addiction is a different matter altogether. Author of *The Heroin Users,* Tam Stewart, gives us a glimpse of what true addiction is like:

The first thing you notice is that you wake up in the morning late, aching all over from sleeping too heavily and too long in one position. Your eyes will be watering. You feel rotten, just rotten... Later you will try to keep in a supply for the morning, but in the early days you may not bother, thinking you may be able to do without, thinking you can hold on until later. Before long, your first waking thought is always heroin and your first act to smoke, snort or inject the amount needed to get you straight, often without getting out of bed if you can manage it.

From *The Heroin Users,* Tam Stewart, Pandora 1996 p52

The urge to light up a cigarette in the morning is simply an urge to light a cigarette, it is nothing like the experience Tam Stewart describes. Real withdrawal symptoms as they are experienced in cases of genuine physical addiction are miserable: as the drug level falls below the minimum "comfort" level, the long-term heroin user is bothered by cramps, sweating and trembling; their mood plunges into listlessness and depression. Comparisons are often made with flu, and although that isn't exactly life-threatening it certainly isn't easy to function if you feel like that. What makes it worse is that the longer you've been using the drug, the more noticeable and frequent the withdrawal symptoms get because the addict builds up a 'tolerance' to heroin, which means they gradually need more and more heroin to get the same effect. The minimum comfort level creeps up and up and up, until the addict is left battling just to attain that, never mind actually get high. Life becomes a struggle just to fend off withdrawal symptoms, to "get straight":

Users may try to keep their habit down to a minimum level but to experience the same feeling of being stoned they will need to continue to increase the amounts they use, taking larger and larger doses. The fact that a person's tolerance continues to grow, and grow indefinitely, is probably the origin of the belief that, in time, junkies cease to enjoy taking heroin. What actually happens is that, once tolerance has developed, the majority of users cannot afford to buy the amounts of junk needed for them to get really stoned. If they are lucky, they will be able to get themselves straight. Often they are on the edge of withdrawal, not because the drug no longer works on them but because the dose they need is prohibitively costly. Life becomes a battle to be normal, to be well enough to carry on. (p53)

That is real drug addiction. So let's compare that with tobacco smoking.

<u>First inconsistency:</u> If smokers' cravings were real withdrawal symptoms, smokers would feel them at their most acute when the drug level was at its lowest, which is first thing in the morning. The nicotine level in the smoker's blood is lower at the moment when they first open their eyes than at any other time. Are all smokers beset by terrible cravings then, crawling out of bed desperate for nicotine? Are they climbing the walls?

In truth they are not. There are a few smokers who have got into the habit of lighting up before they get out of bed, but that's just their personal habit. The vast majority don't do that at all. Most smokers do not even keep cigarettes in the bedroom. So there is normally a significant time-lapse between getting out of bed and lighting their first cigarette of the day. It may be five minutes, or it may be over an hour for some people - during which time they get up, go to the bathroom, get dressed, go downstairs, feed the cat, make a drink – all the time *feeling perfectly normal.*

So where are those disturbing 'withdrawal symptoms'? The smoker hasn't had any nicotine for hours, they should be desperate for a smoke but no, there is a total absence of distress in the vast majority of habitual tobacco smokers. No cravings at all. It is only when they reach the point when they would normally have their first cigarette that any urge to smoke appears. (Or if some other trigger crops up first, such as anxiety or stress.) Cravings therefore cannot possibly be the direct result of low nicotine levels or else every habitual smoker would wake up to the worst cravings they ever experience and feel strongly compelled to respond to that before they could handle anything else. Every smoker knows how stressful and compelling cravings can be once they really kick in, but that is not how most of them feel first thing in the morning.

Second inconsistency: Real withdrawal symptoms are only produced as the drug 'withdraws' from the system, as the level in the blood falls low. But smokers know they can repeatedly get the impulse to smoke when they have already smoked recently, such as when they are socialising. Or worried. Or at a loose end. They are getting these urges to smoke at a time when the level of nicotine in the blood must already be high, because of the recent smoking. That urge, then, is not caused by a low level of nicotine, so it is not a withdrawal symptom. Nothing to do with nicotine levels at all.

Third inconsistency: True withdrawal symptoms will *always disappear* when the drug is taken again, but smokers trying to quit using nicotine patches and gum often report that they still experience urges to smoke. Some will even remove the patch, have a cigarette and then replace it! This proves that the urge to light a cigarette is not an urge to take nicotine because they were taking nicotine already.

Fourth inconsistency: Likewise, smokers know that there are times when they routinely go for some time without smoking, yet get no cravings because of what they're doing, such as: gardening, playing sport or shopping. Many people never smoke in the open air or in public, so they can comfortably spend quite some time in that situation and never feel any urge to smoke, despite the fact the level of nicotine is falling lower and lower. Some smokers find that when they visit family members who don't smoke - or who don't know their visitor smokes! - they have no desire to smoke whilst they are visiting, even though they might have smoked a number of cigarettes in that amount of time if they were at home. That is because the urge to smoke has nothing whatever to do with the level of nicotine in the body. The urge to smoke will only kick in again when smoking once more becomes accessible or appropriate according to that person's usual habit. That pattern may vary enormously from the habits of other smokers in a way which real drug addictions do not.

Real drug addictions follow a typical progression over time, from light or occasional use, to regular use involving increasingly larger amounts. In contrast, although nearly all smokers began with occasional sporadic use it is nevertheless common enough to see a long-term smoker habitually smoking less than ten cigarettes a day, and just as unsurprising to find a relatively new smoker who smokes twenty or more, which is not the norm in genuine drug dependency.

The Real Triggers that Fire Off a Craving Signal

In reality the urge to smoke has nothing to do with nicotine levels at all but will be triggered instead by one of the following factors:

- What that particular smoker would normally do, around about this time of the day, ie. their usual habit pattern

- What other people are doing (suggestion)

- The situation and atmosphere: eg. stress, or a party

- How the smoker feels emotionally.

Any of these factors can trigger an urge to smoke and also sometimes influence the frequency of smoking, yet none of them have anything to do with the presence or absence of nicotine, or its high or low concentration in the blood.

Compelling? Certainly. Withdrawal? No!

All of the unpleasant symptoms smokers experience when they try to abstain from smoking through their own efforts – the main one being an overwhelming urge to light up at certain moments - are real. And it has seemed plausible to smokers that these are genuine withdrawal symptoms, thus indicating drug dependence, for the following reasons:

1. They have been told these things by the medical profession, and many people assume they know what they are talking about.

2. The 'withdrawal' suggestion has been repeated thousands of times now and many smokers have never heard it being challenged at all, so it is familiar, it *sounds true,* or at least plausible. Also (crucially) many other people apparently believe it too.

3. The 'withdrawal' suggestion seems believable on the face of it because abstinence - or to be more precise, attempted abstinence when you normally *would* smoke - seems to cause the discomfort, and lighting up again alleviates that discomfort.

4. No-one has ever previously described exactly what is really going on, so the 'withdrawal' idea seemed broadly believable enough until now, simply in the absence of a better explanation.

Time to change medical history. And destroy the nicotine myth forever.

Interlude: Case Mysteries No.2

First of all, there is what appears to be going on. Then there is what is really going on - the two can be significantly different during the process of hypnotherapy. On a conscious level the client has no idea what is going on in their own Subconscious mind and the therapist often doesn't know much about that either during the session itself. There are some indicators but they are not necessarily reliable and the real success of the session – especially where smoking is concerned - only becomes apparent later.

However, the client is always aware of what is going on in their conscious mind and they cannot help thinking that their conscious assessment of the proceedings is actually a reliable indicator of how the session is going. They do not realise that it scarcely matters what their conscious mind thinks about the trance part of the session, only what their Subconscious makes of the case for change being argued by the therapist. The Subconscious has its own agenda, its own views and acts independently of the conscious mind completely, as is wonderfully demonstrated by the case of:

The Angry Satisfied Customer

This chappie (who we shall call Horace, just because we can) was quite easy to get on with, a hearty fellow in his early forties who was quite positive about stopping smoking but a bit dubious about hypnotherapy. This never bothers me at all, it is perfectly normal. Sometimes people say to me: "You have to really believe in hypnotherapy, don't you, for it to work?" which always makes me smile because nothing could be further from the truth. Many people who come along have doubts about it, some are even quite skeptical but this is only their conscious view, it doesn't affect their Subconscious response.

During the first part of the session when I was explaining everything, Horace seemed very interested in the subject and we had quite a lively conversation during which he asked a number of challenging questions but he wasn't being difficult, just testing the validity of what I was saying. So when we got to the trance bit he seemed positive enough and content with the process so far, so everything looked as if it was proceeding well.

As we got into the trance section he seemed comfortable to begin with but after about fifteen minutes he started shifting about a bit in his chair, as if something was bothering him. Now, one of the things you have to be a bit careful about, as a hypnotherapist, is making assumptions about how the session is going from the way people behave in trance. You might assume - from seeing 'hypnosis' on the TV or in films - that a person in trance simply looks asleep and remains still, and indeed many do, at least most of the time. But some people shift about from time to time, and there are even a few that move around a lot, as if they are most uncomfortable about something. I'm sure there will be hypnotherapists reading this who have encountered this sort of thing early in their career, assumed there was a problem and halted the session - only to be told by a surprised client that they were perfectly happy and comfortable, and nothing was bothering them at all! Appearances can be deceptive.

So when Horace began frowning and shifting his position I just carried on without a pause. Halfway into the session though he seemed more disgruntled and I wondered about halting the usual procedure, but I always trust my gut feeling on these things, and my gut feeling on this occasion was to ignore it. By the end of the session however the chatty, friendly Horace had been replaced by a grumpy fellow who said very little, he just paid and left.

Two weeks later he rang me up: "Well, I've not had a cigarette and I haven't wanted one... but when I left your office I was blazing! I was convinced I had completely wasted my time and money, I went and had a row with the wife because she'd talked me into it, and it took me hours to even notice that I had not wanted a cigarette!" In other words, he had been completely successful but his conscious mind was convinced it was all a waste of time. (You can see another very similar account of this misunderstanding from Allen Carr's own account of his successful hypnotherapy session, quoted in Section 4.)

Horace just assumed that his conscious assessment of the session – which was that nothing was really happening, and it was all a waste of time - was an accurate assessment, when in fact it was 100% wrong. His Subconscious, blissfully unaware of his conscious skepticism had made its own decision, acting entirely on the basis of how he felt about *tobacco*, not the process of hypnotherapy. It had shut down the smoking habit, cravings and all, but it was a while before he even noticed that on a conscious level. In the end he was pleased with the result, but also rather confused because the conscious mind assumes that it makes all the significant decisions, which of course it does not.

The lesson for the hypnotherapy practitioner is this: Making assumptions from clients' reactions whilst in trance can be very misleading. To emphasize that the above case is not just a one-off, here is a fairytale rendition of a true case which demonstrates that the client who appears to have some difficulty at first can turn out to be the actual success, whilst the one who seems on the face of it to have no problem at all...

Hansel and Gretel

Once upon a time, Hansel and Gretel set off into the enchanted wood to find the wizard who could help them stop smoking tabs. [This narrator's from Newcastle.] The wizard was a kindly fellow - happy to help - and he first asked Hansel to go off and read a magazine or something whilst Gretel sat in the Magic Recliner and enjoyed a detailed explanation of what wizards do, which she wasn't really expecting but it was all very informative. Then he cast a spell, which took about a hour and was really quite ordinary and a bit of an anticlimax, not at all the sort of thing Gretel thought it was going to be. There was no wand, no book of spells, no cauldron or anything like that. In fact she couldn't help feeling it was all a bit of a waste of time, and wondered if he was really a wizard at all! He certainly didn't look like one.

The wizard noticed that Gretel seemed a bit disgruntled and that she just couldn't seem to sit still. He saw that Expressions of Doubt flickered across her face over and over again, but he had seen all this sort of thing before and took no notice. Many years ago when he was a young wizard with only a provisional sorcery licence he would probably have been quite concerned about whether she was relaxed enough or something, but now he was older and wiser. He knew that a spell is a spell whether you are relaxed or not, and that disgruntlement is neither here nor there when you are in the Magic Recliner.

There is what appears to be going on, then there is what is really going on. Gretel told the wizard afterwards that her mother would be paying the two gold pieces for herself and Hansel, because her mother really wanted them both to stop smoking. Then she headed home, still looking rather doubtful.

Hansel breezed in, and the wizard began again. Hansel seemed perfectly comfortable with the whole thing and took to the Magic Recliner like he'd been in a recliner all his life. He didn't seem to have a care in the world as the wizard first explained and then cast the spell, and this time there were no Doubtful Expressions – in fact there were no expressions at all, really.

The following week Hansel was back. The magic spell had worked wonderfully for Gretel and much to her surprise she had never felt remotely tempted to inhale acrid fumes at all since leaving the Magic Recliner. But Hansel had been troubled immediately by a Niggly Twitch, which soon developed into a Grumbly Thwarg and he was unable to be unsmokey. So he had been encouraged to return, by Other People Who Meant Well - but all attempts that day by the wizard came to nothing, which was actually no surprise to the wizard at all.

You see, the wizard knew something that neither Hansel, nor Gretel, nor any of The People Who Meant Well knew: that the spell was actually not the thing that made the magic happen. That is why he didn't need a wand, or a cauldron, or any of the other wizarding accessories that some wizards go in for. *It is how you feel about the spell*. That is what makes the magic happen. Not what you *think* about it, not what you *expect* from it nor even whether you think it is all a waste of time and that this might not be a proper wizard at all - none of that matters a bit. It is how you feel about the spell itself. Gretel had her doubts about the wizard and she may have suspected that the

Magic Recliner was really just an ordinary recliner from Ikea, but she had gone there to stop smoking and that's what the spell was all about. She was happy with the spell, just a bit surprised that it didn't seem particularly magical. Deep down, then, positive response was activated.

Hansel had not gone there because he wanted to stop smoking. He had only gone there because someone else wanted him to stop smoking. He hadn't even had to pay for the wizard's time himself, and if someone else had not done those things Hansel certainly would not have done them because he didn't really want to bother with all this in the first place. But he was quite happy to relax in the Magic Recliner for an hour or two, as long as it cost him nothing and if it would shut everybody up. He wasn't even interested in the spell, he really wanted to remain just the way he was – so that is what he did.

<u>Could Hypnotherapy have helped these people further?</u>

Since two of them (Horace and Gretel) were completely successful anyway, the question only really relates to Hansel. At that point in his young life hypnotherapy to stop smoking would produce zero response whoever was conducting the session because the outcome of the session is entirely controlled by the preference of the client's Subconscious, which in this case was to please himself and remain how he was. There is nothing wrong with this - and in fact I would have to say that by taking charge and sending them both along for therapy Gretel's mother was being a bit pushy, albeit with the best of intentions. But hypnotherapy is not like getting your teeth capped or your hair cut: your emotional involvement is an essential part of the process. Hansel had not asked to be 'fixed' and although he did not display any, he may well have had some resentment towards Gretel's mother for being too dominant a character and patronising him to some degree. If so, this too would have been working against change during the session.

Later in life - if he came to feel differently about tobacco himself, as is the usual development - then he would certainly have been able to respond properly just like anyone else. But the tragedy is, his first experience with hypnotherapy may have led him to assume hypnotherapy does not work on him, or that he cannot do it - assumptions which make it less likely he would try it again. This is one very good reason for letting people make their own decisions about when to choose hypnotherapy.

Section Four

Introducing: The Subconscious Mind

If we are going to fully understand what is going on in the mind of a client during a hypnotherapy session - and how our own minds ordinarily work - it is crucial to have a proper understanding of the Subconscious. The key factor that makes a hypnotherapist different from any other kind of therapist or mind specialist, is that we are the only people who work directly with the Subconscious mind of the client as a priority, *as well as* with their conscious mind. To any other mind specialist the mental activity that goes on beneath the obvious levels of consciousness (the subconscious, or unconscious) is generally regarded as observable, but not easily changed. To a skilled and well-trained hypnotherapist this is not the case at all, in fact we would regard the Subconscious mind as a very helpful partner to work with provided the client is comfortable with the proposed change, or can reach a point where they are comfortable with it, even if they are not so at first.

It is important to recognise however that hypnotherapists can only work *with*, not *upon* the client's Subconscious mind. The general popular notion that people in trance will obey commands and blindly follow instructions is absolute nonsense. The Subconscious is not robotic or programmable. It is highly intelligent, totally independent and can easily understand and respond to subtle and complex information. However the Subconscious mind does not do what it's told. It does what it likes, when it chooses. It does not do anything without an understandable motivation. Nor does it hesitate or refuse to do anything without an understandable objection. These are first principles when it comes to working with the Subconscious.

It is also important to understand that what I am writing here is not mere theory. It is not regurgitated from some hypnotherapy text book, but an accurate picture carefully put together from many thousands of hours of therapy with thousands of clients, the majority of whom achieved their goals quickly and with little or no struggle or effort on their part. Mere theory cannot produce that kind of consistent and rapid success. I didn't get that kind of success at the beginning of course, but developed it over time through a process of trial and error, training and retraining until I developed an expert knowledge of how these things actually are - just like any other successful hypnotherapist, in fact. The point that I am making is that in my explanations I am not speculating. My confidence that these explanations are an accurate reflection of the mental reality results from a great deal of personal experience of the consistent success of many clients, especially in the last few years. If I speculate at all, I will make it clear that I am speculating.

N.B. I do not mean to suggest that any fool who learns how to 'hypnotise people' can get results like this, because the results are not achieved simply by doing that. However, I am certain that most clients, with the right instruction and guidance can achieve these rapid and effortless results if that is what they want to achieve.

Most people scarcely realise that they have a Subconscious mind at all. Perhaps the majority of the population has heard of a thing called the Subconscious mind by now but don't really understand what it is, or its role in our daily behaviour so I'm going to explain here in more detail.

First of all, although we talk about "the conscious mind" and "the Subconscious mind" as if they are separate things, it is all one mind really and part of the whole physical being, therefore all one integrated system. But the human organism is highly complex and different parts of our minds take care of different responsibilities for us, so with a view to explaining some of this we artificially divide it into two. There is no actual divide, it is more of a division of labour than any simple physical separation in terms of the brain. These two parts of the mind are really like two different mental 'departments' operating different systems and strategies.

Yet it can be useful, especially from the point of view of therapy, to allow the concept of a separation to exist. For hypnotherapists do not have to concern themselves with such questions as the neuroscientists are engaged with - matters like 'locating' the mind, looking at the anatomy of the brain and studying the biochemistry of human thought-processing. Hypnotherapy is, and always should be 100% practical. Theory is useless unless it can be shown to work again and again, creating obviously impressive success as fast as possible.

What we do - what we deal in - is something largely unmeasurable at present, which is why scientific studies into hypnosis so often seem laughable and misconceived to anyone who genuinely understands hypnotherapy. We deal in thoughts, feelings, ideas, beliefs, conflicts, reactions, fears – experiential things like that. We don't work with a brain, we work with a person. As do counsellors, psychologists, psychiatrists and psychoanalysts, to be sure - but they do not work with the Subconscious mind at all unless they are also hypnotists. So there is a whole world they have almost no access to, the intrareality of our Subconscious world. [I may have just coined a new term by calling it that, I don't know. I'm sure that in itself is not important but I am referring to reality as the Subconscious perceives it, as opposed to 'extrareality' which is reality as it is perceived by the conscious mind. They are not the same.] Therefore that whole arena of mental activity is outside the scope of their therapeutic interventions. A pretty serious limitation, given the relative size of that department compared to the conscious one.

It has been reckoned – though we needn't be too serious about the figures - that the conscious mind represents about 12% of our mental activity, as I mentioned earlier. This suggests that 88% of what goes on in the mind is either outside our awareness completely or we are only dimly aware of it: it is Sub-conscious. This observation - that we are consciously unaware of a good deal of what is going on in our minds - has struck fear into people ever since it was first raised in the popular imagination by Sigmund Freud's early published writings over a century ago. This ignorant fear still persists and the way stage hypnosis performances affect audience perceptions actually contributes to that persistence in a way that has undermined the development of hypnotherapy considerably during the last century. All these fears, though, are quite unnecessary.

You know it all already

If one of my clients seems a little nervous about the hypnotherapy process, I will ask them what they feel nervous about. The most common response is a comment suggesting that the session is – for them – a journey into "the unknown". I immediately point out to them that the session is all about their mind. Since their mind consists entirely of everything they have ever *known,* how can any of it possibly be unknown to them? This simple fact is instantly reassuring to most people.

Obviously there is a lot going on in a human mind at any one time. If we were consciously aware of it all we would be paralysed with information - unable to focus on anything, utterly overloaded. In fact the fewer things that are crowding into our conscious awareness the better, providing the Subconscious is managing everything else well enough. So all the time, every waking moment, the Subconscious mind strives to take as much work off the shoulders of the conscious mind as humanly possible. Or to put it another way *conscious awareness* is focused as precisely as possible, leaving anything that is outside the task at hand to *Subconscious awareness.* But if the Subconscious judges it to be necessary, at any moment it is able to instantly bring something into our conscious awareness. For example: when a person steps into the road, consciously thinking about something else... and then suddenly has an overwhelming feeling that they should look around. The lorry speeding towards them was not noticed by the conscious mind because it was otherwise occupied but the Subconscious used emotional leverage – feelings – to avert disaster. Notice how easily the Subconscious is able to assume dominance, overruling whatever conscious thoughts were being processed at the time. It is a life-saving 'realisation' which is obviously more urgent than whatever conscious processing was engaged in doing.

Introducing: The Subconscious Mind

It was the French philosopher Rene Decartes who famously declared: "I think, therefore I am." But what he did not realise was:

We are Thinking More than We Think We Are

What we refer to as "the conscious mind" is really just the part of the mind with which we are most familiar, because that is *the thinking we know we are doing*. But this is only a tiny proportion of our actual mental activity. Neuroscientists have speculated that the human mind as a whole can process anything up to two million separate bits of information per second. God knows how they go about working out something like that but it gives us some idea of the scale of mental activity. At any time of the day or night there are billions of neurons all busily working away. Can you imagine being conciously aware of all that? You would be lost in a blizzard of information.

So in order that we can think clearly on a conscious level, the rest of the brain takes care of as much as possible for us - without bothering us about it at all, unless it is really necessary – and we call all that mental activity "the Subconscious". Now, we are not totally unaware of that, as some people seem to imagine. For one thing the Subconscious is entirely aware of it, which is really just a different level of awareness. But there are also various activities of the Subconscious mind that we are dimly aware of consciously anyway, and I'll mention a few of them as we go along so you will recognise them from your own experience. Then there are some Subconscious activities we are very much aware of from time to time, like the emotions for example. Our emotions are entirely controlled by the Subconscious mind but we can be keenly aware of them on a conscious level too from time to time, especially as they become intense.

Yet there is a great deal of other activity going on in the Subconscious as well, to which the conscious mind has no access. Therefore from a conscious perspective most of what goes on in the Subconscious apparently does not exist, hence the commonplace skepticism about hypnotherapy amongst those who have never had it properly explained to them. What they are actually skeptical about is the very existence of about 88% of their own mind, which means they are a lot smarter than they think they are. Though paradoxically still dumb enough to assume that people who believe in things like hypnotherapy are credulous fools. But this is only the myopia of the conscious mind, caused by the fact that we were all raised and educated as if the Subconscious does not exist.

So the conscious mind is rather in the dark when it comes to real Subconscious activities but your mind *as a whole* is aware of it all. Every part of your mind knows what it is doing and why, it's just that the conscious part has a limited insight into that. This is due to the fact that in Western culture the prevailing orthodoxy is still retrospectively reverential towards 'The Enlightenment', so Science and Reason form the backbone of our education. Almost the totality of our education is aimed at the conscious mind as if that is the sum total of our intelligence. Consequently your conscious mind does not know that your Subconscious mind exists. Or even if it is aware of the theory that it does, it doesn't actually believe it or expect it to have any real significance in practice. Nor does your conscious mind understand what the Subconscious does or why conscious efforts often fail to prevent behaviour the Subconscious mind is directing. Such as: smoking, eating, gambling, drinking, womanising – or indeed its equivalent, which is presumably 'manising'.

In order to understand the struggles of the conscious mind - the fears, the confusion, stress and denial - and its unreliable attempts to control the organism as a whole, it is essential to grasp this simple fact:

THE SUBCONSCIOUS IS USUALLY DOMINANT

Inevitably, the Subconscious part of the mind is ordinarily dominant in much of what we do - it is by far the bigger player. But that is not the only reason. It is all one mind, in the sense that there is no physical divide, but it is not all one department, so to speak. Think of it as the Department Of External Affairs and the Department Of Internal Affairs.

The Department of External Affairs

We have all been encouraged to believe that the conscious mind is effectively the centre of all operations in the mind, like a sort of mental headquarters which is supposedly in charge of everything. Actually the conscious mind is not the centre of all mental operations at all, it is simply the part of the mind we are most aware of. And of course it is quite important. But the conscious mind is really best understood, if we are simply going to be accurate, as a particular faculty with a particular purpose – outside of which, it is frankly not much use. The conscious mind is only truly effective in dealing with The World Around Us and Other People - which is enough of a task to be going on with, of course – and it is good at that, using logic and rationality to work out what to do with external reality in real time. That is its real job, and that is what it does best, what it is designed and fit to do. The more we are able to stick to that, the happier the conscious mind tends to be, provided of course that our external reality is manageable and we are not living in a war zone or something like that. It is noticeable that many dis-eases of the conscious mind are caused by it straying from this remit too much, perhaps by focussing inward on the Self too often or dwelling excessively upon past or future. For more details about those mental troubles and their solutions, see *Poor Little Conscious Mind* by the same author.

In defining external reality as primarily the conscious mind's domain, I am not suggesting the Subconscious has no part in dealing with the world around us because that would be far from the truth, but it is only over matters pertaining to the world around us that the conscious mind often dominates. Even then, it only has power and influence in so far as the Subconscious mind permits. The Subconscious is by far the more influencial player, always. It's just that it frequently doesn't feel the need to pay much attention to our surroundings if the conscious mind is already handling it well enough. How does the Subconscious know whether the conscious mind is managing everything well enough? Simple: if a state of relative ease and calm pervades the body and mind – or at least no more than the usual levels of stress and everyday tensions – the conscious mind is apparently coping and the Subconscious can largely ignore our surroundings.

So the focus of conscious attention is ideally directed outwards. Whenever it is not – for example when the conscious mind turns attention inward and considers the Self - that is usually with some doubt, hesitation or even anxiety. The conscious mind then typically loses confidence in the prospect of positive change, because it is painfully aware of its own miserable record when it comes to changing *anything* about the Self. (N.B. This is a generalisation which is pretty universal but obviously true to a greater degree in some than in others. No human has total and consistent confidence in every aspect of the Self unless they are seriously and worryingly abnormal. In short, anyone who has no conscious self-doubt at all is insane.)

Ideally the conscious mind should avoid turning inwards and dwelling upon aspects of the Self, and certainly not for lengthy periods as it is inclined to be over-critical and feel powerless. This is the analytical part of the mind we are talking about here and it is really designed for analysing The World Out There and Other People, not ourselves. In fact the less time we spend analysing ourselves the happier we are likely to be, and the more successful too. There are no mirrors in the natural world, excepting the reflective pool which in mythology destroyed Narcissus, so I am not the first to point this out. Indeed it could be convincingly argued that the invention of the mirror has done more to waste peoples' time and make them feel dissatisfied than anything else. At least until satellite television was invented.

Just as an aside, this 'mirror' thing is also one of the main factors responsible for the gruesome carnival of the cosmetic surgery boom, accelerated dramatically by the distortions of that extended 'hall of mirrors' that is the trashy end of the media and the freaky fashion world. I was recently told (by a cosmetic surgeon, in fact) that the most common reason for taking out a personal loan was now cosmetic surgery. Not so very long ago in the UK, we collectively laughed at the bizarre fad in the USA for carving up a perfectly healthy body, but now more and more ordinary people here in the UK - with nothing really wrong with them at all in terms of their physical health - are borrowing thousands of pounds, risking disfigurement and infection just to meddle with their outward appearance. They also risk dissatisfaction and even death - and all just because of suggestion, mistaken beliefs and the sheep-like following of fashion. The suggestion is that they *should look different* from the way they naturally look. The mistaken belief is that low self-esteem can be cut out with a scalpel and confidence implanted, and fashion just comes down to this: both my friends have had it done, so I want plastic bags sewn into my body as well.

A few relaxing sessions with a good hypnotherapist can change your negative beliefs and self-perceptions completely with no risk, no mutilation, no pain, no damage, no scarring, no painful healing process - and at a fraction of the cost, leaving you happy and confident with the way you were made in the first place. I know, it sounds crazy doesn't it? We hypnotherapists are just way out there, aren't we? It's like we're from a different planet, or something. Maybe the fashion freaks are right and we should all just go with the Jack the Ripper Roadshow and the botulism injections in our faces, perhaps that's the Road to Happiness and Fulfilment right there.

Oh-oh, I've gone too far, haven't I? I've just suggested that cosmetic surgeons are like Jack the Ripper, which is completely unreasonable since he carved people up without their consent. On the other hand he probably had the mitigating factor of being psychopathic, wasn't in it for the money and he did stop short of injecting deadly poisons into the faces of living people just because they were apparently ageing quite naturally.

Botox injections are sometimes offered free with other cosmetic surgery, and since they seem to make it difficult for people to form normal facial expressions it has occured to me that maybe when the bandages come off and the patient says: "Oh my God, what have you done to me?" the Botox ensures that their expression is not quite so horrified.

So anyway – now I've got that off my chest - the conscious mind is most comfortable and successful when tackling aspects of the Here and Now, managing external reality as it occurs in real time. It is less comfortable - and far less effective - when dwelling too much on the past or the future. It can deal with concepts of past and future perfectly well of course, but if it gets into the rut of going over the past again and again, or worrying frequently about the future - what we in hypnotherapy call: playing the "What if?" game – then mental stress can build up over time, sometimes to a most unpleasant degree. Obsessive thoughts along the lines of "What if I had only done that differently?", or "What if such and such a thing happens?" can lead to endless over-analysis, indulging many possible scenarios that are fruitless and uncomfortable to consider. As a therapist I really enjoy helping people to stop doing this, especially since I used to do it rather a lot myself.

So the conscious mind is usually far more positive than that (and more productive) when focusing on a particular aspect of external reality in real time, a task it can practically grapple with. This is of course assuming that the Here and Now is bearable. In extreme circumstances, when it may not be – such as prisoners held hostage under threat of death, for example – *then*, the conscious mind may find useful escape into the past or future, to *avoid* intense mental stress. Under normal circumstances though, 'living in the moment' is the healthiest and most stress-free state for the conscious mind. Live for today, cross each bridge as you come to it, forget the past and cheer up it might never happen – and indeed probably won't.

The conscious mind can be powerful and effective when used properly but it certainly is limited, and not just by its size. Maintaining consciousness apparently takes effort and we cannot sustain that effort 24 hours a day. Trying to sustain it for too long at a stretch, or taking stimulants to do so artificially both cause malfunctioning, distress and discomfort, so conscious faculties need to be shut down regularly and rested. We call this 'sleep' but most of the mind is not asleep at all, just taking care of other matters whilst we take a break from the effort of maintaining alertness to external stimuli: 'consciousness'.

Introducing: The Subconscious Mind

"The conscious mind" is simply the label we attach to the mental processing of which we are most keenly aware. It is the focus - or pinnacle - of our general awareness and we prefer always to direct it towards a singular, particular point of interest. For example: if you are talking to one person on the telephone but then someone else starts asking you questions, that is only two things calling for your attention at the same moment but it is annoying and you want it to stop. We find it almost impossible to divide our conscious attention in that way, it is far more comfortable to get one party to wait until you had dispensed with the other, so you could then give them your 'full attention'.

Unfortunately we have all been misled into believing, on a conscious level, that the conscious mind is in charge and encouraged to expect that if we make enough of a conscious effort, we can do anything. All very encouraging, I'm sure. But this is not very accurate. In fact it is quite wrong where certain matters are concerned, and the conscious mind keeps bumping up against that fact regularly and feeling all frustrated and inadequate - not to mention powerless - when in fact this is just an uncomfortable illusion caused by a lack of true understanding.

Poor little conscious mind. It takes on so much, and gets itself all in a muddle. Our education makes it Emperor, and it then has to try to control and direct *everything* as a result. Not just handling the outside world and other people - its real job - but everything else as well. Consequently, it worries a lot. Sometimes it breaks down, like any other overloaded system. Does it get properly understood then? Does it get expert assistance to get back to normal in next to no time?

Well, that largely depends upon which way you turn for help.

The Department Of Internal Affairs

The Subconscious Mind mainly deals with our internal, personal world. It controls the body in every detail, and to the finest detail too. All of our survival systems are safely under the control of the Subconscious mind so we don't have to 'think' about them at all, in fact they operate much faster than conscious thought can be processed. The conscious mind has no influence over these things. The Subconscious also directly operates all our habitual behaviour, established skills and talents; it is our passionate and creative side, dominated by those two great powerhouses of the human mind, the Emotions and the Imagination. It is also the locus of our self-esteem, which is what we really think of ourselves when no-one else is present. In hypnotherapy we believe that all healing is directed by the Subconscious mind - whether physical, emotional, mental or 'spiritual'.

The Subconscious understands logic and reason alright but it is not bound by them, as the conscious mind is. It can go beyond – via the potentially unlimited dimension of the Imagination. Every leap forward in technology, every great achievement, every human endeavour that dramatically superceded anything that went before owes much to the power of the Imagination to conceive of that which has never been, which goes further than our experience of the Real and ventures out into the unmapped country of the Possible/Impossible. The conscious, rational mind certainly plays a key role in turning that new concept into reality - by practical problem-solving, getting rid of the various obstacles that may stand in the way of achieving it - but it never produces the new concept itself. That takes imagination and a free-flow of ideas that is unrestricted by pre-existing patterns or established maps.

Take dreams, for example. Dreaming is pure Subconscious processing which seems sometimes to be directed at our conscious awareness, although it is by no means certain that it is purposely or deliberately made conscious. As all hypnotherapists know, the Subconscious can easily hold back knowledge and memories from the conscious mind, so why should we be consciously aware of anything we dream at all, unless it is intended to serve some purpose? There is apparently some emotional significance in dream content, even if the 'literal' content often seems bizarre – in the same way that there is sometimes emotional significance in Alice In Wonderland, though the actual events and conversations are often nonsensical. Does the conscious mind *accidentally* pick up fragments of dream content? Or is there sometimes a message in it for the conscious mind? We simply don't know.

The fact that dreams *are* Subconscious processing is beyond doubt because the hallmarks are all over it. Logic can be present within the experience but can also be subverted at any time, it doesn't dominate. For example, in a dream you can fall off a roof, terrified of smashing to the ground (logical), yet actually land unharmed (illogical). Things can appear together in bizarre juxtaposition, for instance you can 'know' that the house you are in is your house but in the dream it has the appearance of a castle. Someone from your primary schooldays may be with you, for no apparent reason. On an emotional level there can be a kind of time-travel - in dreams you can be back with an old partner, and once again experience all the *feelings* you had then. Or you might be sexually involved with someone in a dream that you have never consciously thought of in that way, which can be a confusing experience! Or living at an old address, yet there may be inconsistencies as well. And the clearest indicator of all is that you don't recognise the illogicalities until you re-activate the conscious, logical mind in the morning. The dream can then be reviewed – but does the conscious, logical, unimaginative, skeptical, unemotional part of the mind know how to read it?

Now, I'm not into the practice of interpreting dreams. Proposing universal theories of dream symbolism seems laughable to me because everyone has their own personal dictionary of signs and symbols and their conscious mind doesn't know where to find it anyway, so let's not waste any time on that pointless endeavour. The point is, these two different mental departments take care of different business and actually talk different languages as a result. And although your Subconscious mind knows how to get through to your conscious mind, your poor little conscious mind has never had the reality of the situation explained to it until now. Hang on in there, little conscious mind! All will become gradually clearer and clearer to you as we go on.

The Subconscious mind generally allows the conscious mind to get on with dealing with The World Out There – that's what it is for – and doesn't pay too much attention to external reality ordinarily, as long as everything is trucking along as usual. It trusts the conscious mind to handle the everyday details, and so the Subconscious can get on with governing the Internal World instead. As well as controlling the body, the Subconscious also directs rather a lot of our behaviour for us as well. This is a point that most people do not realise: the Subconscious mind directly controls a good deal of our everyday behaviour for us. All of our habits, skills and various activities that we have developed the ability to do *without thinking* are directed by the Subconscious mind, and people generally refer to this as "doing things on autopilot". And of course we do a lot of things on autopilot because most of what we do is really just repetition - of what we did yesterday, and the day before that etc.

We begin the day by switching on the conscious mind, we 'wake up'. The Subconscious does not sleep at all, it is very much a 24-hour culture in the Department of Internal Affairs. In contrast, the conscious mind does shifts. During each conscious shift, which for most people is about sixteen hours, the conscious mind spends some time actually being focussed usefully upon what we are doing at the time and the rest of the time on call. Whilst on call it may be amusing itself with any number of idle diversions, some of which are more pleasant than others. Worrying and daydreaming are common examples.

Sharing the Driving

As we go through the waking day, there will be times when the conscious mind is 'in the driving seat', as it were – directing our behaviour – because we need to *think* about this particular activity in order to do it. Then we might arrive at some task or activity that we have done a thousand times before, so there is no need to think about that. The conscious mind rests - 'takes a back seat' - and the Subconscious takes us through the usual pattern of behaviour 'on autopilot'. This state of mind is called *trance*.

Now, this often confuses people at first because most people think trance is something much more exotic than that, or you need to have a hypnotist present. But in reality trance is a normal state of mind we are often in and we certainly don't need a hypnotist to get us in or out of it. Whenever your conscious mind is not required and the Subconscious is directing your actions, you have dropped into trance. In fact we are so accustomed to drifting in and out of trance that we scarcely notice whether we are in trance or not most of the time.

For example: people who drive a vehicle regularly will often be driving in trance. In fact operating any familiar machinery, not just cars, can become 'second nature'. In other words your Subconscious is controlling that, you can do it without thinking consciously about it. This is not remotely dangerous, it is actually safer because the Subconscious can easily handle several things at the same time, which the conscious mind finds almost impossible.

Trance states are both normal and scarcely noticeable – even deep trances are common experiences. Daydreaming is a trance state, for example. If we go very deep into a daydream, we say we were "miles away". Sunbathing, especially for real 'sun-worshippers' can be a very deep trance state, with deep relaxation too – very much like hypnotherapy in fact, only warmer. There are various other common trance states. In the above example - of carrying out a familiar behaviour on autopilot - trance is being used to repeat a previously-learned action *without thinking*. If you have become able (through repetition) to do something successfully without thinking, then you usually do. Thinking is a mental effort, so if you can avoid it, that saves effort. Your brain is being energy-efficient: you drop into a sort of 'cruise control' mode and repeat the usual performance on autopilot simply because it is easier.

Now whilst you are doing that, under the direction of the Subconscious, your conscious mind has a choice. It can either hang around and observe this behaviour anyway, even though it is not actually *driving* it – as a sort of onlooker – or it can do what it usually does, wander off and think about something entirely different. So very often we are physically doing one thing whilst consciously thinking about something quite different and it is the Subconscious mind which is controlling the physical behaviour.

Those of you who drive regularly will recognise this easily from your normal experiences of driving. It doesn't seem like that for new or inexperienced drivers, but once driving has become habitual much of it is done on autopilot especially on familiar routes. Experienced drivers will frequently arrive at their destination with only partial conscious memory of the journey because they were only paying conscious attention to the driving for some of the time. On a familiar route it is not necessary to think about the driving so the conscious mind wanders off from time to time and thinks about something else. As a result of this, at journey's end the conscious mind will probably have a memory of what it was thinking about but little or no memory about driving the car.

Every now and then the conscious mind worries about this because *it has already been led to believe it has to do everything*, it doesn't really recognise the fact that the Subconcious mind exists. So if the conscious mind recognises all of a sudden that it hasn't been focused on the driving... *who was driving the car back there?* thinks the conscious mind. *I could have gone through a red light, or anything... I wasn't paying proper attention!*

Actually that is not the case at all. We have many levels of awareness and the Subconscious had it covered. This is why you arrived safely at your destination and didn't end up in a ditch. But if you consider for a moment what your Subconscious is actually doing during such moments – whilst your conscious mind has wandered off, left the scene – the Subconscious is not only controlling the vehicle with the vehicle's controls - which is complex enough - it is also watching all the other road-users, judging speeds and distances correctly, watching out for obstacles, reading road markings, watching your mirrors, signals, lights, signs... and navigating... all with no apparent effort, while you think consciously about something completely different.

Introducing: The Subconscious Mind

It's quite impressive really isn't it? That is your Subconscious mind driving a car. And of course, you trust your Subconscious with your life and the lives of everyone else on the road, which you are quite right to do because it very rarely makes mistakes, especially with driving. The human Subconscious mind is amazing: it can do lots of things at the same time with no apparent effort and get them all right too!

Now - all you experienced drivers out there - just contrast that effortless driving performance with the awkwardness with which you first learned to drive. That was a different ballgame, wasn't it? This is because whenever we learn an entirely new skill like driving, at first we have to do it consciously, there is no way to avoid that. The conscious mind really struggles to get the hang of driving too because the conscious mind always prefers to focus upon *one thing at a time*. The first time you try to drive a real car down a real road it is a very stressful experience because you are attempting to think consciously about six or seven things at once, which is almost impossible. It makes your head hurt, you get all snappy and you wonder if you'll ever be able to master it.

What changes that is repetition. The more you repeat the behaviour, the more the brain gets a chance to recognise patterns, and the Subconscious gradually takes one thing after another off the shoulders of the conscious mind, so by the time you take your driving test you are really only having to *think* about the gears, the road and the instructions. Even that is quite difficult, but the rest of the activity is already becoming automatic. Once you have passed your test, if you drive every day, within six to nine months the whole thing is on autopilot and you can drive a familiar route whilst chatting about something entirely different or singing along to the radio, a combination you could never have managed at the start.

If you are an habitual smoker, then smoking has been one of those activities your Subconcious has controlled for you for some time. But it wasn't at the start. The first thing the new smoker has to do is to learn how to smoke, because it is not easy and it is not natural. You have to inhale a cloud of poisonous gases into the lungs and try to look relaxed and comfortable at the same time. There is a bit of a trick to that.

So it was a conscious decision to begin with, to try one of those smokey, smelly things. Most of us tried not to inhale the smoke at all at first because it was obviously pretty unpleasant, hoping to get away with just blowing it straight out again. Then some kind soul pointed out that we were not doing it properly and we were then obliged to attempt inhaling smoke for the first time. The first reaction of the Subconscious was to violently object. There was instant recognition in the brain: *That is not air!* We just inhaled a cloud of poisonous gases, and so powerful reflexes are kicked in by the Subconcious to get rid of it. The smoke catches in the throat and to the delight and amusement of our friends we choked, coughed and some people even threw up. This was most uncomfortable and of course it put quite a few people off so they didn't feel like doing it again.

This coughing reaction was our Subconscious mind's first comment on the whole idea. We attempted to inhale smoke, so it kicked it back with some force. But some of us are not immediately dissuaded by this, perhaps regarding it as a challenge and we may become determined to master this business of breathing smoke in and out as if it were nothing. So if we have any kind of motivation to overcome this obstacle the Subconscious has raised, we know we *can* overcome it because we have seen other people do it. If we persist and persist trying to breathe smoke in, what happens after a fairly short delay is that the Subconscious mind – which is intelligent, by the way - comes to the conclusion that we are going to do this anyway no matter how much resistance it kicks up. So it drops the resistance in the end because we are paying no attention and reluctantly adjusts the reflexes so we can do it without coughing.

"Now the ace up our sleeve here today," I tell my smoking clients, "is that your Subconscious mind thought that was a stupid idea - breathing smoke in - and of course was right, but ever since then it has been proceeding on the assumption that you still want to do it. Perhaps you have changed your mind since then – a few times, maybe? –

consciously. But each time you decided to stop smoking or cut down, you made a new conscious decision, followed by a big conscious effort (willpower), which your Subconscious knew nothing about. And since the Subconscious was controlling the *habitual behaviour* by then, that was very significant. So when we explain to the Subconscious, later on during the trance part of the session, that you no longer wish to inhale poisonous fumes we get a delighted response from that part of the mind, because it never wanted you to do it in the first place. Not only that, your Subconscious never changed its opinion. It just didn't know about the new conscious decision, did not know this was under review. And so it caused a mental conflict: you ended up in a conscious battle with your own Subconscious mind! Smokers don't realise this, they think they're fighting a battle against tobacco or nicotine. No they are not, they are fighting a conscious resistance against their own Subconscious mind, and since the balance of power is heavily in favour of the Subconscious, the new conscious effort is highly unlikely to win out under ordinary circumstances."

Now many of you reading this may have noticed that when I was 'talking to my client' as it were, about what the Subconscious mind does or what it thinks... that the conscious, rational part of *your* mind did not really believe a word of it - as if I was just feeding my client a load of half-baked waffle that only some mug who was daft enough to believe in airy-fairy nonsense like hypnotherapy could possibly be taken in by. This negative *conscious* assessment (skepticism, disbelief) is actually common to most of us, because:

The conscious mind does not believe in the Subconscious, except perhaps in theory. (Getting the hang of it now?)

So the conscious mind, by extension, does not believe in hypnotherapy either - except perhaps in theory. Therefore it would not be at all surprising if *your* conscious mind is still struggling to believe some of what you're reading here. Don't let this bother you, it is normal. Your Subconscious knows it's all true. Your conscious mind will probably get there too, in the end. It has simply been completely misled for years.

You see, your conscious mind was already accustomed to the idea that *it* decides and controls everything and it quite liked that idea, even though it wasn't true. So it may not like the sound of this thing called the Subconscious Mind at first. Especially if the Subconscious Mind gets to have Capital Letters and the conscious mind doesn't. This makes the **Subconscious Mind** seem alarmingly significant, possibly even **DOMINANT.** The conscious mind doesn't like the sound of

THE SUBCONSCIOUS MIND

...one tiny little bit, at first. At least, until it gets to understand it better. Takes a while. Don't expect to become an expert in these matters overnight.

Of course it is all one mind really. It's just that the conscious mind thinks it's all one conscious mind, which is *very* wide of the mark - and the Subconscious is largely unaware of the beliefs and opinions held by the conscious mind anyway. The conscious mind does tend to believe it controls all choices and actions, or that it *ought* to be able to, when actually it doesn't. Also, we do know that the Subconscious mind can completely fool the conscious mind if it chooses to do so, and that conscious perceptions are often subject and secondary to what the Subconscious intends, or believes.

For example: you fear that you have lost your car keys, so you search everywhere. They're not in the hall, the kitchen or the lounge – they are never in the bathroom but you check anyway, and they aren't in the bedroom or your coat pocket either. You search everywhere again, and again. Gradually you are becoming more desperate and panicky... then all of a sudden there they are, on the hall table. But that's the first place you looked! Three times, you looked and they weren't there, you'll swear to God.

But now they are. So what happened? Did some little leprechaun hide them away for a bit, just for a laugh? Or did the strength of your **fear** that you had **lost** your keys dominate the search process, overruling conscious perceptions entirely at first? The fear is an emotion generated by the Subconscious as a reaction to the Subconscious belief that the keys were not there to be found, that they were actually lost. This fear is the dominant experience, actually denying conscious perception at first.

An even clearer demonstration – albeit with very different emotions in play - is the one favoured in the past by many stage hypnotists, in which a person in trance is presented with a raw onion for consumption along with the suggestion that it is "a delicious apple". Anyone witnessing this will see that it cannot be faked (just try to fake it yourself, if you think it can) and it is obvious the person in trance is not consciously experiencing the normally overwhelming taste of raw onion but something much more pleasant than that.

Now don't go assuming that the Subconscious is being fooled in that demonstration. The Subconscious is being invited by the stage hypnotist to play a practical joke on the conscious mind and is entering into the spirit of the thing just for fun. It is the conscious mind that is deceived because all sensory perception is processed by the Subconscious before it is presented to conscious awareness. So if the fun-loving, imaginative Subconscious agrees on this occasion that it might be a bit of a laugh to switch one experience for a completely different one from the vast memory-banks of the Subconscious before presenting it to conscious awareness, it can do that easily.

This means that as long as the desire is to enjoy the experience suggested, the person with the onion is not just trying to pretend they are enjoying an apple – they really are! Just look at the kind of vivid 'perceptions' we experience in dreams. They seem very real at the time, do they not? Whilst dreaming, people can reach sexual climax or wake up screaming in terror when nothing is actually happening 'in reality' as it were. Well, not in the external reality anyway. There's a lot going on internally of course, and the part of it that reaches conscious perception just prior to being fully awake can be very convincing indeed.

To sum up, thanks to the way we are 'educated' the conscious mind can be completely wrong about a lot of things. For example, the conscious mind has been led to believe that the only way to change our usual behaviour is by a firm conscious decision followed by a sustained effort of conscious will, and that if that doesn't do it then the thing cannot be changed. Which is wrong, fortunately.

<u>Question:</u> If you want the Company to change its policy or procedures, do you talk to the receptionist about it?

Receptionists often end up imagining they control everything. Look at Doctors' receptionists, who commonly have an amazingly inflated notion of their own importance. Not all of them are like that, but some are astonishingly full of themselves. GPs are bound to notice when their receptionist has an exaggerated sense of self-importance, yet at the same time the Doctor recognises that having a confident and assertive receptionist is essential unless you want to be constantly having to deal with the world out there and other people yourself.

Since the conscious mind's primary responsibility is to deal with The Outside World And Other People, it is effectively the mind's Receptionist. That is it's real job, it just *thinks* it is the Director, because it is largely unaware of the Subconscious. In reality the conscious mind is merely the interface between the true self and external reality, but it thinks it is the self. It is quite funny in a way and the Subconscious does enjoy making the conscious mind look foolish from time to time. Basically that is what stage hypnosis is all about - the hypnotist colluding with the volunteer's Subconscious to make their conscious mind get confused or ridiculed just for a giggle, because the conscious mind has little power to overrule behaviour being directed by the Subconscious. Sure, we can make all sorts of conscious decisions and resolutions to change something – but does it *change?*

So you see when people think they are fighting a battle with tobacco or nicotine they are actually wrong, they are fighting a conscious battle against their own Subconscious mind. It is an internal conflict which the conscious mind is not likely to win because the Subconscious is usually dominant, especially with regard to our habitual behaviour. In fact the Subconscious is largely unaware there is a battle going on because all the stress and struggle is going on at a conscious level. This makes the conscious mind *feel powerless* over so many things, and since nobody told the conscious mind that the Subconscious does control those things your conscious perception is that you have limited control over yourself or are being 'controlled' by some external factor - like a slot machine, tobacco or cocaine - which is just not true at all.

The Subconscious simply does not recognise that there is a problem, it is just repeating the usual behavioural pattern - controlling it all fine, actually - and is usually happy to change any of it once we explain to the Subconscious that the behaviour is now under review. Provided we explain clearly to that part of the mind *what changes are required* and *what benefits that will bring/what dangers it will avoid* - and providing the Subconscious has no objection to any of that - it will go ahead and change it. When it does change, it happens with no apparent effort and the results amaze the conscious mind, which didn't do a thing. If at first there is no change, then there is apparently a Subconscious objection or hesitation, and we would then need to negotiate around that. But the Subconscious is intelligent, we can usually work out a deal. This is called "hypnotherapy". Most people alive today have never experienced it, which is a shame really, since it has to be just about the most useful phenomenon ever. It is not the Power of Suggestion. It is not the Power of Hypnotism, or the hypnotist. It is the phenomenal power of the human Subconscious mind, and we all have one.

In addition to changing habit patterns the Subconscious can also change emotions and emotional reactions easily. All of our emotions are controlled and operated by the Subconscious, which is why the conscious mind doesn't always understand why you feel the way you do. "I know it's silly," people often say, meaning 'not strictly rational', "but I can't help the way I feel!" In fact it is fairly commonplace to hear someone say defensively: "I can't help my feelings, can I?" as if their feelings were controlled by somebody else. But that is the conscious mind talking, freely admitting that it doesn't control emotions because they are all controlled by the Subconscious. And it can adjust them any time you like, slightly or radically. But it needs a good reason, so when I request such changes when I'm addressing the Subconscious mind of a client, I have to do some artful negotiating, or else it will probably just ignore the request. Skills of advocacy and diplomacy are needed in equal measure when talking to the Subconscious, as are the abilities to inspire excitement and enthusiasm in another person regarding the prospect of change. Hypnotherapy is inevitably an emotional business because the Subconscious is the emotional part of the mind. A hypnotherapist who is timid or hesitant in the stormy field of human emotions will inevitably be an average agent of change, at best, and may resort to working with the conscious mind rather too much – which is not really hypnotherapy at all, but counselling or psychotherapy.

Actually the conscious mind tends to regard emotions as a bit of a disruptive nuisance, mainly because we learn from experience fairly early on in life that if we become emotional, then the conscious, rational part of the mind is knocked rudely out of the way and is not allowed to dominate again until we have calmed down. So the conscious mind naturally tends to regard emotions as unpredictable, disruptive and sometimes apparently illogical. The conscious mind often cannot understand or influence the emotional intensity or direction - but the Subconscious can.

So in the ordinary course of your day, there will be times when your conscious mind is directing your behaviour, and times when it is the Subconscious. It cannot be both, so if there's a conflict over control, the conscious mind can only manage to dominate with a considerable effort of will - and even then, only provided the Subconscious motivation is not very strong at that moment. If there is a strong Subconscious motivation, forget it - the conscious effort will be futile virtually every time. You can put up a struggle but really you are just delaying the inevitable... and it feels like that, too!

So if that doesn't appeal – and really, why would it? - you can choose instead to visit someone like myself, who properly understands this thing called "hypnosis" - possibly the most consistently misunderstood phenomenon I have ever encountered - and knows how to put the conscious mind's point of view over convincingly to the Subconscious. Then the Subconscious can adjust behaviour accordingly, without any conflict, and without any conscious effort being required. Many things are up for negotiation with the Subconscious mind. Just remember where the power really lies – and it *isn't* with the hypnotist.

Interlude: Case Mysteries No.3

Misunderstanding hypnosis and hypnotherapy has been the norm throughout history and to illustrate this, I'm going to directly quote a man who has been repeatedly described – mainly by himself and his publishers - as the world's greatest authority on smoking: Allen Carr. This is a Case Mystery which does not feature one of my clients at all, but a man I never met and who recently passed away. I will let him describe his own experiences by quoting directly from his published works, then I will comment upon his statements and his claims.

Some of you may not have heard of Allen Carr but he certainly was a very well-known chap, author of numerous self-help books, at least six of which are about how to stop smoking. The success of these books led to the development of many Allen Carr Clinics, a franchise system promoting his trademarked 'Easy Way' method, not just in the UK but everywhere from Iceland to Ecuador! These clinics claim "a success rate of over 95%". (See *Success Rates* in Section 14, Volume II.)

I am quite familiar with Allen Carr's work, having read four of his books including two on smoking. In fact the general theme of the smoking books were remarkably similar, which is perhaps not surprising when you consider that his published works on that subject include:

Allen Carr's Easy Way to Stop Smoking

The Only Way to Stop Smoking Permanently

Packing it in the Easy Way

How to Stop your Child Smoking

The Little Book of Quitting

and *Allen Carr's Easy Way for Women to Stop Smoking.*

Case Mysteries 3: Allen Carr's Success Stories

Presumably already in the planning stages were: The Only Way for Men to Stop Smoking, How to Never Smoke Again, The Easy Way for Redheads to Stop Smoking, How to Stop Women Smoking Permanently the Easy Way, How to Easily Stop Smoking Again and The Easy Way to Not Start Smoking. Sadly events have robbed us of those titles and the world's smokers will just have to try to save themselves with the six introductory volumes and the many disciples running the franchises all over the world.

Allen Carr's Success Stories (Are you sitting comfortably?)

In the first book, *Allen Carr's Easy Way To Stop Smoking*, originally published in 1985, the following notes are written under the heading 'About The Author':

"A successful accountant, Allen Carr's hundred-cigarettes-a-day addiction was driving him to despair until, in 1983, after countless failed attempts to quit, he finally discovered what the world had been waiting for – the Easy Way to Stop Smoking".

Now, what is most interesting about this 'thing' he discovered is that most people who read the book apparently don't remember it. Many times when people come to me for smoking therapy, they mention that they have read this book, so I ask them: "Do you remember how Allen Carr himself stopped smoking?" and so far, only a few clients have actually been able to tell me. So for all of you who have never read the book, and also those who have, but don't remember precisely what Allen Carr "discovered", I will quote the book directly and let Allen himself explain (Page One, by the way):

"Eventually my wife sent me to a hypnotherapist. I must confess I was completely sceptical, knowing nothing about hypnosis in those days and having visions of a Svengali-type figure with piercing eyes and a waving pendulum. I had all the normal illusions that smokers have about smoking except one – I knew that I wasn't a weak-willed person. I was in control of all other aspects of my life but cigarettes controlled me. I thought that hypnosis involved the forcing of wills, and although I was not obstructive (like most smokers, I dearly wanted to stop), I thought no-one was going to kid me that I didn't need to smoke.

"The whole session appeared to be a waste of time. The hypnotherapist tried to make me lift my arms and do various other things. Nothing appeared to be working properly. I didn't lose consciousness. I didn't go into a trance, or at least I didn't think I did, and yet after that session not only did I stop smoking but I actually enjoyed the process even during the withdrawal period."

So the thing most people who read this book don't remember by the time they've finished it, is that what Allen Carr actually "discovered" was hypnotherapy. Not that it was lost in 1983, but it was the first time Allen Carr had encountered it for real. And it certainly is the easiest way to stop smoking, as well as the quickest and the safest. But if he just wrote:

"Go and see a hypnotherapist – worked a treat for me, even though I spent most of the session thinking it was a waste of time!"

...it would have made a very short book, and he couldn't have opened all those Easy Way Clinics on the back of that simple piece of advice. So Allen Carr did something entirely different. Look how he dispenses with hypnotherapy in the next paragraph in order to claim the success of hypnosis for himself, and then actually warn you off the therapy that saved him. Allen Carr again:

"Now, before you go rushing off to see a hypnotherapist, let me make something quite clear. Hypnotherapy is a means of communication. If the wrong message is communicated, you won't stop smoking. I'm loath to criticise the man whom I consulted because I would be dead by now if I hadn't seen him. But it was in spite of him, not because of him. Neither do I wish to appear to be knocking hypnotherapy; on the contrary, I use it as part of my own consultations. It is the power of suggestion and a powerful force that can be used for good or evil. Don't ever consult a hypnotherapist unless he or she has been personally recommended by someone you respect and trust."

(*Allen Carr's Easy Way to Stop Smoking,* Penguin 3rd edition, 1999)

Isn't that amazing? It's all right for Allen Carr to go rushing off to see a hypnotherapist, but not you. Clearly the right message was communicated to his Subconscious, because his habit was suddenly removed easily. His conscious mind didn't understand it though, and it later decided that he must have managed somehow, after many years of futile attempts, to suddenly solve the problem logically - coincidentally during a hypnotherapy session, and "in spite of" the assistance of the therapist! Well if I were his hypnotherapist I'd feel like hitting him with a shovel. As for the last two sentences from Mr Carr, those ignorant suggestions are obviously just a cheap attempt to scare you off going to see a professional hypnotherapist. But it's all right for you to go to one of Mr Carr's clinics of course, where hypnotherapy is used for good, presumably, and not evil.

In fact, if you ever feel inclined to ignore Mr Carr's grim warning and risk ringing a Real Hypnotherapist - instead of the disciples of Mr Carr, who are not real hypnotherapists, even if they claim to use something he calls "hypnotherapy" as part of his patented method - it might be worth asking the Real Hypnotherapist if he or she is using hypnotherapy for good, or evil purposes? Just as a precaution, you understand. Good hypnotherapists won't mind answering the question at all, whilst evil ones will scream: "Curses! Foiled again!" and slam the phone down.

What is an evil hypnotist? Has there ever been one? Can you name one? No problem naming an evil doctor: Josef Mengele, Dr Crippen, Harold Shipman - to name but three - although actually poor old Crippen shouldn't really be bracketed with those other monsters, that's a bit unfair. He only killed his wife, and although that is a terrible thing to do it is at least arguably understandable, so it doesn't put him on a par with Mengele and Shipman, far from it. And there have been quite a few other fairly evil medical persons too, like that mad nurse who poisoned all those young children in hospital. But can you name one evil hypnotist?

Can you name two or three *famous* hypnotists, anyway? And have any of them ever been accused of being evil or using hypnosis for evil purposes? If not, why not? If hypnosis really was a way of controlling other people wouldn't hypnotists simply rule the world? Surely life would be one long battle between the Good Hypnotists and the Evil Hypnotists, each side commanding great armies of hypnotised people, a bit like the Lord of the Rings. Well why not, it would obviously be more thrilling than helping people to stop biting their fingernails or get over their morbid fear of escalators.

The Hypnotist Controls Nothing!

Obviously hypnotists don't control people. If we could, we would control everything via that influence and I'm sure that would be tremendous fun but the reality is nothing like that at all, which is why I still have to turn up at the office Monday morning just like everybody else. I don't mind that so much these days because I get to make all the decisions and don't have to answer to anyone - but it's not quite the same as ruling the world, now is it?

So Allen Carr didn't think he was in a trance because he didn't lose consciousness. This is a very common misconception. People in trance are not unconscious or asleep, they are actually in a heightened state of awareness. Or to put it another way, a highly focused state. This doesn't feel strange in any way because we are often in trance, so it is common for people to think they aren't in trance at all because they were not expecting the trance state to feel normal. They were expecting to *feel hypnotized* – even if they weren't quite sure what that would actually be like.

From what Allen Carr has written it is obvious to me he had a very confused notion of what hypnosis is, which makes me wonder what exactly passes for 'hypnotherapy' in his clinics. But the most ridiculous aspect of the passage quoted above is this: if he really "discovered EasyWay" and solved his own smoking problem independently in spite of his hypnotherapist, as he claims, then why would he want to incorporate hypnotherapy in his own consultations? Isn't that a contradiction? Either hypnotherapy helped him or it didn't. If it did, then all you need is good quality hypnotherapy, just as I am advising throughout this book. But if Allen Carr honestly believes it didn't play any significant role in his sudden liberation, why on earth would he be going down that road with his own clients?

Actually what Allen Carr did is by no means new, because what he really did was re-package hypnotherapy and give it a different name, in this case "EasyWay". But he also changed it, and not for the better either. He took the message, extended it and put too much emphasis on convincing the conscious mind, with nowhere near enough emphasis on persuading the Subconscious to make the change. Since the Subconscious controls all habitual behaviour and generates all 'craving' signals, this is a serious error.

His clinics do group therapy too, more lucrative than one-to-one sessions but it is not easy to get spectacular results with smoking if you work with people in groups (see Case Mysteries 9 in Section 16, Volume II). Not only that, but Mr Carr - or rather his franchised practitioner nowadays - only spends about twenty minutes out of the four-hour session addressing the Subconscious. Most of the session is aimed at the conscious mind. This may well affect the clients' *conscious intentions* but all smokers know their habitual smoking pattern has very little to do with their conscious intentions. Cravings are signals fired off by the Subconscious mind, and all habitual behaviour is handled by that mental department. Allen Carr's method is likely to leave too many people with cravings still happening, which makes them much less likely to succeed long term. Also, in presenting the case for change it is important to make all the same points to the Subconscious mind that you make to the conscious mind, not a much-shortened version which cuts nearly all of the detail out. If anything it is far more important than convincing the conscious mind, although actually the ideal outcome is to have fully convinced both.

How Allen Carr came to misunderstand in the first place

Allen Carr was an accountant by profession. It is not surprising he should overestimate the significance of the conscious mind – everyone does, but especially people whose work heavily relies upon analytical processes. Accountancy is one of a number of professions which demand sustained conscious analysis of boring detail regarding matters the Subconscious would not be remotely interested in, which happens to be money in this example. When people are in the habit of thinking analytically all day long, they often continue that mode of thinking outside of work as well. Allen Carr would inevitably have been in the habit of assessing matters analytically, so he would be likely to have great confidence in his rational processes, and indeed he comes across in his writing as a man who prides himself on his ability to use reason and logic to approach a problem in a way he describes himself as "scientific". Therefore it is easy to understand why his conscious mind quite quickly decided to take full credit for what his Subconscious actually did during his own hypnotherapy session – in denial of the existence of the Subconscious in fact, and completely misunderstanding what hypnosis is:

I thought that hypnosis involved the forcing of wills... I thought no-one was going to kid me that I didn't need to smoke.

Notice how that outlook is completely conscious-centred, revealing the common assumption that conscious mental processing IS the human mind, as if mental processing outside of that simply isn't there. Since the operations and activities of the Subconscious are sub-conscious, of course he was not consciously aware of what his Subconscious did during that session. But he certainly noticed the remarkable results:

"I actually enjoyed the process, even during the withdrawal period."

In other words there was no 'withdrawal' experience, obviously it is impossible to enjoy withdrawal. This is consistent with our usual findings in hypnotherapy. After the sessions in which success is total, the client simply feels great.

<u>The conscious mind always assumes the therapist is talking to IT</u>

During a hypnotherapy session the client is always unaware of what their Subconscious is doing. It is mental activity beneath the usual level of consciousness, that is what subconscious means. Whilst in trance you are perfectly well aware of what your *conscious* mind is doing though, and since the conscious mind thinks it controls everything - or should be able to - the conscious mind's assumption during the trance part of the session is that the hypnotherapist is still talking to *it,* as if expecting the conscious mind to make the changes. Of course the conscious mind can hear the hypnotherapist, as normal, but he is actually addressing the Subconscious. It's just that the conscious mind doesn't understand that. It doesn't really believe in the Subconscious anyway and is already a bit confused by the fact that all this feels perfectly normal, almost as if nothing special is happening at all.

Of course the hypnotherapist is not talking to the conscious mind! If the conscious mind could make the change it would have done so already and the hypnotherapist would not be required. The hypnotherapist is directly appealing to the Subconscious mind. But since the client is not consciously aware of the real existence of that mental entity, doesn't feel any different in trance anyway *and* their conscious mind assumes the hypnotherapist is still talking to *it,* Allen Carr's conscious confusion about his session is both normal and commonplace. His Subconscious *desire* to be rid of the habit was all that really mattered though:

"I was not obstructive (like most smokers, I <u>dearly wanted</u> to stop)"

so his Subconscious, judging exclusively by the deeper *desire for change* and oblivious to any conscious doubts, went ahead and made the change:

"...after that session not only did I stop smoking but I actually enjoyed the process..."

This is so markedly different to all his previous experiences of trying to stop smoking, not to mention his very low conscious expectations of going to a hypnotherapist:

"I thought no-one was going to kid me that I didn't need to smoke..."

...that it is obvious, really, that the crucial difference was indeed hypnotherapy. The fact that Allen Carr later added a hypnotherapy angle to his EasyWay method when he started opening clinics hints at the fact that he knows this, actually, and while he was alive a number of critics raised exactly this point, much to his annoyance. The addition of the hypnotherapy part at the end of the standardised sessions in his clinics also created a problem for him in the promotion of his method. Did he not warn everybody off hypnotherapy in the first book? Although he freely admits to being astonished to find that his smoking habit seemed to have disappeared sometime during his hypnotherapy session, he did not want to give hypnotherapy the credit for that. In fact, all of his own subsequent success and fame entirely depended upon him not giving hypnotherapy the credit, but finding a way to convince himself (and hopefully the world) that he did it all by himself, coincidentally during a hypnotherapy session.

The Attempted Cover-Up

I sincerely hope you enjoy reading this part as much as I know I'm going to enjoy writing it. Originally I was going to go easy on Allen Carr because the books he has written, and his clinics, have helped a lot of people and I thought it was fair to acknowledge that – although of course he did make an absolute fortune out of it all and ended up crediting himself with being some sort of guru. Also because, for a long time I had just assumed that he simply misunderstood what had happened in his hypnotherapy session, and he did not fully realise that he had actually stolen the credit from his therapist and built a lucrative empire by capitalising upon that theft. Or that if he did realise it later, it was a bit late to correct it and he just decided to keep quiet and hope no-one noticed.

However, that is not what happened at all, and this is a fact I was largely unaware of until very recently. Once I began writing the final draft of this Case Mystery, I became more curious about what Allen Carr had written about this matter in all the other books on smoking he published later, only one of which I had read. So I went and did some research. What I discovered made me so angry, on behalf of my beloved hypnotherapy profession, that I lost all sympathy for the man. To be quite frank, if his reputation is seriously tarnished by the next few pages he thoroughly deserves it, and brought it upon himself. His deception turns out to be quite calculated and his denial of the true value of hypnotherapy – which saved his life – so mean and self-serving that it shows Allen Carr in a very poor light, a man whose ambition completely overrode his objectivity and his judgement... well, see what you think. If you are not involved in the hypnotherapy profession, you can be more objective than I can. I am just angry. Later I'll clear it with a bit of self-hypnosis, but not before I've finished writing this. In fact, setting the record straight is a vital part of the therapeutic process!

I am going to quote from four different books in which Allen Carr gives various accounts of how he stopped smoking. Presumably he hoped that no-one would bother to critically analyse and compare them all. The first is the one from which I quoted already, which Allen Carr originally published himself in 1985 under the title *The Easy Way to Stop Smoking*. I believe this to be the only version that honestly attempts to be accurate, and it clearly shows that Mr. Carr was astonished and confused about what had happened. It is also clear to anyone with a proper understanding of hypnosis that Allen Carr doesn't know the first thing about it, despite the fact that he claims here to have read lots of books on the subject after his session:

I didn't go into a trance, or at least I didn't think I did, and yet after that session not only did I stop smoking but I actually enjoyed the process even during the withdrawal period.

Then further down the same page:

... Let me make something quite clear from the beginning: I am not a mystical figure. I do not believe in magicians or fairies. I have a scientific brain, and I couldn't understand what appeared to me like magic. I started reading up on hypnosis and on smoking. Nothing I read seemed to explain the miracle that had happened. Why had it been so ridiculously easy to stop, whereas previously it had been weeks of black depression?

The answer is simply because the hypnotherapy worked, but having taken up the position that the session was a waste of time, Allen Carr had to come up with a different explanation, first for himself, and then later so he could write a book about it. In this first version, he admits that this mental journey took a long time, and indeed it must have been quite a while if it truly included enough time to read up on hypnosis to any useful extent. Quite why he should bother to do that if he really believed that the session had been a waste of time, he doesn't say.

It took me a long time to work it all out, basically because I was going about it back to front. I was trying to work out why it had been so easy to stop, whereas the real problem is trying to understand why smokers find it so *difficult* to stop. Smokers talk about the terrible withdrawal pangs, but when I looked back and tried to remember those awful pangs, they didn't exist for me. There was no physical pain. It was all in the mind.

This is a fundamental misunderstanding. The discomforts experienced by smokers who try to abstain from smoking using willpower are real physical experiences, but they are created and controlled by the mind. Allen Carr's Subconscious mind simply shut them down during the hypnotherapy session, removing all motivation to smoke, but to believe in something like that was as alien to Allen Carr's 'scientific brain' as magicians and fairies. Note the *arrogance* of his conscious mind, in total denial of the existence of a Subconscious.

Now, according to the myth-making of the later books, Allen Carr arrived home from his hypnotherapy session declaring confidently to his wife that he was going to singlehandedly "cure the world of smoking", having had some blindingly brilliant notion, coincidentally during a hypnotherapy session. But that is not how he described it in the section I quoted above. His poor little conscious mind – which describes itself as a "scientific brain", presumably because it sports a white coat and thinks the terms *skeptical* and *intelligent* are interchangable – was clearly confused and troubled by a "miracle" which it knew it did not perform and could not explain. So the conscious mind did what it always must: it made up a plausible explanation which allowed it to take the credit for the change in due course. Now just watch how that evolved over time, as Allen Carr's analytical mind tried to hide the contradictions and manipulate the thinking of his readers. This next account of the same events is taken from the second book on smoking, *The Only Way to Stop Smoking Permanently,* first published in 1994:

I knew that the hypnotherapist would not be able to help me. But I thought that if I go through the ritual, I could come home, conscience completely clear, and say, "You see, it was a complete waste of time and money!"

... "I'M GOING TO CURE THE WORLD OF SMOKING!" Those were the actual words I greeted Joyce with on my return.

Hang on, that's not what he said in the first book, is it? What happened to:

I couldn't understand what appeared to me like magic. I started reading up on hypnosis and on smoking. Nothing I read seemed to explain the miracle that had happened....It took me a long time to work it all out...

Now, nine years later he is apparently suggesting that he managed to get all of that done on his way home from the hypnotherapy session. His wife was very dubious too, it seems:

She couldn't have looked more aghast if I had hit her on the knee with a hammer... I was on such a high at the time that I couldn't understand her disbelief... I think she believed that the hypnotherapist had put me into some sort of trance and had forgotten to take me out of it.

Notice how he has now transferred the confusion and astonishment to his wife, and claims to have been 'on a high' himself, which is significantly different from his original description of the aftermath of his session. He then continues thus:

What you will find difficult to believe is that before I extinguished that last cigarette, I was already a non-smoker and already knew that I would never have the need or desire to smoke again.

Allen Carr expects that you will find that difficult to believe, and in saying that he is unconsciously giving himself away. He fears that you will not believe it for the simple reason that it isn't true, and he knew it wasn't true when he constructed that sentence, anticipating your disbelief. It is the same mistake a liar makes when he begins a sentence with "You're never going to believe what's just happened..."

My visit to the hypnotherapist was on 15th July 1983 and was the most important day of my life. From here on I will refer to it as Independence Day. You might well be tempted to rush off to the nearest hypnotherapist. Please don't! I am loathe to run down the man that I consulted, because I would be dead now if I had not made that visit. But I succeeded in spite of and not because of that visit. Later I will explain more about the mysteries surrounding hypnosis which will enable you to decide whether or not it can be of sevice to you.

Although I did not fully comprehend everything that happened to me on that day, I was fully aware that I had made a discovery that every smoker was secretly searching for: AN EASY WAY TO STOP SMOKING!

Yes Allen, it's called hypnotherapy and you did not discover it. In fact you tried your very best to bury it later, as we shall see. Notice again how he claims here to be "fully aware" of his method at this point, directly contradicting what he said in the first book. Also notice how he has dropped the bit about reading up on hypnosis, because that would suggest he was still prepared to entertain the idea hypnosis might have caused the change. However, he still cannot help admitting at this stage that he does not (yet) fully comprehend what had happened on that day. He is still in the process of formulating a story that will award him full credit, a myth upon which Easy Way can stand firmly. As for explaining any "mysteries" about hypnosis later on in that book, well, if he mentions hypnosis at all after that point I certainly cannot find any trace of it. So the reader is merely left with a warning - "Please, don't!" - and the sly suggestion that hypnotherapy is mysterious, which is enough to put some people off.

From this point in time onwards he becomes more and more dishonest. Oh, what a tangled web we weave, eh Allen? This next group of quotes are taken from *Packing It In The Easy Way,* first published in 2004. Again he begins by describing his wife's attempts to get him to seek help:

She implored me to consult the hypno-therapist who had helped a friend of ours to quit. I was very dubious. Our friend didn't seem completely cured. He had that lack-lustre appearance characteristic of smokers who are using willpower... I was certain hypnotherapy was not the answer and that the whole excercise would be a waste of time and money. No-one could kid me that I didn't need to smoke. But I agreed to go, purely to placate Joyce. I wanted to be able to say to her: "Look, I've done what you asked, but it hasn't worked!"

I didn't set out with the deliberate intention of resisting the hypnotherapist's influence...

What? After what you just said? Come off it Allen, you've just stated that you fully intended to prove your own conscious assumption that hypnotherapy was not the answer. What really confused you afterwards was that it worked! You were totally thrown by that, as you admitted in your first book, but later on you started to change your tune, and it became necessary to invent a different tale in which hypnotherapy is cast in a more and more negative light. Far from explaining any mysteries surrounding hypnotherapy, watch how he plays upon the fears and likely ignorance of his readers in denying the role of hypnosis in his successful session:

If he could have cured me I would have been prepared to pretend I was a chicken or suffer any indignity he might suggest...

This from a man who claims to have read widely on the subject of hypnosis and also claims to use hypnotherapy as a part of his own method. There is no indignity in hypnotherapy, although some might feel that there is in stage hypnosis. Does this fool not know the difference? How on earth is he proposing to enlighten his readers about hypnotherapy if this is the reality of his own ignorance and prejudice?

What is perhaps most significant is that in the first book he merely comments that nothing significant seemed to be happening in his hypnotherapy session, yet seems content to credit that session with being the occasion of change, prompting him to go reading up on hypnosis afterwards to see if he could arrive at an understanding of what exactly happened. Bear that in mind as you read what he says two decades later about what happened immediately after the session, now that he has become a millionaire and self-styled smoking guru. By 2004 it is as if he is describing completely different events. He has by this point invented a "process of realisation" that involved a number of factors coming together:

Two distinct factors were introduced, they combined and then fused in my consciousness.

I was not aware of either when I dutifully made my way to the hypnotherapist's clinic.

I had anticipated being met by an individual straight out of a Hollywood film, with bushy eyebrows, piercing eyes and a goatee beard. To my relief, what I got was a bright, earnest, clean-shaven and articulate young man...

You were lucky. Most of us are really scary monsters you wouldn't want to meet on a dark night. One of my heads actually has fangs. Now just listen to this new edition of the tale. According to Allen Carr, this next detail is central to the original conception of his method, a moment of such significance it changed his life and led to the salvation of millions of smokers worldwide. This is his third book on how he developed his method, yet it is the first time he has ever mentioned this:

Before the therapy we had a friendly chat about smoking generally, during the course of which the smidgen was added: "Do you realise that smoking is just nicotine addiction and if you quit for long enough you will eventually be free?"

I cannot remember another statement he made during our chat, but that smidgen – that smoking is just nicotine addiction – remained lodged in my brain.

He then goes off into a long ramble about nicotine and heroin which is actually a load of claptrap, but the gist of it is supposed to be that this was a great moment of insight for him, which he sums up thus:

Like many smokers I couldn't understand why I smoked. The therapist's statement actually explained the reason – drug addiction. For the first time I saw myself as akin to a heroin addict, and not merely as an habitual smoker. The part of the statement that really stuck in my mind was: "if you quit for long enough you will eventually be free."

Hm. Where to start? Well for one thing, no hypnotherapist would be likely to say that because it would imply that the hypnotherapy we are about to do is pretty insignificant, but if you can abstain from nicotine for long enough, the problem will be resolved eventually via a natural detoxification process. Is Allen Carr seriously trying to suggest that this notion struck him as a revelation? How is it different from the standard medical assumptions that spawned NRT? And if all this were true, then an unpleasant withdrawal experience would be absolutely inevitable, wouldn't it? Finally, if this was such a blinding flash to him, which changed his perception of smoking so markedly, why did he never think to mention it in either of the previous books? Why did he originally claim that he immediately started reading up on hypnosis? That course of action would make no sense at all if this 2004 version of the tale were the truth.

But look how he further changes his story in an attempt to rob the hypnotherapy process of any credit. In this version of the event, the significant moment is placed in the conversation before any hypnosis is involved, and he now claims to *know already* that a change has taken place:

Now, seeing myself in this new light, as someone addicted to a drug, I believed the goal of quitting was achievable. I didn't care how long it would take. I wasn't expecting it to be easy. On the contrary, I knew I could expect at least six months of misery... I had about five cigarettes left in the pack and decided there and then that they would be the last I would smoke.

It seemed a bit late to be springing news of my conversion on the hypnotherapist, and so I kept quiet. The session was now pointless, but as long as he didn't become aware of this fact there would be little harm in going through with it.

The session was now pointless, says Allen Carr. And it now becomes essential, in the construction of the myth that will safeguard EasyWay, for him to emphasize just how pointless it was in every respect. So in this version he takes the trouble to go into some detail about the supposed incompetence of the therapist, details which actually allow real experts in hypnotherapy only two possible interpretations. This description either demonstrates how dull and inert Mr Carr was in failing to respond to really basic methods of inducing trance, or else he is exaggerating the cluminess of the occasion, but with the use of a poor imagination that has no real understanding of hypnotic procedures upon which to draw.

Yet none of that actually matters, because even if this new and very negative description of the trance part of the session were true to the letter, hypnotherapy can still succeed. When you read the details in Section 6 about what really happens in hypnotherapy, and compare it to the details coming up, you will see that the last fifteen minutes of the session contains all the ingredients necessary for the Subconscious to do the job: a genuine desire to be rid of the habit at an emotional level, suggestions that smoking is futile and negative, presented to the client whilst the Subconscious is paying attention because he had his eyes closed for that period. Not being relaxed is irrelevant, but Carr didn't know that - and the fact that his conscious mind was convinced it was all a waste of time is also irrelevant, as we saw with The Angry Satisfied Customer and many other cases too.

All the therapist's induction suggestions - about arms lifting, and eyes closing by themselves - are exactly the sort of thing I never bother with because they are unnecessary and can be very hit and miss, as I explain in Section 6. But notice how Allen Carr uses his non-response to those things to help him present the whole process of hypnotherapy to his readers as a waste of time – ridiculous even. Hypnotherapists take note: 'convincers' can easily create exactly the wrong impression. But look how Carr first strikes a note of compliance, to suggest once again that he was not being obstructive:

> I was asked to close my eyes and imagine I was walking through a beautiful garden. This I did and very pleasant it was too. Then I was told my left arm would begin to feel very light, it would become lighter and lighter and eventually weightless and float in mid air. Ten minutes of cajoling didn't make it feel any lighter and my growing embarrassment for the therapist blocked out all possibility of relaxation. I seriously considered cheating just to get a result but decided against it.

All of this bears out my comments about such unnecessary methods in Section 6, and does suggest that this therapist might not have been any great expert in the art of hypnotherapy. Carr also described him as "earnest" and "young", which might suggest limited experience. Why bother with any of this arm-lifting stuff anyway? But the next bit simply doesn't ring true at all, because Carr claims the therapist asked him to open his eyes again, only to attempt an induction aimed at achieving eye closure:

> Eventually he gave up and asked me to open my eyes. He decided on another tack, explaining that certain techniques worked better with some people than with others. This time he held a pencil about a foot from my nose and in a monotonous chant told me how my eyelids would gradually become heavier and heavier until I could no longer keep my eyes open. I'd never felt more awake in my life.

Why attempt to achieve something you already have? Eye closure is eye closure by any means, which is why I simply ask people to close their eyes, and then explain why. I never encounter resistance to trance from any client nowadays, mainly because I've stopped bothering with convincers, pencils, pendula and overcomplicated techniques that do indeed seem mysterious or annoying to the client. Just explain it! Works a treat.

So the order of events as described here is nonsensical and smacks of invention, but by a mind that understands none of this. People in trance *are* awake, but Carr obviously didn't have any clear understanding of that. Was the hypnotherapist just as ignorant about the realities of hypnosis as Allen Carr? It is not impossible, but it isn't likely. Did all this really happen? Some of it does tally with the original description, but it is telling that now he is trying harder to convince his readers that the hypnotherapy certainly could not have been the cause of the change, a possibility he accidentally left open in book one. But unbeknown to Allen Carr, through his ignorance of how hypnosis really works he leaves it open here too. Because even when hypnotherapy is presented poorly, it can be totally successful anyway. The outcome is controlled by the client's Subconscious, not their skeptical, analytical conscious mind – and not by the hypnotist either. Here's the twist:

Seeing the consternation on the young man's face as this technique went the way of the first was excruciating. I decided to bring the farce to an end as quickly as possible, and closed my eyes...

Compliance. Coupled with sympathy for the poor young man, which will do for rapport from this point onwards. Don't forget that Carr's real hostility toward hypnosis developed much later. In 1983 he was merely skeptical and dismissive on an analytical level, which certainly does not prevent it from working. He had no axe to grind until years later, so on an emotional level – where it matters – he probably had no negative feelings about the therapist or the prospect of being rid of tobacco. Five seconds or so into eye closure, and the Subconscious gets curious about what is going on and tunes in to the conversation.

Now, I usually only refer to what is going on in the mind, not the brain. To me they are not precisely the same thing, but obviously so closely linked that the conventional scientific view would be that the brain is the mind. I have no expertise with regard to the brain, but for those that do have an interest in the physicalities, here is a link that backs up what I have stated about eye-closure and also states of fixed attention, both of which become trance states within a few seconds, with or without relaxation. It concerns the brain waves known as alpha rhythms, first recorded by Berger in 1929. In a book called The Craving Brain (Perennial, 2000), Ronald A. Ruden notes that behavioral states:

> ...have been related to certain alpha rhythms, specifically low levels of arousal and altered states of attention. The areas of the brain which are activated when alpha is generated are the limbic and associated structures on the right side of the brain which feed into the stress response system... Alpha rhythms are also observed under conditions of profound attention. Archers, when sighting a target, appear to produce an alpha rhythm just prior to releasing the arrow.... Alpha rhythms are best observed under conditions of physical relaxation with the eyes closed. The alpha rhythm is diminished or blocked by opening one's eyes.

Obviously, whether your brain produces an alpha rhythm or not is a matter of which you would not be consciously aware. In other words, it is sub-conscious brain activity which the conscious mind does not realize is happening, related to behavioral states and the stress-response system, and also linked to highly developed skills such as archery, and therefore also similar skills like driving which become highly developed, or 'second nature'. Smoking, of course, quickly becomes 'second nature' too. Notice how the above description recognises relaxation as helpful to the production of alpha waves, but not essential. This bears out my own observations about that matter in Section Six.

Allen Carr didn't know any of this, of course. In fact there are quite a few hypnotherapists who are still under the impression that working with the Subconscious is far more complicated than that, and of course they convey this impression to their clients also, in everything they say and do. This creates complications that need not be there.

> It took a further fifteen minutes for him to deliver a string of platitudes about the futility of smoking.

Notice how his conscious mind still thought the therapist was talking to it. Platitudes, it says. Meanwhile his Subconscious, picking up on his emotional attitude to tobacco:

CASE MYSTERIES 3: ALLEN CARR'S SUCCESS STORIES

I was not obstructive (like most smokers, I <u>dearly wanted</u> to stop)

...took a different view. And that is exactly why Allen Carr describes the aftermath of this session thus, in the *first* book:

> I didn't go into a trance, or at least I didn't think I did, and yet after that session not only did I stop smoking but I actually enjoyed the process even during the withdrawal period... I have a scientific brain, and I couldn't understand what appeared to me like magic. I started reading up on hypnosis and on smoking. Nothing I read seemed to explain the miracle that had happened. Why had it been so ridiculously easy to stop, whereas previously it had been weeks of black depression?
>
> It took me a long time to work it all out...

Now look at what he says in 2004, and see if you can spot what I am angry about:

> ... a string of platitudes about the futility of smoking. All I could think about was escaping outside for a smoke.
>
> I lit up the moment I left the clinic and made my way home...

Members of the jury! I put it to you that Allen Carr evidently became a liar to try to protect his reputation, method, status and income. In a book which sold over two million copies he plainly described how he stopped smoking during a hypnotherapy session, but found himself at a loss to understand why that happened. Simply because he did not believe in hypnotherapy in the first place, his "scientific brain" was unable to accept that it really worked and concluded – with amazing arrogance – that he must have done it all by himself. By his own admission in the first book, it took him a long time to work out just how that might have occurred. As he developed his own method, he mysteriously added the very thing which he insisted had nothing to do with his own success: hypnotherapy.

Irritatingly for Mr Carr, critics kept asking why that should be, and repeatedly returned to the now-awkward fact that his smoking cessation coincided with a hypnotherapy session. So in 2004, for the first time he claims that it did not, which directly contradicts his original account. For the first time, he now claims that he smoked cigarettes after that fateful session. Ladies and gentlemen of the jury, as I have clearly demonstrated Mr Carr keeps changing his story, dropping inconvenient details from his original statement and introducing a completely new angle to account for how he came by his celebrated method. Shall we read on? I have a feeling that if we give him enough rope he'll hang himself, don't you?

...and made my way home, that statement – my catalyst for quitting – still going round inside my head. Sometimes I wonder what would have happened if John, my eldest son, had not provided that second piece of vital information, the substance with which my catalyst would mingle and harden into an unbreakable resolve.

To lie. The new statement tells how John brought round "a medical handbook which contained a chapter on smoking". This is materially different from "I started reading up on hypnosis" in the original statement, where the aim was to find an explanation for "the miracle that had happened". In this 2004 version, the session had come and gone, but the miracle had not happened yet. This alteration is damning. What Carr now suggests is that the reading for enlightenment actually preceded the miraculous change, and that his smoking was allegedly still going on:

After John left, I sat down with my remaining cigarettes and that book...

The cigarettes are mentioned here so pointedly, and so unecessarily, that they function like a prop in a dramatic scene, carefully being placed "in shot" as it were. He is going out of his way to remind the reader that he is supposedly still smoking at this point, so it cannot possibly have been the hypnotherapy - just in case anyone was still wondering about that. (You see, I'm not called Holmes for nothing!)

...and turned to the relevant chapter. I found the language incomprehensible. Clearly the book was intended for those well versed in medical-speak. I was determined to make sense of it and get something out of that chapter. I read it again and again. Gradually something very weird started to happen.

Did it, Allen? Did it really? Do tell us about the weirdness, so we can judge for ourselves just exactly how fucking weird it was.

If you stare at the pattern made by a hologram and allow your eyes to go out of focus, suddenly an identifiable image appears as if by magic in 3D. Blink your eyes and it disappears. As I re-read that chapter, a startling fact began to emerge. Can you imagine spending your entire adult life studying Egyptian hieroglyphics, being absolutely fascinated by the subject but completely clueless as to their meaning, and then discovering the one clue that removes all the mystery? The startling fact I discovered was that when nicotine leaves your body it creates an empty, insecure feeling. By smoking another cigarette you replace the nicotine and get rid of that feeling, which leaves you feeling less nervous or more relaxed than you did the moment before you lit up.

What a startling 'fact'. So let's put it all together now. First the therapist revealed the astonishing new theory that smoking was nicotine addiction, and then later the medical book, through some sort of mystical hologram effect involving ancient Egypt added the final clue: that withdrawal isn't pleasant and so the addict takes more of the drug to fend off withdrawal. Thus the illusion is that the drug brings relief when really it causes the discomfort, and abstinence will allow a return to natural harmony. And this is how Mr Carr now claims that:

The catalyst and seed of what would become Easyway had fused in my brain.

Well something had fused in your brain, mate, if you think we're going to believe that load of old twaddle. So you've got rid of the miracle and turned it into a moment of inspirational genius arising from the 3D effect of a medical book, but to make that change you had to invent new details about smoking *after* the session that were not in the original account. The therapist has now been turned into a clown who is to be pitied for his utter incompetence – and don't forget to throw in the obligatory reference to chicken-like behaviour, so we can keep the tone about right for scorn and skepticism about hypnosis - but there is still one small problem, Mr Carr. How on earth are you going to account for the introduction of hypnotherapy into Easyway, having painted it like this? Here is Allen's scientific brain again:

Some people, when they had discovered that I had quit smoking after consulting a hypnotherapist, naturally concluded that the therapy should take more of the credit than I was prepared to give it.

Naturally. And they didn't really need to "discover" anything, you told everybody that yourself in the original book when you were still being relatively straightforward about the whole thing, before you had a business empire to protect. Go on then, let's hear why hypnotherapy should get no credit, but your method includes it anyway. You've had a couple of decades to work on your story now, let's see what you've come up with.

I knew the attempt to hypnotise me had been a farce, and that in no way could it have been responsible for turning me into a non-smoker.

You certainly didn't know that in 1983 Allen, because your immediate response at the time was:

I couldn't understand what appeared to me like magic. I started reading up on hypnosis and on smoking. Nothing I read seemed to explain the miracle that had happened.

Farce... miracle... it's so hard to tell the difference isn't it? Anyway, back to the statement of 2004. He goes on:

However, it is impossible to argue effectively from a position of ignorance, even if the people you are arguing against are your equals in ignorance...

If I was to argue the case that an appeal to someone's subconscious can't rid them of a particular phobia or, as in the case of nicotine, an addiction...

You would be wrong in every respect sir, because I routinely make such appeals every working day of my life and they are usually successful, which makes me wonder if *anyone* is quite your equal in ignorance regarding hypnotherapy. Ok, I'll stop interrupting now. It's just so hard not to, when ignorance and pomposity are vying for supremacy thus.

...I would have to prove it, and to prove it I would have to know how hypnotherapy works. I began by reading every book on the subject I could find...

Sorry... really didn't want to interrupt again, but I felt the need to point out that he has just changed his story yet again, this time regarding exactly *when* he addressed his ignorance by reading up on hypnosis.

Originally he said it was straight away, because he couldn't understand the miracle. Now he says it was sometime later, because he needed to try to prove that the miracle was actually a farce.

These were not particularly illuminating, their authors seemingly more interested in dreaming up new types of gimmickry by which to serve up the basic technique. Unfortunately many practitioners are ex-stage hypnotists who perpetuate the image of the therapist as some sort of Svengali figure.

No, that's what *you* are trying to do Allen, and you are quite wrong. The vast majority of hypnotherapists in the UK have never done stage shows, in fact many of them argue that they should be banned. You didn't really read any books on hypnotherapy at all, did you?

When the opportunity of attending a half-day seminar was offered, courtesy of a sympathetic doctor, I took it. I came away disappointed that the medical profession seemed as seduced by the delusion techniques associated with hypnotherapy as the stage hypnotists.

Ignorance upon ignorance. Really this is too much. Hypnotherapy does not involve delusions, and the suggestion that the medical profession generally have anything at all in common with stage hypnotists almost amounts to raving. Of the lunatic variety, I mean. Now just listen to this pretentious piece of scaremongering:

I am convinced that hypnosis is a mis-used tool, and potentially dangerous in the wrong hands. I regard it as the equivalent of a hypodermic syringe. By itself it can not kill or cure, but fill it with an agent that has either of these capabilities and it can.

When has hypnosis ever killed anybody? In statements like these, Allen Carr's scientific brain is clearly being 'the equivalent' of a horse's ass. And you know what they are filled with. Here comes some more of it now:

The one aspect of hypnotherapy I could appreciate was its usefulness as a method of relaxation. All of us are better able to absorb information when we are in a relaxed frame of mind. Give somebody a piece of information when they are in a panic or fearful and they will in all probability not even hear you, let alone absorb the implications...

I was certain that if smokers were to absorb my method of quitting, they would have to be in a receptive frame of mind. That was where hypnotherapy would play its part, initially to remove whatever problems are crowding the smoker's mind and help them to reach a state where they feel relaxed, warm and secure, and able to absorb the content of the method.

Aha! After only two decades, Allen's brain has finally figured out a dodgy suggestion to account for the contradictory inclusion of hypnotherapy within his own method. Relaxation! Hmm. Funny how that apparently wasn't required for success in your own case Allen, if your later version of events is to be believed, and yet you felt there would be an advantage in finding some premise to include it for your clients despite the obvious disadvantage that it doesn't square with your increasingly hostile attitudes to hypnotherapy generally. Why not just have them stare at a medical book, Allen? That seemed to provide a perfect solution for you, *and your remaining cigarettes.*

It won't wash though, because what Mr Carr is talking about here is merely relaxation. He is revealing his ignorance again, as well as recycling a common myth, because hypnotherapy is not "a method of relaxation". Relaxing is a method of relaxation, and the only natural one I know of. Hypnosis is all about trance and suggestion. Hypnotherapy can easily be done without relaxation, and relaxation can easily be utilised without hypnosis being involved at all. Often in therapy we may choose to *combine* those things, but the truth is that levels of relaxation are usually of little consequence when it comes to the process of change in hypnotherapy, so for Allen Carr to suggest it is the most useful aspect of hypnotherapy is just daft. But here's the thing. Mr. Carr specifically said in the first book:

Neither do I wish to appear to be knocking hypnotherapy; on the contrary, I use it as part of my own consultations. It is the power of suggestion and a powerful force that can be used for good or evil...

That sounds a bit different from relaxation to me. I mean you can relax in a deck chair, without any powerful forces being involved. Except gravity of course. Actually, that's what relaxation is: utter submission to gravity. But should we be doing that? Should we ever risk utter submission to the forces of gravity? After all, gravity is undeniably a force that can be used for good or evil. A child can drop a coin into the begging-bowl of a blind man. A mobster might hurl a victim from a rooftop. Does that make gravity a force we should be dubious about? Or does it really all come down to the way we, as individuals choose to interact with any Force... hold up, this isn't fucking Star Wars. I'll be hearing voices soon, if I carry on like this.

How to Rub Someone Out

As we allow Mr Carr the last little bit of rope, he doesn't seem to notice that the more he speaks, the more it curls into a loop. Meanwhile, the jury strains to hear the defendant's final testimony above the sound of hammering in the execution yard. Scientific Brain Mk.4 is now called to the stand, which first made its statement in 2003, but I have saved it to last because in this version of how he "discovered Easy Way", Mr Carr fails to mention his hypnotherapy session at all, as if that event just never happened. If you want to check this out for yourself, read pages 19 and 20 in 'Chapter 3: Miracle or Magic?' from *Allen Carr's Easy Way for Women to Stop Smoking*. It's quite funny if you compare it with pages 1 and 2 in the first book, which is still available because it is an international bestseller - so you can check this out in any major bookstore without having to buy either of them. In this version, aimed particularly at female smokers for no valid reason I can fathom, he never mentions hypnotherapy at all. He simply says:

"Then it happened, as if a thick and ever-present veil had been lifted from my eyes: I could see smoking without the brainwashing. Even before I'd extinguished my final cigarette, I knew I was already a non-smoker. I knew for certain that I would never, ever have a need or desire to smoke again."

Hang on - where's your hypnotherapist gone, Allen? He has vanished! Not only can you suddenly see smoking without the brainwashing, you can see quitting without the therapist too. It's a miracle! You made the guy disappear, as if obscured by a thick and newly-present veil.

It gets better. He continues:

"What I didn't understand immediately was why it was so easy. Why didn't I have the terrible withdrawal pangs I'd suffered previously when attempting to stop? I had no withdrawal symptoms whatsoever and actually enjoyed the entire process of quitting."

It's not difficult to understand, Allen, if you just lift the veil obscuring the hypnotherapist you chose to edit out of this latest fantasy version of how you quit smoking. Or did you just forget about him, perhaps? But the really funny bit comes next:

"At this stage, you may have several questions you'd like answered. I've no doubt the first one is: "Just tell me what happened to you, and how can you make it happen to me."

How can I make it happen to you? I can't. But you are, in fact, already doing it by yourself. All you have to do is complete the book with an open mind. This means you shouldn't meekly accept everything that I tell you. On the contrary, it is essential to question everything I tell you..."

Good idea. And you're right Allen, I do have several questions I'd like answered at this stage but you are wrong about the first one, which is actually: "Where did you bury the hypnotherapist?" It was bad enough in the first book when you claimed to have stopped smoking during his session "in spite of him". Later you added insult to injury by making him out to be a clown, but now you've rubbed him out altogether!

The Truth About Allen Carr

I can tell your readers exactly what happened to you Allen, even if you would prefer to perpetuate the myth of your own sudden moment of inspirational genius. You went to see a hypnotherapist just as you described in your first book, and like many clients you didn't understand what happened even though it worked perfectly because it seemed as if nothing was really happening. That is in fact a commonplace hypnotherapy experience, it's just that you didn't know that.

Then you wrote a book about stopping smoking as if you did it all by yourself, invented a dubious way of taking the credit and unconvincingly rubbishing hypnotherapy - yet in an obvious contradiction to that, you later adopted hypnotherapy as part of your own method. The book sold millions all over the world, and being an accountant you saw a franchising opportunity that was potentially global.

Not content with that you repackaged the same method in several further, quite unnecessary books about smoking because your real ambition was to become The Man Who Saved The World From Smoking, but you found that people kept inconveniently bringing up the hypnotherapy and questioning your story, so you felt inclined to change the story. And it went on changing, until at some point you decided that mentioning the hypnotherapist was a mistake in the first place so you killed him off, which is why that character does not appear at all in the sequel from which I quoted above. You had to get rid of him because he knew too much about what really happened that day.

That's what Allen Carr really did. And he would have got away with it too, if it hadn't been for ...another pesky hypnotherapist! But hey, all you smokers, don't go rushing off to see a hypnotherapist now. We're an evil bunch, as everybody knows. Going around helping people - who do we think we are? Better off going to see an ex-accountant really, aren't you, if you want therapy.

So, ladies and gentlemen of the jury, there I rest my case against Allen Carr. No need for you to return a unanimous verdict, you can all please yourselves on that one. Some may think I have been a bit harsh, but actually he started it, suggesting that people should be wary of hypnotherapy. That really is cheek, since by his own admission – well, he admits it in the first book anyway - he would have died by around 1985 if he hadn't visited that hypnotherapist two years before. No, if his reputation ends up dangling from a rope, he wove every fibre of it himself.

But actually, it shouldn't. Not entirely. Everything I have pointed out so far is true enough, and needed to be said. Yet it is still probably true to say that Allen Carr has done more than any other single ordinary individual - so far - to help smokers all over the world to quit and therefore partly realised his ambition, and for that he does deserve acknowledgement. I won't say praise, for obvious reasons, but acknowledgement for sure, because contrary to the suggestion in the title of one of his books, there are actually quite a few ways of stopping smoking, and Easyway is one of the better ones. I just wish he had fully realised from the outset the vital role that hypnotherapy played in his own success in stopping smoking, and put as much energy into promoting this wonderful profession as he put into promoting himself.

I don't want to cure the world of smoking, or anything else. That's the biggest difference between myself and Allen Carr. Let the world do what it wants – it will anyway. Lots of things kill people in pointless and unnecessary ways: look at mountineering. I wouldn't join a crusade to put an end to it, would you? And although I'm a therapist, I'm not a health guru. But to any individual who wishes they had never started smoking, or has decided they are just sick of it now or whatever, I would say this. There are many hard ways to quit, and there are one or two easier ways. Allen Carr's way can be pretty easy for some, although its success rate is nothing like 95%, let's be realistic. Still I would bet on it beating NRT by a very respectable margin. But hypnotherapy is the easiest way of all, because you don't even have to read a book. Having said that, anyone who has read this book, and especially if they feel it has enlightened them, will find success with hypnotherapy a breeze – assuming it is properly conducted, of course.

'EasyWay' can work well enough for some people because it really functions as a mild form of hypnotherapy. It uses some of the principles of hypnosis, especially the frequent repetition of key phrases to drive them deep into the psyche, and also what we call 'reframing' which is basically getting you to look at something from an enlightening new perspective. Even his books can function as a sort of self-hypnosis process, although it is rather hit and miss, as are all self-help books, because we can either read consciously or Subconsciously.

Yes, your Subconscious may be reading some of this! And if so with great interest, because this is a book which is mainly about the power and significance of the Subconscious mind, written by a person who evidently understands the Subconscious mind pretty well and thinks it is terrific. Of course the conscious mind is wonderful too in its own way, but the idea that it controls all decisions and activities – the myth of conscious freewill in all things – must now become a quaint historical delusion just like the four bodily 'humours' and the notion that the heart is the emotional centre. Truth will out, after all.

Could hypnotherapy have helped Allen Carr further?

Hardly. Quite apart from eliminating his 100-a-day smoking habit easily, I suspect Allen Carr's personal fortunes were more dramatically boosted by one session of hypnotherapy than anyone who ever lived. Hopefully hypnotherapy can now actually get due credit.

Section Five

Why the Nicotine Addiction Theory is Wrong

First of all let us recognise the inevitably high level of pre-conditioned doubt with which some persons will be reading this, for that factor would be subverting those readers' objective analysis of my explanations at a Subconscious level if we do not bring it forward into the light - make it conscious. Any doubts or disbelief you may be experiencing in reading any of this is quite normal at first, don't let it throw you. I have to *prove* my case here, I don't expect you to believe me just because I say so.

On the other hand, if you find that you seem to be easily recognising the validity of each point immediately here, you may already have noticed some of the anomalies in the 'nicotine addiction' theory, in which case I'm sure you'll enjoy finding out in detail later what is really going on with the smoking habit and what cravings really are.

But for many readers I would not be at all surprised if there is a part of your mind that struggles to accept that I could possibly be absolutely right *just because* of the enormous amount of suggestion to the contrary to which you have already been subjected – even though you may never have really questioned that – coupled with the implication that myself being right would automatically make thousands of scientists and medical people the world over wrong.

I mean, come on! Which is more likely: thousands of well-educated and highly-qualified experts wrong and one lowly hypnotherapist right, or the other way around? Seriously, just consider it now. Everybody has heard all about nicotine being highly addictive, and smokers obviously find it very hard to stop even with nicotine replacement therapy. Hypnotherapists make all sorts of dramatic claims, but it all sounds too good to be true. There have been lots of scientific trials involving nicotine, but we are often told that there are hardly any by comparison involving hypnotherapy. Why would anyone in their right mind believe me? Who do I think I am?

Earlier in the book I did point out that a wise man once said:

"It is easier to go on believing what you have always been told, than to recognise the truth you have never heard before."

I'm sure you can recognise and acknowledge the wisdom of the observation, and you may have wondered which wise man said it because I never credited him by name. Actually, it was me! Little old me, not anyone particularly special at all in fact. And if the statement no longer seems as wise now that you know that I said it - and not Ghandi, Bhudda or Nelson Mandela - then the question really should be: Who do *you* think I am? How much credibility do you think you should lend to my explanations here, and has that begun to change already since you started reading the book?

At this point I would like to quote a kindred spirit by the name of Dr Malcolm Kendrick, whose recent book *The Great Cholesterol Con* (John Blake Publishing, 2007) explodes the myth about cholesterol and accuses the drug companies and the medical hierarchy of seriously misleading the public, with the result that millions of people are on cholesterol-reducing 'statin' drugs that they don't need, because raised cholesterol levels in the blood are not the real cause of heart attacks. He pulls no punches:

... the misguided war against cholesterol, using statins, represents something very close to a crime against humanity. So close that you may not be able to spot the difference. (p xvii)

Like myself challenging the nicotine myth, Dr Kendrick is aware that the official line on cholesterol is so widely accepted that he may have trouble getting anyone to listen to him at first, and he addresses this point thus:

Everywhere you look, everybody is in agreement about the need to lower your cholesterol level. How can almost everybody be wrong?

In fact, almost everybody being wrong has been a quite normal phenomenon throughout human existence. So the fact that there are only a few dissenting voices out there should not bother you unduly. And medical scientists (an oxymoron if ever there was one), have a long and distinguished history of grabbing entirely the wrong end of the stick, closing their eyes tightly shut, holding on grimly and refusing to listen to anybody else...

The list of stupid, damaging and plain wrong things that doctors have been taught over the years makes rather depressing reading. It has certainly depressed me from time to time. We can all be wrong. Even me. But for some reason the medical hierarchy is exceptionally reluctant to admit their mistakes. (p xv)

Although he pulls no punches, especially in passages like those above, Dr Kendrick's book is not a depressing read in any way. In fact it is very enlightening, lively and although the subject is complex, the frequent joviality of the writing style guides the reader through, and I recommend the book to anyone who has ever been told their cholesterol level is too high. I was told that, and my GP was muttering about medication only a few weeks before I read Dr Kendrick's book. The book is not mere opinion, it steadily builds up into a case that is so convincing, there is no way I will ever take that kind of medication. Even if you never read the book yourself, just imagine a text of about 270 pages composed of startling information like this:

The protection provided by statins is so small as to be not worth bothering about for most people (and all women). The reality is that the benefits have been hyped beyond belief... Statins have many more unpleasant side effects than has been admitted. Side-effects up to, and including, death and the creation of horribly deformed babies. (You think not? Then read on.)

...I am not alone in my beliefs. There are many hundreds of doctors and researchers who agree that the cholesterol hypothesis is bunk. Many keep their counsel, others have been stomped into silence, but a few have had the guts to speak out. However, their voices, unlike those of the implacable medical 'statinators', are not supported by multi-billion-dollar pharmaceutical budgets.

...In a world created by PR-controlled spin, critics of the cholesterol hypothesis get very little airtime. If they did, this world would change, and I hope this book starts the process of change.

I hope so too Malcolm, and that is exactly why I have included excerpts from it in this one. The more people get to hear about all this, the better. And yes, of course it is easy enough to go on believing what you have always been told, but that does not make it impossible to do otherwise. Humans remain able to see the truth when it is presented to them clearly, even if it is absolutely contrary to what they previously understood to be the case. As a hypnotherapist I have learned over the years to have great faith in the human capacity to learn and change, even where clients have little faith in that themselves. And so, dear reader, regardless of all that has gone before, and whatever you may have believed before you ever picked this book up, and whatever anyone else believes, I believe in you.

Part 1: The Smokers who Don't Believe They are Addicts Anyway

I should begin by acknowledging all those smokers who actually didn't need me to tell them any of this because they worked it out for themselves logically, because of the nature of their personal habit. They may still need cravings explaining but they already figured out that cravings cannot possibly be drug withdrawal symptoms and so they don't believe they are addicted to a drug at all. Habits vary a great deal, and clearly if someone smokes 80 cigarettes a day - maybe even has a cigarette if they wake up in the night, and always has tobacco within reach even when they are in the bath - well, it is easy for them to believe in nicotine addiction. But what about all the people who only smoke a few? There are thousands of smokers who are obviously not in the grip of some pernicious drug addiction because they only smoke when they go to the pub, or in the evening. Some people just smoke occasionally, and have been doing that for years.

Nowadays in the UK most workplaces are smoke-free, so there are plenty of habitual smokers who spend most of their working day not smoking at all and this does not cause the majority of them any great distress. Then they go home and smoke ten cigarettes sitting in front of the television. So some of these people have naturally figured out for themselves that they cannot possibly be 'unaddicted' all day long, then suddenly 'become addicted' in the evening. Yet they find it difficult to abstain from smoking in the evening. This book explains exactly why, and it has nothing to do with nicotine.

Part 2: The Fundamental Error

Addictions and compulsive habits are very different things. The bottom line is the same – you can't stop doing it – but for totally different reasons. A real drug addiction, such as an established heroin addiction for instance, cannot be shut down by a single session of hypnotherapy. It is treatable but would take many sessions because that problem is more complex, and other expert support and intervention would probably be needed as well as the hypnotherapy. Not only is the physical addiction genuine with heroin but it is a compulsive habit too, and also the emotional attachment to heroin is usually far greater than it is ever likely to be with tobacco.

Part of the mistake in regarding tobacco use as drug addiction is that the meaning of the word 'addiction' has become so blurred. Nowadays, almost anything that a person apparently can't stop doing can be loosely called an addiction. But the impression smokers are under – generally – is that they are *physically addicted to a drug called nicotine,* that nicotine is what they are smoking for and that cravings are literally withdrawal symptoms i.e. a physical bodily need for nicotine.

The main reason many smokers believe that is because they have been told to believe it - not just once but thousands of times, directly and indirectly. Also, they are aware that this view has the official sanction of the medical profession. That is enough to convince most people, especially if they have never heard anyone offer a better explanation anyway. Another reason is that the addiction theory *seems* to account for the fact that smokers apparently find it very difficult to stop smoking just with a conscious effort. On the face of it, 'nicotine addiction' seems broadly believable in the absence of a better explanation, so it is not surprising that a lot of people came to believe it.

Rather than just accept that unquestioningly for all the common reasons above, let us examine the drug addiction theory in more precise detail. According to the British Medical Association's Illustrated Medical Dictionary, nicotine is:

"A drug in tobacco which acts as a **stimulant** and is responsible for dependence on tobacco."

Now if this were true, then a single session of hypnotherapy could not possibly eliminate smoking behaviour because any physical "dependence on tobacco" would be exactly the same at the end of the session as it was at the beginning, wouldn't it? If the body needs nicotine to stave off withdrawal symptoms, then it needs nicotine. Talking to the person about it would not change that, would it? All I do in a hypnotherapy session is talk. Surely that should not make any difference at all in any case of real drug addiction, not even temporarily. After a couple of hours in my office the client should be dying for a smoke, in fact.

Fortunately - for smokers, at least - the BMA are completely wrong about this. Nicotine is not responsible for compulsive smoking behaviour, cravings are. That is precisely why people wearing nicotine patches still get cravings. The urge to light up is not an urge to take nicotine but a compulsive urge to light up a cigarette, to repeat the habitual behaviour. And anyway, the vast majority of smokers are under the general impression smoking relaxes them, or helps them calm down when they feel under stress. At the risk of stating something blindingly obvious, stimulants don't relax people. They do the reverse.

The BMA again:

"Nicotine acts primarily on the autonomic nervous system, which controls involuntary body activities such as the heart rate. In habitual smokers, the drug increases the heart rate and narrows the blood vessels, the combined effect of which is to raise blood pressure."

So far so true, and based on good old-fashioned scientific measurements. But is the BMA really suggesting that smokers are 'using' nicotine in order to make their hearts beat faster and raise their blood pressure? That would be a particularly crazy thing to do at moments of *stress*, wouldn't it? And again, smokers generally believe tobacco relaxes them, which is the very opposite of nicotine's effects as described here by the BMA. Even to the simplest of simpletons, this is a glaring inconsistency in the theory of tobacco smoking as 'drug use'.

The BMA's Medical Dictionary then continues:

"Nicotine also stimulates the central nervous system, thereby reducing fatigue, increasing alertness, and improving concentration."

Wait a minute! Which does nicotine do for the smoker: help them relax, as smokers usually claim - or make them more alert? Calm them down after something has upset them, or help them to concentrate on it more? These are polar opposites, aren't they? Clearly nicotine cannot possibly do *both*.

Now, all you readers who have ever tried smoking tobacco, cast your mind back to that first cigarette. When you inhaled tobacco smoke for the first time, did you notice it improving your concentration at all? When you sampled the delights nicotine had to offer, did you feel more alert? No of course not, it made you feel dizzy and sick just like everyone else. Whatever idea first prompted you to try smoking tobacco, it wasn't to 'feel more alert and concentrate better' that's for sure! And anyway, look around you – who looks more alert and focused, smokers or non-smokers? Smoking deprives the brain of oxygen and gives you a sickening dose of carbon monoxide too. That can hardly be aiding mental focus.

When a smoker extinguishes the dog-end of a cigarette, the feeling is one of tiredness and lethargy rather than anything else. Feeling a bit rough, rather glad to put the horrible thing out in fact. If someone was offering tablets that made you feel like that, just how many would you buy? It is obvious that the actual experience of smoking a cigarette is a world away from the effects of taking real stimulant drugs. The truth is that the habitual smoker's cravings are distracting, which *disturbs* concentration. The smoker has to light up repeatedly to get rid of the distraction so they can then concentrate normally, that is what is really going on. But Science is so determined to describe the poison nicotine *as if it was a drug,* which smokers are deliberately 'using' for its effects, that it ends up crediting nicotine with effects it does not have.

Smokers are not Attempting to Stimulate Themselves!

Nicotine is not a stimulant drug that people are deliberately consuming in order to 'be stimulated'. There are a few real stimulant drugs in common use: cocaine, ecstasy, amphetamines (speed) – and sure enough, these will all make your heart beat faster and your blood pressure increase too. But that is not why people take them, those are dangerous side-effects. People take those drugs because it gives them a high. They just try to ignore any *other* effects. Nicotine does not get anybody high. It might make the smoker feel slightly faint or dizzy occasionally – especially when they first try smoking – but that is certainly not a high, it isn't even pleasant. It is nausea really, and is partly caused by carbon monoxide anyway because that reduces oxygen levels in the blood, and therefore also in the brain. A similar effect would result from inhaling fumes from your car's exhaust pipe. (Don't try that, by the way. It is potentially lethal and nowhere near as pleasant as it sounds.)

If the smoker is young and fit they probably will not notice their heartbeat increasing, and nobody knows what their blood pressure is even if it is dangerously high. So the two so-called 'stimulant' effects of nicotine are not even noticed by the smoker, who is certainly not aiming to make those particular changes happen.

So the *heart* might be stimulated to beat a bit faster, but the smoker does not notice that and does not 'feel stimulated' - hence the smoker's confusion about what nicotine does. The truth is, smokers do not notice what nicotine really does at all. This explains why smokers cannot correctly answer the simple question "What does nicotine actually do?"

I have personally asked thousands of smokers that question and so far not one of them has ever given me a full and factually-correct reply. Most of them frankly admit they have no idea, although they often tentatively say: "I think it relaxes me, or something." This is because there is no way a smoker could figure out what the actual effects of nicotine are, merely from their own habitual experience of smoking tobacco. In fact it would be true to say that many smokers started smoking without knowing of the existence of nicotine, still would not know of it if they had not been told all about it by the medical profession, and even though they've now had the nicotine theory drilled into them, still don't know what it does. The same could never be said for anyone taking a real drug.

Smokers may well notice other recognisable aspects of their typical smoking experiences however, and comment upon them. For example: the common observation that they tend to smoke less when they are busy (because it gets in the way) but smoke more frequently at moments of repose. So it becomes easy to imagine that they are 'smoking to relax', just because they are often smoking at the same time as they are also relaxing, or when they have stopped exerting themselves. Many of the smoking episodes, then, happen to be relaxing moments but certainly not because of the effects of nicotine. Rather in spite of it, in fact.

Thus it becomes obvious that tobacco-smoking behaviour is not a wilful act of self-stimulation using the poison nicotine as if it was a drug. In short, nicotine is not a stimulant drug. The BMA are wrong. Habitual smokers are simply repeating their usual behaviour automatically, regardless of how it makes them feel. And they are not choosing to do it purposefully, as an optional act of freewill, once it has become a habit - but compulsively.

If you doubt this, consider the example of the smoker who has a bad cold and tells you just how terrible they feel, and then says: "...but I'm still smoking! It's killing me to smoke with this bad throat!" So, what is the point of that behaviour then? Is nicotine helping them to be more *alert* to how much their throat hurts, better able to *concentrate* on feeling terrible? Or is it just meaningless repetition of the old habitual behaviour which is being endlessly repeated compulsively, regardless of how it makes them feel? Obvious really, isn't it?

Now clearly it is possible to challenge this. Consider these two scenarios:

1. If someone wishes to pretend they are still smoking purely voluntarily, like we all were to begin with, they can easily make a big show of lighting up deliberately and then extinguish the cigarette, saying: "Look, I am choosing when to smoke, and when to stop! Therefore I am in control."

2. If any smoker placed a cigarette in their mouth, and then suddenly someone put a gun to their head and convincingly threatened to blow their head off if they light it, they would suddenly feel no inclination to smoke at all. Consequently the smoker *appears* to be in conscious control of the behaviour, which is why non-smokers fail to see why smokers cannot simply stop at will.

But in the first case, the smoker is merely proving that the conscious mind can *also* instigate and control a demonstration of smoking - which we all know anyway because that is how we started. That fact alone does not mean it would be just as easy for the same habitual smoker to *choose* not to smoke at all for the next 48 weeks. And in the second case involving the gun, the Subconscious simply freezes the usual smoking action because there is a temporary and immediate hazard, as it will always hesitate if danger threatens. Once the lunatic with the gun has disappeared over the horizon, he'll smoke that cigarette for sure! And the smoker may well be under the illusion it is helping him to relax too, when the thing that is really assisting him to calm down is the fact that the anti-smoking lunatic with the gun has left.

Smokers are not smoking for the effects of nicotine, and indeed never were. Smokers do not even know what nicotine does. If you doubt this, ask a few. They will either admit that they do not know, or guess wrong. If by some amazing fluke you stumble upon a smoker who does give you the following full and correct answer:

"If you take nicotine into the body in tiny amounts - like through smoking, or sticking a nicotine patch on - it will make your heart beat faster than it should, which is both useless and dangerous. It will reduce blood flow to the skin and the extremities, which is bad for your circulation, and the combination of these two changes will raise your blood pressure. Obviously, this does not help anyone calm down at times of stress, when heart-rate and blood pressure are already climbing. Instead it makes a sudden heart attack or stroke more likely."

"Nicotine also raises fat levels in your blood which is not only useless but also leads to clogged arteries, heart attacks and strokes. As if that were not enough, nicotine also inhibits the production of an enzyme in the body which normally breaks up blood clots, directly causing a higher incidence of thrombosis and strokes in smokers."

"If you take nicotine into the body in any more than tiny amounts it will kill you stone dead because it is a very deadly poison indeed."

...you can ask them directly if they imagine for a moment that they are smoking tobacco for the effects of nicotine.

These effects listed above are the only real effects of nicotine. So whatever smokers think they are smoking for, it obviously isn't for the actual effects of nicotine. They have simply been told that they are smoking for the effects of nicotine thousands of times, and assumed that must be true because the information comes from the medical and scientific community. We assume they know what they are talking about, don't we? But are they not simply repeating what they were told to believe themselves as part of their training? And don't fashions in medical training change, as new generations notice the errors in the training of previous generations? If you look at the course of medical history, as well as all the wonderful successes you will find some howling errors from time to time, because these people are only human. Assuming that tobacco smoking must be a drug addiction just because people cannot easily break the habit was a mistake from the start, and there have always been a few people who have said so, too – it is just that the addiction idea got into the mainstream of medical opinion, and then they drilled it into the public.

The General Effects of Suggestion

If humans are told the same thing thousands of times and no-one contradicts it, they usually come to believe it is true unless they have some specific reason to doubt it. This is simply the cumulative effect of repeated suggestion. The more often a suggestion is repeated the more convincing it becomes, generally speaking, especially if it is not contradicted. It becomes "common knowledge". The individual Subconscious mind comes to assume that it must be true – because if it wasn't true, why would we keep on hearing it reaffirmed time and time again? This is particularly the case if the 'fact' is suggested by 'experts' such as scientists and the medical profession. Admittedly this is not quite so true today as it used to be, and there are always a few oddbods who openly denounce medical people as outright 'quacks', but it is still true that the majority of people have a kind of blind faith in medical science and are a bit surprised when it is proven wrong.

Actually scientists will reject the idea that science can ever be proven wrong because the scientific principal is that proof that can be repeatedly demonstrated establishes truth, so any scientific tenet that can be proved wrong is an example of science correcting itself scientifically and therefore continually validating itself as an infallible way of disproving falsehoods and endlessly marching on in the direction of pure knowledge. This would make me a scientist too, and a pretty good one given that I am correcting the errors of every scientist that has ever concurred with the idea of smoking as a drug addiction. Which would be all very amusing if it were not for:

The Vast Financial Cost of this Fundemental Medical Error

Tens of millions of pounds per year is currently being spent in the UK on 'nicotine replacement therapy'. The manufacture of NRT products is now a vast global industry worth an estimated 1.2 billion dollars annually, and it is entirely based on a myth. Smoking is a compulsive habit. Cravings are real, but they are produced by the brain and have nothing to do with nicotine or anything else in the smoke. The Subconscious part of the brain can easily shut them down completely, turning a person from a smoker into a non-smoker in one or two hypnotherapy sessions with no effort or conflict. I will happily demonstrate this, with as many real live smokers as it takes to convince the world that everything I am explaining is true. And you have to admit that if I was wrong about all this, and these smokers actually were physically dependent on regular 'doses' of nicotine - then

Why the Nicotine Addiction Theory is Wrong

I would not be able to demonstrate this even once, much less succeed easily most of the time.

What is more, this is not a temporary effect. Most clients quit permanently and never need another session. This is particularly true in a culture like ours, here in the UK at the start of the 21st Century where tobacco smoking continues to be in general decline, because there are now fewer incentives to start smoking again than there used to be, so 'relapse' is an ever-declining factor. Even if someone does start again it is even easier for them to stop a second time with a further session of hypnotherapy, provided of course they choose to do so and they actually bother to take that positive step. (See *Relapse is Not Failure* in Section 14, Volume II).

I know these things to be facts because I deal with these matters on a daily basis, but understandably many people would want to see proof. They would reasonably wish to see convincing numbers of ordinary smokers stop smoking easily with one or two hypnotherapy sessions, and they would also wish to hear from these smokers that they had not felt any urge to smoke after that and had not gained weight or noticed any other unwanted side-effects. Since most people are reasonable enough they would not expect miraculous success rates of 100% or 95%, but regard anything over 50% success as giving all smokers a better-than-even chance, which beats any other method by far. Just how much higher than 50% it would turn out to be would be very interesting to find out.

The obvious question would then be - once this fact had been demonstrated to everyone's satisfaction - what happened to the smoker's 'nicotine addiction'? Where did it go? How could I talk it away? Either their body needs nicotine or it doesn't. So if it doesn't need it at the end of the session it obviously didn't need it at the beginning, because talking is all that happens in a hypnotherapy session. There's no magic, there's no medicine. There's no equipment. No tapes you need to listen to. No exercises you need to perform. No situations you need to avoid, no efforts you need to make at all. The habit is gone and there are no side effects.

So where's the addiction, Doc?

Part 3: More Evidence that Smoking is Not Addiction

a). Nicotine is often described as a very addictive drug, "more addictive than heroin" we often hear some fool say. Well if nicotine really is such a physically-addictive drug, why do smokers find it so damn easy to stop using patches, or chewing nicotine gum? The same person who finds it so difficult to kick the cigarettes has no problem at all abandoning the patches. How many people do you know who cannot stop using NRT products? Why aren't there thousands of people addicted to the patches or the lozenges?

b). There are of course a very small number of people – compared to the overall number of smokers - who transfer their smoking habit to a nicotine gum habit, or even a lozenge habit. But nobody has a long-term patch habit! Why not? Because smoking, sucking and chewing are all something to do, a nervous activity which can also become a habit, so it is quite possible to swap one with another. It has nothing to do with the presence or absence of nicotine, except insofar as the user believes it does (suggestion). Wearing a patch isn't something to do. It is not an activity, so no-one develops a habit of 'patch-wearing'.

c). The vast majority of smokers do not stick with any of those products anyway. They go back to smoking, even though it would surely be more convenient to stay on the gum if all you really needed was nicotine, since you can chew gum or suck a lozenge anywhere.

d). The truth is that the vast majority of people who try nicotine gum or patches do not succeed with those methods, mainly because they are barking up the wrong tree in the first place. But even the small proportion of smokers who do successfully quit whilst using nicotine gum is not valid evidence for the theory of nicotine addiction. There have always been smokers who successfully quit by transferring their smoking habit to a chewing habit with ordinary gum, or sweets - so of course this phenomenon has nothing to do with the contents of the gum. It is a nervous activity, just like nail biting. Simply another compulsive habit, exactly as habitual smoking is in reality. The only difference is in the beliefs and attitudes attached to those habits.

e). Why do we never see adolescents or teenagers using nicotine patches, gum, lozenges etc. if they really are smoking for the effects of nicotine? Why is there no black market in these products, selling them to minors who are not allowed to buy them? The answer is: because they are not remotely interested in nicotine. They might have a smoking habit, or they might not have developed that into a habit yet – but none of them are addicted to nicotine so they naturally have no interest in other products that contain nicotine. This is never the case with real drugs of addiction or abuse, where any product that contains the drug will be of interest to the addict, even if they have to be quite ingenious to figure out a way to access or abuse it.

The fact that some young smokers may later come to *believe* they are nicotine addicts - because: a) they have been told all about it many, many times, and b) they have accidentally developed a compulsive habit by then and honestly do not know how to stop smoking - does not change the reality. Some people honestly believe that they are talented, psychic or destined for great things. Beliefs and reality can be quite different matters.

f). Why does no-one ever *steal* patches, gum or lozenges – like they do with alcohol and drugs of abuse? Nobody ever bursts into a pharmacy and nicks all the nicotine! Why not, if there are so many desperate 'nicotine addicts' about? When people do break into pharmacies - to steal real drugs of course - do they ever bother with the patches? Did you ever bump into a dodgy character in a pub, offering you knock-off nicotine? No? Well why not - the place is full of 'nicotine addicts', isn't it?

The truth is no-one in the pub wants the bloody things, you'd have trouble giving them away. No real drug is that unpopular, not even speed. Knock-off *ciggies* though – now you're talking! So it isn't nicotine smokers 'crave', but their usual habitual object.

g). Why are habitual smokers not habitually using gum or patches on a daily basis as well as smoking... to get through meetings, long train journeys or just the working day? Why wait? Why put up with the morning shift on the hospital ward without nicotine if you could just stick on a patch and have a cigarette later? I know that a small minority do this on occasion, like once a year when they fly – and of course smokers might do this when they actually try to quit, but my point is why don't the majority of smokers do this whenever they cannot smoke? That's what real drug addicts do, they don't go without unless there's no supply available. If this was really a drug addiction, addicts would make sure they had various types of supplies to cover them for every situation.

Smokers try to make certain they don't run out of cigarettes, whether there is likely to be an opportunity to light up or not. So why don't they just make sure they don't run out of other sources of nicotine too, to supply their 'need for nicotine' in between smoking opportunities, which are becoming rarer? These things are on sale in every pharmacy and supermarket, even petrol stations now. So why go without nicotine *at any time*?

The explanation is simple. It is because smokers are not 'taking nicotine'. They are compulsively smoking cigarettes which just happen to have a lot of toxins in them, one of which happens to be nicotine. That is also why the smoker wearing a nicotine patch still needs willpower, as the drug companies acknowledge. They still have cravings, because cravings are nothing to do with nicotine in the first place. Nicotine is just one of the many poisons in the smoke.

The Illusion of No Control

Habitual smokers are no longer simply choosing whether or not to smoke on any given day. Ever since their Subconscious mind took over responsibility for the activity they have felt compelled to reach for tobacco at certain moments of the day, and because of the compulsion smoking has become something they feel as if they 'can't help' doing. Habitual *s*mokers are either in denial about this - claiming they are doing it on purpose for various 'reasons' - or else they recognise their lack of conscious choice but are under the impression that this is because they are addicted to a drug. Neither is true at all. Smoking begins as a casual, voluntary activity which can soon become compulsive-habitual behaviour *controlled* by the Subconscious mind. It isn't outside the smokers control, it is only outside their conscious control. Their Subconscious is controlling it fine, and simply has no idea that the conscious mind made a decision to change that, so the Subconscious continues driving the usual behaviour. Hence the conflict. The smoker who is trying to quit is not fighting a battle with nicotine or tobacco, as they have been told so often. They are fighting themselves. It is an internal conflict in which the conscious mind is attempting to repress by force (willpower) behaviour directed by the Subconscious, and the Subconscious is unaware of that fact.

It is worth mentioning once again, at this point, that the conscious mind does not typically believe in the Subconscious except perhaps in theory, until it is explained at some length. And even after that, the conscious mind still tends to be doubtful about the Subconscious as a reality. If this factor is still making it difficult for you to accept the reality of all this, please be patient because it is simply an unfortunate effect of the way we were all educated in the first place – as if the Subconscious mind does not exist. So any conscious doubts you may still have are entirely normal, don't let them trouble you. They certainly don't surprise me. Hang on to them as long as you like, but you will probably find that more and more difficult to do as the evidence piles up. The conscious mind may be skeptical and it has certainly been misled in the first place, but in most cases it certainly isn't stupid. That will be true of anyone who has got this far into the book. In fact anyone who is reading a book written by myself is manifestly not stupid, whatever they believe.

Part 4: Compulsive Habit, not Addiction

What is addiction anyway, what do we really mean by it? Is it enough to say it is simply something you can't stop doing? That certainly seems to be the modern *casual* use of the term. But there are so many things that people cannot stop doing once they get started that this rough definition of addiction ends up being meaningless: smoking tobacco, snorting cocaine, chocolate-eating, gambling, playing computer games, watching horror movies, drinking beer or coffee, 'shopaholic' behaviour, comfort-eating, bodybuilding, cola drinks – people are described as being addicted to all these things, and many others. Yet the notion of addiction as a physical or chemical dependency is clearly unrelated to examples like gambling or playing computer games for hours on end, yet seemingly 'unable' to stop.

Recent scientific theory has focused on brain chemicals, suggesting that experiences of tobacco, gambling, cocaine and chocolate all release similar pleasure-chemicals in the brain. There has been much talk of dopamine and seratonin, 'nicotine receptors' and the like. But anyone who has snorted a few lines of cocaine, lost twenty quid on a horse and had a Mars bar will be well aware that these are totally different experiences when it comes to pleasure. Yet these *behaviours* can be equally difficult to quit once they become a regular habit – as can nail-biting, spending money and masturbating, to name but three other very common compulsive habits. None of them are physical dependencies – not even habitual cocaine use. The fact that they are notoriously difficult to cease altogether just with willpower does not mean the person is dependent on that substance or seeking a pleasure rush in the brain, it just *looks like that* if you do not understand the role of the Subconscious in repeating that habitual behaviour.

You see if we put forward a case for change regarding any of these behaviours to the conscious mind (reasoning), we might get concurrence verbally, but usually do not see lasting change. Explain the same case to the Subconscious, through a perfectly straightforward process of communication which has become known as hypnotherapy, and we find that the Subconscious is often quite happy to change that, with no effort and no risk. The fact that we do not see success in every case should not make us any less excited about this: since the outcome is in the hands of the client's Subconscious, we are going to see a range of responses which is bound to include no response at all in some cases. But if it were not within the gift of the Subconscious to change the behaviour anyway, we would never see success with any of these issues, and I have seen success repeatedly with all of them. All of them, that is, except masturbation. No-one has ever consulted me about that, which neither surprises nor disappoints me in any way.

The problem with looking at the brain chemicals alone, as if the lively intelligence of the Subconscious mind doesn't even exist, is that you head off down the scary, scary road that leads to half the population taking Prozac, anti-depressants, Zyban, sleeping tablets - not to mention the poison patches and the poison gum. For drug companies, this is the road to heaven. For everybody else...

Britain becomes a Prozac nation

The number of Britons prescribed anti-depressants is at a record high, despite official warnings that many patients may not need them. More than 31 million prescriptions were written by doctors for anti-depressant drugs last year... the cost to the NHS was £291.5 million.

The Times, Front page May 14th 2007

Now, some of the people who talk about nicotine receptors in the brain and brain chemicals are very learned people and I do not presume to question their observations about the brain itself, only the assumptions and suggestions that are often attached to their observations, and not necessarily by them. But I will say this: if you want to quit the smoking habit easily and quickly, the people who know all about the brain chemicals cannot help you to effortlessly achieve that in a short time. I can help you to do that, and without any reference to brain chemicals at all. Now if it really was the active role of the chemicals that were influencing or controlling the behaviour, that shouldn't be possible, should it? It is the same with all our successful anxiety sessions, insomnia cases and emotional issues which include cases of depression, as well as all kinds of other misery and unhappiness which are not depression, but will still probably get you classed and treated as 'depressed' if you turn up at the doctor's surgery with it.

Part 5: Scales of Dependence and Habit-Forming Mistakes

The following is a quote from the Royal College of Physicians:

'Addiction' and 'dependence' are terms whose definition has a social as well as a scientific dimension. In principle, they may be distinguished, but in practice such a distinction serves little purpose and the terms are used interchangeably here. They are socially and scientifically defined in that their meaning can be, and has been, changed to reflect changing perceptions rather than to indentify unequivocally an invariant, objectively definable entity. Under the current definition, the terms refer to a situation in which a drug or stimulus has unreasonably come to control behaviour.

The RCP then go on to detail at considerable length "three of the most widely used generic criteria for substance dependence", which "comprise the American Psychiatric Association (APA) Diagnostic and Statistical Manual of Mental Disorders (DSM)-IIIR criteria, the DSM-IV criteria (which superseded DSM-IIIR in 1995), and the World Health Organization International Classification of Diseases (ICD)-10 criteria.

But! We needn't bother with any of that. Because all this really means is that these people do not even agree with each other, for the truth is that none of them know what they are talking about. They *think* they do – and will probably be very miffed about my declaring otherwise – but they don't. And it is simply because they are completely misunderstanding what it is that is really controlling our behaviour, be it reasonable or otherwise.

You see, in order to decide that any behaviour is *unreasonable* you have to look at it logically: i.e. it is a conscious assessment. In order to jump to the conclusion that a *drug or stimulus* is controlling a person's behaviour, it is only necessary for a conscious mind – whether it is the conscious mind of the person themselves, or that of their doctor or analyst – to observe:

a) that the behaviour is detrimental from a logical point of view and therefore unreasonable, and

b) that the person concerned apparently lacks the ability to stop it with a conscious effort alone. Given that we have all been led to believe from an early age that the conscious mind is in control of all our choices, decisions and behaviour - despite all the ordinary evidence to the contrary in everyday life - it is easy to see how the analytical mind may come to assume that the *drug or stimulus* has "unreasonably come to control behaviour."

Of course, in order to arrive at this false conclusion it is necessary for that analytical conscious mind to have no detailed understanding and experience of the workings of the Subconscious. But since that factor is almost universal at the present time, that is currently very likely to be the case. Also, there *is* such a thing as real drug addiction, and compulsive habits can look very similar because the bottom line is the same - you can't stop doing it - but for totally different reasons.

The ongoing confusion and disagreement in medical circles over what constitutes an addiction, or a dependence - or whether a substance can be called "habit-forming" - is largely due to the huge void in their understanding and experience that is the Subconscious mind. Medical people have no real knowledge of the Subconscious at all because it is not part of their training, which effectively leaves their perplexed little conscious minds classifying symptoms and arguing over definitions, which is - well, useless. And frankly, if their use of these interchangeable terms:

"...can be, and has been, changed to reflect changing perceptions rather than to indentify unequivocally an invariant, objectively definable entity"

...then they might as well take (DSM)-IIIR, (DSM)-IV and (ICD)-10 and use them to prop up a wobbly table or something useful like that, and leave me to identify unequivocally an invariant, objectively definable entity, because I can. It's called a Compulsive Habit, and I define it in Section 10. You'll find it all makes perfect sense.

So forget the supremacy of the conscious mind - which is mythical - and where all compulsive, emotional and habitual behaviour is concerned, assume the supremacy of the Subconscious. There is no such thing as a "habit-forming" substance or stimulus. Habits are formed by the brain, as a result of regular repetition of the behaviour which the Subconscious recognises as predictable and then repeats, often for no other reason than it has become predictable, although there can be other factors motivating the continuation of the behaviour too. It is most likely to be the conscious mind which first recognises, by logical analysis, the detrimental aspects of the behaviour – provided there is no denial, of course - but the conscious mind is no longer controlling it by then. Since the conscious mind thinks it is in charge and knows nothing of the Subconscious really, it misinterprets the situation and leaps to the alarming conclusion that the tobacco / alcohol / chocolate / cocaine / roulette wheel / slot machine / available women / available men / fast food / stage hypnotist…has unreasonably come to control their behaviour!

This is a bit of a shame, because the Subconscious is usually quite happy to change it, you know. The Subconscious mind is not unreasonable but it is very likely to be completely unaware that the behaviour it is repeating automatically is causing a problem, and certainly unaware of any conscious decisions to change it, or cease doing it. Explain all those matters to the Subconscious - convincingly, and under suitably reassuring conditions - and providing that change is genuinely desired by that individual, you just watch how unaddicted, independent and habit-free they can become. You'll be amazed. They usually are. But I'm not, I've been doing this for years.

Part 6: Where the Mistakes were Made

Ok, so if it's not really nicotine addiction at all, how did everybody come to believe that it is? Well if you happen to be a dogged researcher who is happy to trawl through endless amounts of tendentious scientific research throughout the last forty or fifty years, be my guest - go find precisely where the mistakes were made. What is certain is that nobody was particularly interested in studying nicotine in any comprehensive way until some bright spark – and I use the metaphor with the deepest sarcasm – dreamed up the notion of nicotine replacement therapy. All of a sudden the race was on, to prove nicotine was the key factor so that the idea of a nicotine substitute could be justified. So it was actually the colossal *business opportunity* that nicotine suddenly represented that was driving the explosion of 'scientific' interest, especially from the 1980s onwards.

Don't forget there is no such thing as pure science, not in the real world! Someone is paying for all these experiments involving nicotine, and they are not doing it purely for the benefit of smokers, it is a business investment. For most of the time people have smoked tobacco in Europe, it has simply been regarded as a filthy habit, which was accurate enough. It wasn't until the 1960s anyone managed to prove it was even harmful and there was no common talk of "nicotine addiction" in those days. Smoking was just something people did, like chewing gum or drinking half a pint of bitter. No smoker regarded themselves as an addict in those days, nor did anyone really regard smoking tobacco as 'drug-taking'. And they were quite right, because it isn't.

When is a Poison not a Poison? When it becomes a Product!

The first nicotine replacement product was a chewing gum developed in 1971, and eventually launched in Switzerland in 1978. The U.S. Food and Drug Administration (FDA) approved it as a prescription-only aid to quitting in 1984, round about the same time as the nicotine patch was being developed. The FDA approved patches (prescription only) in 1991, and then scrapped the prescription requirement in 1996. All this talk of 'nicotine addiction' has really risen along with the development of nicotine as a product in its own right – or rather, wrong - and the global market in nicotine replacement products is now worth billions and set to rocket further as tobacco smoking continues to go out of fashion and more smokers want to quit.

So you see, some people have a huge stake in nicotine being regarded as a drug of addiction. If it turns out not to be, then the poison gum, the poison patches and all the other poison products will all become completely obsolete overnight and share prices in those drug companies will tumble. They shouldn't complain though - the nicotine myth has been a huge bonanza for them which never should have happened in the first place, so they have had a good run with their poison placebo. Especially when you look at its appalling failure rate in reality, which we shall be doing in due course (Section 9. You'll be livid, if you are a UK taxpayer).

Even though the nicotine notion has gained general popular acceptance since the 1980s, in reality there has always been scientific argument over whether or not tobacco smoking is a drug addiction, and more specifically over whether nicotine is physically addictive, habit-forming, a drug of dependency or what. But never before has so much money been riding on that question. Vast fortunes now hang on this, so if we are going to deal with realities here, we don't just need to look at "scientific research" that appears to show one thing or another but we now also need to make sure we know who commissioned that research - when, where, who carried it out, who funded it, how much research was actually done and how much of the total results were ever published. Also if some of the findings were not published, what was the reason for that?

It is also time to look again at the original 'research' that won approval for the first NRT products to see how all this got off the ground, because when we consider the estimated figures for the abject failure of NRT as it is currently reported here in the U.K. they are atrocious, and it makes one wonder if the products were really approved in the first place on the basis of dire results like that. (See Section 9.)

One shocking discovery in my research into all this was the fact that the FDA do not actually do any of the testing of new drugs, they let the drug companies themselves organise the trials, collate the results and prepare the reports on all of that. Then the FDA base their decision on whether to approve a product or not entirely upon what the drug companies have chosen to tell them. That is a system which relies heavily upon total integrity on the part of global pharmaceutical corporations. This puts the FDA in the position of a blindfolded driver steering only by instructions from the passenger. It is true that neither wants a disaster because both will be affected, but the point is they may have different notions of where this vehicle should be heading. My suggestion is that the FDA should be directing that, not the drug companies, yet in effect it seems to operate the other way around.

As if that was not bad enough, the standard applied by the FDA to assess NRT products was lax almost to the point of being ridiculous. The results of the clinical trials had to demonstrate that the products apparently showed some level of effectiveness, and were of course within the standard limits with regard to hazardous side-effects. But the FDA decided for some bizarre reason to approve the products if they managed after six weeks to show better rates than placebos for just 28 days of continuous abstinence. That is barely a month, and obviously says nothing about long-term effectiveness. The fact that most of those smokers were smoking again at the end of the year was ignored by the FDA, and the drug companies were allowed to list the quit rates at six weeks on their products.

Whether you call this fraudulent or just misleading really depends on how close to, or distant from the position of the drug companies you happen to be standing... but scientific it is not. Of course the whole business of success rates is problematic, as I review in Volume II, but where smoking habits are concerned, success measured in mere weeks is obviously no indicator of true effectiveness. This is a point to which I shall be returning when I deal with the Department of Health's regular reporting of the 'success' of the NHS programmes in Section 9.

Also – and this is an extremely important point: all you scientists and serious analysts take note of this point particularly - it could be very significant that during scientific trials smokers can easily recognise the *presence* of nicotine as being part of their usual smoking experience. Having been told so many times over the years by 'experts' that nicotine is actually what they need to relieve cravings and that is why they cannot stop smoking, any smokers who believed that would then be likely to get *a more significant placebo effect during a trial* from a product that gave them a detectable nicotine experience than from one which did not. *Noticing* the presence of nicotine would then be likely to increase their *expectation* of a benefit, an important part of the placebo effect. This would not happen in those smokers given a nicotine-free placebo, which would account for the small differences in early reactions which won NRT the official status of "more effective than placebo" in those original trials. But since the placebo effect - particularly in the context of supposedly-recreational habits - would only be temporary for many people, it is precisely the long term results that are truly significant in assessing the 'success' of NRT. The same is true of assessing the success of hypnotherapy of course, which is why we only regard a case as a true success when the person never feels the urge to smoke again. So by getting the FDA to only look at short-term reactions during the trial, the drug companies actually created a completely false impression about the promise of NRT and obtained a licence to print money by producing a useless poison to sell to the world as if it was a medicine.

So did the drug companies really just test one placebo against another, and temporarily produce more of a reaction with the one which the smokers could tell featured a nicotine experience? If so, it was simply the smokers' belief in the myth of nicotine addiction which made the tiny difference. It is time to look more closely at:

Part 7: The Placebo Effect

What follows is part of a report by Barbara Lantin published in The Daily Telegraph in the UK on 25th October 2002. The Telegraph is generally regarded as a sober and conservative publication not normally given to progressive views, so it is interesting that it should appear in that newspaper. Although this article, titled: *Healing can be all in the mind* is not about smoking, some of what it says is pertinent to the points I am making here. I have also included here the references to hypnosis in the article, both as a point of general interest and in support of my claims for hypnotherapy in this book.

"For years, the placebo effect has had a bad press. Those organising clinical trials go to extraordinary lengths to rule it out [sic] when presenting their results, and any medical intervention that is deemed to be "no better than a placebo" is dismissed as worthless. But the truth is that many know it works, and are quietly using that knowledge.

Drug manufacturers have discovered that large pills produce better results than small ones, red ones are more effective than white, blue pills are more likely to improve sleep, and four pills taken regularly work better than two. Although GPs are officially not supposed to prescribe a placebo, 63% of 200 who took part in a survey said that they had done so.

Studies have shown a significant placebo response in conditions as wide-ranging as cardiac failure, peptic ulcers, multiple sclerosis, dementia and schizophrenia. In some conditions, the more severe the symptoms, the better the placebo effect. Irving Kirsch, professor of psychology at the University of Conneticut, claims that data from the original trial on Prozac submitted to the Food and Drug Administration shows that placebo is 80% as effective as the active drug."

Just to interject for a moment: 80% as effective? In a case like that, since the placebo has no side effects, why bother with the drug? More to the point, since the placebo effect is really the effect of suggestion, what does all this say about the potential for hypnotherapy to alleviate these conditions, if conducted effectively? Because that is all that is really happening here: placebos are nothing more or less than the effect of a general suggestion.

The word "placebo" derives from the Latin verb *placere* meaning "to appease or placate" and the term encompasses many intermeshing strands affecting healing. "There are a lot of different things disguised in what happens when somebody who is given an inactive substance seems to get better," says Dr David Peters of the University of Westminster. "It has to do with the patient, the practitioner, the medicine itself and a combination of all of these."

Actually to be more usefully specific, it is entirely a matter of *what the patient believes and feels* about all those things. In hypnotherapy we work with beliefs and feelings all the time, and we find that in changing these things for the better, there is zero requirement to meddle with the chemical composition of the brain.

Even the setting can play a part. In one trial, post-operative patients were assigned either to a room with a view or one facing a brick wall. Those looking on to the meadow had a shorter stay in hospital, made fewer complaints to nurses and took fewer strong painkillers than those overlooking the wall.

If you are more prone to getting a cold when you are stressed, you will know that your state of mind can affect your body – and the effect can work for good or bad. Work by Dr Steven Greer at the Royal Marsden Hospital has demonstrated that cancer sufferers who displayed a "fighting spirit" were 60% more likely to be alive 13 years after diagnosis than those who felt "helpless and hopeless".

In a recent study at Imperial College, London, patients with chronic genital herpes that did not respond to medicine were taught to practice self-hypnosis three times a week for six weeks. "The recurrence rate of the condition halved, which is a phenomenal result in these severe cases," says John Gruzelier, Professor of Psychology at Imperial. "We looked to see what happened when we injected a blood sample with the virus before and after the self-hypnosis training. After training, the cytotoxic [cell-destroying] effect of the body's natural killer cells stepped up immensely in two thirds of the group."

The study of psychoneuroimmunology is in its infancy, but it is thought that the brain can reverse disease via a group of neurotransmitters called neuropeptides. These are triggered by the physiological equivalent of feelings and thoughts, and can lock onto cells all over the body. One is endorphin, the "feel-good" effect released by strenuous exercise. Others can boost the production of killer cells and lymphocytes and reduce levels of cortisol, all of which can strengthen the immune system.

"The potential for mind-body medicine is enormous," says Professor Gruzelier, who is about to embark on trials of self-hypnosis for advanced breast cancer and early-stage HIV. "It's non-invasive, easy to teach and to do, and very cost-effective."

Stop Press: Hypnotherapy Discovered by Medics in 21st Century!

The potential for mind-body medicine has been enormous for the last 150 years, ever since those wonderful pioneers began experimenting with mesmerism/hypnosis for anaesthesia and getting very exciting results (see *Hypnotherapy v Science,* Section 17 Volume II), just like the exciting results described above. Perhaps you are beginning to wonder why mind-body medicine is described by this worthy reporter at the Telegraph as being "in its infancy" a century and a half later. And the medical folk can call it psychoneuroimmunology if they like, but it is actually hypnotherapy, as the words "self-hypnosis" do rather give away in the study at Imperial College. It is just that if the medical world call it hypnotherapy, they begin to look a bit stupid for being generally prejudiced against it for a century and a half. But if they call it psychoneuroimmunology, then the psychology professors can do what Allen Carr did: re-package hypnosis under a different name and claim the wonderful successes of hypnotherapy for themselves as if they just 'discovered' it.

Well I've got news for you, guys: it was never lost. And it has always been the medical authorities that have gone out of their way to make sure people like myself are not allowed to claim we might be able to help with medical problems just like those listed above, which nevertheless respond astonishingly well to the placebo effect – which is nothing but suggestion.

The medical profession owes the hypnotherapy profession the biggest professional apology in the world. That's the truth. But we won't hold our collective breath. We'll just keep doing what we do best – glad you found the time to catch up eventually. But don't go acting as if you've suddenly discovered some marvellous new branch of science – go back a century and a half and read your medical history. Look at what your predecessors did to the mesmerists in your own profession, and hang your heads in shame. Psychoneuroimmunology, hypnosis, mind-body medicine, mesmerism... as the bard said, "what's in a name? A rose by any other name would smell as sweet". Revenge is sweet, they say... and to those of us who feel furious about what happened to the mesmerists because it was so stupid, unnecessary and so unfair... yes, it is sweet to read the words of Professor Gruzelier, and to know that despite all the prejudice, lies and hostility that was directed at advocates of these methods in the past, despite all the horseshit from the pathological disbelievers in the medical profession, hypnotherapy has, of course, come up smelling of roses.

I'll let Barbara Lantin have the last word regarding placebos for the moment because later, when we are looking at the actual failure rates of nicotine replacement products I would like this statement to be easily recalled:

The placebo effect is a powerful medicinal tool: in an average drug trial, 35 per cent of patients receiving dummy pills show an improvement in their symptoms.

35%. Let us plant that figure firmly in the Subconscious mind and stick a big flag over it saying "Placebo: 35%". Now you will always be able to remember, and at any time in the future – perhaps at a dinner party – if someone is being dismissive, saying "Oh, that's just a placebo!" you can coolly remark:

"Actually, in scientific trials the placebo effect can normally be expected to have a success rate of anything up to 35%." All will be impressed.

Interlude: Case Mysteries No.4

If We Could Talk to the Animals, *or* How Nicotine was Framed

We will get back to the proper Case Mysteries in due course because they are rather enlightening, but in the meantime, a man's gotta do what a man's gotta do. Picture the scene: it is high noon, and the streets are deserted as the stranger with the swinging gold pocket-watch and the relaxation CD puts down his shot-glass and strides boldly out of the saloon to face... the one they call 'The Scientist'. Hey, better not play on the stoop now, Junior. Looks like there's a-gonna be trouble. Go inside, and keep away from the window. Go on, now!

Before the exciting gunplay though, a little context. Amongst the clients that come along to my office for therapy there are some medical people from all branches of the profession, including GPs. Of all these health professionals, interestingly enough it is the GPs who are least surprised to hear what I have to say about nicotine, and I think that is because they have been at the sharp end of handing out patches and gum for years and they know what to expect from that in terms of success. Privately, on a one-to-one basis most of the doctors with whom I have discussed this will freely admit that they don't believe in all that addiction stuff anymore, but collectively, as a profession they have gone so far down that road that they can hardly come out and say: "Whoops, forget all that stuff about nicotine addiction! Looks like we were wrong there. Everybody just go back to regarding it as a filthy habit - just like we all did right up until the 1970s, in fact."

One young GP was very surprised though, and he told me about some experiments involving mice that proved - he seemed quite sure - that nicotine was an addictive drug. When I pressed him, he acknowledged that hadn't studied the experiments himself but he thought the study involved mice choosing a nicotine option repeatedly, suggesting that it had addictive properties, so I guess this is what is being taught in medical school now.

At the time I told him I could not explain the behaviour of the mice because I am an expert in the behaviour of humans, but I did point out two things: firstly, that those scientists conducting experiments involving nicotine probably could not help him at all with his smoking habit, so what was the practical value of all that? And secondly, if the experiments truly showed nicotine was highly addictive then how can hypnotherapy eliminate the problem? That doesn't make sense.

This poor medical chap was on the horns of a dilemma. Should he keep faith with the training that justified his new-found status as a professional with specialist knowledge... or trust a hypnotist? Of course, being inexperienced he stuck with the mice story, preferring to reject contradictory suggestions and he carried right on smoking, and I can't say I was surprised. It was too early in his career for him to start questioning what he was taught. It's a matter of confidence. (Most medical people I see for smoking do not do this by the way, they just stop smoking. They might be a bit surprised, but it doesn't give them a crisis of confidence. It just broadens their perspective a bit.) But the mention of the mice did prompt me to take a look at the experiments to which he referred, because this is a significant strand of the "scientific evidence" that is underpinning the official medical line on nicotine which has spawned the global market for nicotine replacement products – or was it the other way round? And so for anyone who wishes to judge for themselves, here is one official medical account of these animal experiments involving nicotine. First I will let someone else tell you all about it, and then I will comment ruthlessly upon their foolishness and ineptitude.

Unreliable Evidence: Monkey Junkies and Coked-up Rats

A key example of the sort of scientific research that is supposed to serve as satisfactory evidence in support of the notion that nicotine is an addictive drug is the rather sick phenomenon of 'Animal Self-Administration' via an intravenous (IV) link, the so-called IVSA experiments. This is an experimentation model that aims to get different species of animals to apparently dose themselves with various dangerous substances - some of which are held to be physically addictive - to see whether they apparently 'become addicted'.

The information I am using in this section has been provided by the Royal College of Physicians ("Setting Higher Medical Standards", as it says on their website), hereafter referred to as the RCP, and it may become apparent as I am tearing this 'evidence' to shreds using good old-fashioned logic that I am very much opposed to animal experimentation on the grounds that it is:

a) no different from what Josef Mengele was doing in Auschwitz, except the animals he was using were human - to *us* that is, not to him - and

b) stupid, for reasons which will become obvious as I point out the glaring chasms of doubt and uncertainty in these trials that animal experimentation always seems to involve.

Now I don't wish to come over as some sort of maniacal extremist here. Opposing vivisection (experiments on animals) on moral grounds is one thing. Assessing the actual value of any particular experiment is another, and most of this section will be the latter. Of course I understand there will always be arguable opposing views about vivisection that can also claim a moral basis, so this is by no means a simple matter if we are going to allow democratic principles to hold. I remain prepared to listen to any serious argument that might prove an example of the 'justifiable' use of animal life as if it were disposable laboratory equipment. Maybe somebody will one day convince me that animal life is inferior to human life and therefore always expendable in any service of human interests, who knows.

Humans dominate the globe at present, so it is not surprising that some cocky individuals regard all other creatures as essentially inferior, an attitude which is really just species-fascism. Usually these types will challenge anti-vivisectionists with queries like: "Do you wear leather? Do you eat meat?" To them, there is no difference between one type of disposal and another – a view which leads to live goats being hurled from church towers in Spanish fiestas, just for fun. Or in the name of Jesus, whatever. Or just because we can, and we're curious about what a goat would look like, after... It's a scientific interest, if you like, about what happens to a helpless body when such enormous forces... Oh Jesus, will you look at that? That's one goat that won't be offending Christians again. Eh, Father? That's one in the eye for the Devil, right?

Nature, not Torture

My view is that animals eating each other is part of the natural order of things, and making practical use of the hide, bones or other inedible bits has been normal human behaviour for thousands of years, so I would say that is natural to us. In order to survive day to day, and feed the family, I reckon I would be prepared to do all of those things myself if necessary, although I respect the feelings of those who would not. Likewise, if I were killed by a crocodile or eaten by a bear, I would regard that as extremely unlucky, but not unnatural, as we are fair game to those creatures.

But if I were taken up into a UFO without my consent, and experimented upon, I would be exceedingly pissed off. I don't care if there *is* stuff the freaky fuckers want to find out. No probes. Put me back, and leave the livestock alone too. In fact don't land, at all, if you've got nothing useful to tell us. And quit drawing on the crops. Oh, that wasn't you? Ok.

Meanwhile, back on Earth...

I believe that the people who defend vivisection on the grounds that it is of indispensable value to humans should make their case more publicly by demonstrating to us all - on TV perhaps - exactly what essential work is being done, and just how it is done. For if it is truly valuable and necessary, surely we will all appreciate that. Give us a chance to view and follow these procedures in detail from the conception of the experiment right through to the conclusions, so that we can see for ourselves the true value of the work, instead of it being hidden away all the time.

One of the main themes proposed by vivisectionists is that if a close member of your own family was dangerously ill, you would suddenly be prepared to sacrifice any number of defenceless dumb animals to the God of Human Life in order to attempt to save your loved one. Quite apart from the fact that no human is ever going to be faced with that outright choice so it is a ludicrously emotive suggestion, just how much of the vivisection that has so far occurred has had anything to do with saving people from deadly disease? In the past a great deal of it has been about launching a new shampoo or something equally inane, which had to be routinely rubbed into the eyes of numerous doomed quadruped slaves before it could be promoted on TV by some girl under a waterfall.

So come on, let's see the proof it won't make our eyes sting! We already have cosmetic surgery on television - that's pretty graphic and yet it is acceptable now as entertainment, so why not this sterling work? Show us your heroic efforts on our collective behalf in close up detail, and don't forget to let us know who is magnanimously funding the experiments and what sort of vital, indispensable products that company has previously put on the pharmacy shelves as a result of such procedures. Things we couldn't possibly have managed without, like cough mixtures and hand creams. It could be a huge TV ratings hit, a sort of "Their lives, for your hands" inspirational medical documentary. These scientists are probably not getting the recognition they deserve, and the self-sacrifice of the animals involved will fill us all with teary gratitude, especially if any life-saving drugs actually were involved. I've even got a snappy title for the show: "You Dirty Rat – You Saved My Brother!"

I'm quite proud of that joke. It's just a shame so many people would now need the movie reference explaining. By the way, just for the record, although I am strongly opposed to vivisection I do not support force or any form of terror campaign to end it. I believe such methods damage the moral case against experimenting on live animals and lose public support, which is essential if change is going to come. And I am not just saying that, I have no time for self-appointed bunny-vigilanties, they are playing right into the hands of the drug companies.

But putting the moral case aside now, just look at this particular example of quite indefensible animal-bothering, as I point out just how useless and stupid these procedures can be, and just how dodgy the conclusions often are. What follows is directly quoted from the RCP. It is perhaps best to read it first as it actually appears - part of their longer website article "Nicotine Addiction in Britain" - and then I will offer a critique. If you want to read the original and all the rest of the stuff they have to say about nicotine, visit the website www.rcplondon.ac.uk

Animal self-administration and nicotine addiction

The concept of addiction has at its core the idea of compulsive use, as reflected in powerful drug-seeking and drug-taking behaviour. In IV self-administration (IVSA) experiments, animals learn to administer drugs to themselves. Typically, the animal has the opportunity to press a lever; when it does so, it receives an automatic IV infusion of a drug (through a chronically-indwelling venous catheter). Several animal species, notably rats and monkeys, will press levers to obtain injections of the 'classical' addictive drugs such as morphine, heroin, amphetamine, cocaine, barbiturates and benzodiazepines. Large amounts of these drugs can be self-administered in this way. Furthermore, animals will work very hard to obtain the drugs, for example, pressing a switch thousands of times, for hours on end, to obtain drugs. This drug-seeking and drug-taking behaviour can dominate the animals' behavioural repertoire to the detriment of normal behaviour, just as in cases of serious drug abuse in humans. In fact, under appropriate conditions, animals will administer to themselves most of the drugs abused by humans. IVSA in animals is therefore a suitable animal model for the study of drug dependence in humans.

It has been established that monkeys, dogs, rats and mice can all exhibit nicotine IVSA. Monkeys have pressed levers for nicotine at rates similar to those at which they pressed levers for cocaine. In these experiments, the nicotine or cocaine was paired (associated) with brief flashes of light, which in this model were functionally equivalent to the smell and taste stimuli associated with smoke inhalation. Both the nicotine and the light stimuli served as rewards for these animals, the latter by virtue of association with the nicotine. Nicotine IVSA has also been demonstrated in monkeys using simpler procedures without associated light stimuli, although rates and consistency of responding for the drug were less striking. Dogs have also learned to press pedals to activate IV injections of nicotine. Up to several hundreds pedal presses were made to obtain a single injection of nicotine, indicating that its rewarding effect, although powerful, was less strong than that of cocaine. Nicotine

IVSA has also been reported in mice both with an 'acute' procedure in which stress may be a confounding factor, and in chronic IVSA experiments of the usual type. There is also some evidence for IV self-administration of pure solutions of nicotine in human subjects, but these studies do not seem to have been reported in full. The animals studied most extensively in nicotine self-administration experiments have been rats, and these results will be considered next.

Nicotine self-administration in rats

In 1989, Corrigall and Coen succeeded in developing a rat model for nicotine IVSA. The rats learnt to press levers to obtain IV infusions of nicotine, but did not press an inactive (control) lever in the same test chamber. The rate of lever pressing was related to the dose of nicotine, and the lever pressing ceased if nicotine was no longer available. As in the experiments in monkeys and dogs mentioned above, the lever-pressing produced nicotine and no other substance. The nicotine served as a goal object (positive reinforcer) for these animals, much in the same way as other drugs of abuse and natural rewards.

These observations have been reproduced and extended in numerous published experiments from many different laboratories. All these studies demonstrate that rats will self-administer solutions of pure nicotine in the absence of any other reward. The validity of the observation is supported by the finding that the plasma concentration of nicotine in rats during IVSA experiments can be close to that in heavy cigarette smokers who inhale.

Some studies have failed to find robust nicotine IVSA. To understand these results, it is essential to recognize that the extent to which a drug is self-administered depends on a multitude of procedural, environmental and genetic factors. As discussed elsewhere, it was at one time difficult to demonstrate even the self-administration of opiate drugs. Some studies have failed to show nicotine IVSA, but these used a strain of rat shown subsequently to be poor in performing this task; strain differences in animal studies may reflect genetic factors that influence human use of tobacco. Nearly all successful studies in rats used rapid 'bolus' injections, and data suggests that rapid infusions support self-administration more effectively than slow infusions. Other studies used relatively slow infusions of nicotine and obtained equivocal results. It is, however, apparent in most experiments that nicotine is a weaker reinforcer than cocaine, its self-administration is acquired more slowly and maintained under a narrower range of conditions. It is unclear whether this reflects on either the appropriateness of the animal procedures to model the richness of the human environment or on the importance of other reinforcers in human tobacco use. Non-pharmacological sources of reinforcement may be significant, and recent studies provide indirect support for the presence of other psychoactive substances in tobacco in addition to the nicotine.

Summary

IVSA is the primary animal model for studying drug-taking behaviour. The species thought to self-administer nicotine (and other drugs of abuse) in this way include mice, monkeys, dogs and rats. The combination of broad cross-species similarity of these animal data, plus the exceptionally high validity of drug self-administration procedures, generally strongly suggest that they are a reliable guide to the human condition. Studies have also shed light on the brain mechanisms underlying nicotine IVSA. Nicotinic receptors are found in many areas of the mammalian brain, and their involvement in nicotine IVSA is supported by observations that the non-competitive nicotine agonist......

Can I just interject, here? I'll let the RCP continue with this in a moment, but I just wanted to draw your attention to the way this suddenly shifts onto completely different ground. This is supposed to be a "Summary" of what you already read! Quite apart from the fact that the first three sentences are not what I would call an accurate summary of what went before but rather a summary of what they *wish* it demonstrated, what follows next is not only quite different from the earlier content but also dissimilar in terms of language. The rest of the text adopts a scientific jargon that would be likely to lose any readers who were not involved in that kind of work themselves.

I know this is a scientific website so there is no reason to exclude scientific jargon, but the rest of the text hardly seems intended to de-mystify but rather to give a reassuring impression of 'hard science', as it were, to bolster that which has gone before, which actually wasn't very convincing in itself, as I will show.

I suspect that at this point in the text and for the rest of the article the average reader is supposed to be completely blinded by science and drift away, thinking: "Oh well, they've lost me there, but they seem to know what they are talking about, so I guess it's alright... I certainly was impressed with those thousands of lever-presses, for hours on end. That nicotine sure is addictive stuff!"

So what comes next is actually a completely different level of commentary, which aims to be convincing because it is using technical terminology regarding the "mammalian brain". To borrow the advertising expression 'here comes the scientific bit', which *implies* precision but which is really full of suggestion and generalizations, which I have highlighted in the text below because otherwise you might not notice them. I have also drawn attention to two instances where the findings for real drugs - which are naturally a bit more convincing - have been 'stitched together' with nicotine in the text, so that the case for nicotine itself can hopefully be carried by the unconnected, but stronger evidence:

> ...the non-competitive nicotine agonist mecamylamine **can** attenuate lever-pressing for nicotine. The competitive nicotinic antagonist DhbE blocks nicotine IVSA by an action on nicotinic receptors in the VTA of the mid-brain. Nicotine acts in the VTA to activate the ascending mesolimbic dopamine system. This neural pathway is also critically **implicated** in the reinforcing action of abused drugs such as amphetamine, cocaine and opioids. **Like these substances, nicotine enhances** the release of dopamine in some of the projection areas of the mesolimbic dopamine system, notably the nucleus accumbens. **All these drugs, including nicotine**, produce dopamine release mainly in the shell area of the nucleus accumbens rather than in the core.
>
> Dopamine agonist drugs and selective neurotoxin-produced lesions of the dopamine-containing neurons of the nucleus accumbens strikingly attenuate nicotine IVSA. **Recent studies suggest** an impairment of both dopamine release and nicotine IVSA in transgenic mice lacking the b2 subunit of the nicotinic receptor; nicotinic receptors containing the alpha4beta2 subtype are the most prevalent in the mammalian brain, and these **important** observations **suggest** that they **may be** required for nicotine IVSA. The roles of nicotinic receptors containing a and other b subunits **have yet to be evaluated** in a similar manner. Overall, the results to date **suggest** that the ascending mesolimbic dopamine system is essential for nicotine IVSA. This is also the major known neuroanatomical and neurochemical mechanism of reward for the classical addictive drugs. **Therefore, both the behavioural effects and the mechanisms of action of nicotine in the IVSA model <u>resemble</u> those for classical drugs of abuse such as heroin and cocaine.**

The last sentence is highlighted because it is nothing but a suggestion, posing as an objective conclusion. The key word in that suggestion I have underlined: "resemble". I will now demonstrate why this is at best just a slight resemblance but the attempt here has been to pass it off as a close resemblance. Whoever wrote this article either has no acute critical faculties of their own, or they were deliberately setting out to arrive at that conclusion no matter how difficult it proved to be. Having reached the end, I could just imagine them turning to a colleague and saying: "Phew! Do you think I managed to pull that off? Did I succeed in trying to make nicotine seem pretty similar to real drugs, even though the actual evidence is patchy and inconsistent? Will we get away with that, do you think?"

Will They Get Away With It, Do You Think?

Not if I have anything to do with it, they won't. Now let us analyse this critically, from the top. The first sentence of the article confuses two quite separate things: "addiction" and "compulsive" behaviour, and it is largely the project of this book to clarify the difference:

> The concept of addiction has at its core the idea of compulsive use, as reflected in powerful drug-seeking and drug-taking behaviour.

I would immediately refute the suggestion that compulsive use is at the core of the concept of addiction, and posit instead that *need* is the characteristic experience there. Many people compulsively bite their fingernails or eat chocolate, and seem unable to resist doing so, but even they would not seriously claim that they have any *real need* to do that, just a powerful urge to do so. By contrast the heroin addict has not only a compulsive urge to take heroin, but also a desperate feeling of *need* that leaves them profoundly bereft, even ill. Nobody feels ill if they don't bite their fingernails, so compulsive urges are not the defining factor in real addictions - merely an additional factor, for addictions are invariably compulsive habits too. This does not mean compulsive habits are addictions, as is clearly indicated by many ordinary compulsive habits like nail-biting.

> In IV self-administration (IVSA) experiments, animals learn to administer drugs to themselves.

Actually that is an assumption, and of course a suggestion. All that is truly *observed* is that some animals - but not others - learn to trigger the mechanism. It is not unreasonable to suppose that some of this behaviour, especially where the results are dramatic such as those involving heroin or cocaine, is drug-seeking and therefore truly self-administration. Still it will always remain a likely supposition, nothing more. But the results are certainly not dramatic where nicotine is concerned, and indeed the article later mentions that some studies failed to report any conclusive evidence of nicotine self-administration. So we must not let the more striking results for heroin and cocaine carry the case for nicotine, as the writer of the article seems to be attempting to do. The true motivation of some of these animals in playing with the mechanism is never questioned. It is taken as read that it can only be drug-seeking and the fact that some animals show little interest or do not play the game at all does not trouble the writer, who tries to dismiss that problem by admitting:

...the extent to which a drug is self-administered depends on a multitude of procedural, environmental and genetic factors.

In other words, it is pretty difficult to get any of this to look convincing, so we shouldn't be surprised when some studies do not.

Several animal species, notably rats and monkeys, will press levers to obtain injections of the 'classical' addictive drugs...

Why not all species? This curious phenomenon does not seem to trouble the writer at all, but the whole point of these experiments is to attempt to draw useful conclusions about human experience from the behaviour of the animals involved. If we are to assume that these particular creatures, the rats and monkeys, are getting the same sort of experience as we do from these substances - which is questionable of course - why don't all creatures that are capable of learning to press levers, like cats for instance, behave the same way? If the nature of the substance is the cause of the behaviour, why should it fail in other species?

Only two answers seem likely, both of which negate the point of the experiment. Either different species experience the substances in different ways, so we can draw no certain conclusion about humans from the behaviour of any of them - only make assumptions, which doesn't get us anywhere if we are going to be rigorously scientific. Or, only a few species will oblige in playing laboratory games with levers and flashing lights - a likely explanation for the disinterest of cats - which raises the question: How often is it really the substance which is prompting this behaviour?

Case Mysteries 4: If We Could Talk to the Animals

Now, I don't want to be unduly dismissive of *all* the findings mentioned by the RCP. I note with interest that some animals "will work very hard to obtain" such drugs as morphine, heroin, amphetamine, cocaine and barbiturates - sometimes "pressing a switch thousands of times, for hours on end, to obtain drugs." But take careful note: that bit of background information never mentions nicotine. Yet it is presented here in support of an argument about nicotine addiction specifically. Put simply, how these animals react to heroin, cocaine etc. has nothing to do with the properties of nicotine, yet this is not made clear. The reader could easily get the impression that various animals are working very hard for hours on end to obtain nicotine also, pressing a switch thousands of times - when in fact no such results for nicotine *alone* are claimed anywhere in the article. The studies which are later dismissed as 'flawed' because they found no results for nicotine at all are not mentioned until later on, so our first impression in this article - which is specifically about *Nicotine Addiction in Britain* - is of levers being triggered thousands of times. Looking at it as pure suggestion this is actually quite clever, if the attempt was to mislead. If it is simply clumsy that is less impressive, but no less *effective* in creating the impression of dramatic IVSA results for "All these drugs..." Including nicotine more by implication than any concrete findings detailed here.

This drug-seeking and drug-taking behaviour can dominate the animals' behavioural repertoire to the detriment of normal behaviour, just as in cases of serious drug abuse in humans.

To the detriment of "normal behaviour"? Just what degree of normal rat behaviour is permitted to laboratory rats? There is nothing normal about their situation, and this goes for all the other creatures mentioned too. This is not a bleeding-heart point, but a rigorous analysis of the findings as they are reported here since the scientists are focusing on *behaviour* in these experiments. If the rats and the monkeys were not pressing levers and getting themselves smacked-up or high on coke, just what else would they be doing that day? Was the monkey allowed a nice female companion to amuse himself with, instead of being stuck in a cage by himself? No. Did he have a pal with him? No. Did he have anything *else* to do all day but press levers? No of course not, this is a scientific procedure, so it has to be a controlled environment. All other distractions would have to be eliminated so they don't risk confusing the picture when results are analysed.

So what normal monkey or rat behaviour were the scientists expecting to see under these "appropriate conditions"? Because this is exactly the point, you see - for whom are these conditions supposed to be appropriate? Not the bloody monkey, that's for sure. He should be swinging through branches in Botswana, not huddled in a cage in some freaky laboratory with nothing to do all day and night but press levers. Do you see what I'm getting at? How can the scientist - who is very unlikely to be any expert on natural monkey behaviour anyway - distinguish between 'normal' and 'abnormal' under such blatantly abnormal and distressing conditions for the animal?

Now before somebody suggests that the animals are not distressed or bothered about any of these environmental factors because they are just dumb animals - that we should not assume they would feel similar to us, if we were undergoing a parallel experience of incarceration, isolation and alienation from our natural surroundings - let us not forget that the whole point of these experiments is to find out more about human problems via the assumption that these animals are getting the same 'reward' experience from the active substance, ie. *feeling the same way as us.* So you cannot have it both ways: either they are *not* experiencing similar things to us, in which case the whole thing is a waste of time, or they *are* - in which case distress, loneliness and the complete lack of alternative stimuli must be taken into account to at least partially explain the desperation and obsessive-compulsive aspects of their behaviour. Forget normal, that is nowhere to be found in this mad scenario.

So when the RCP concludes glibly that:

> IVSA in animals is therefore a suitable animal model for the study of drug dependence in humans.

Case Mysteries 4: If We Could Talk to the Animals

I would have to say: No it bloody isn't, unless you are comparing the results with the behaviour of humans who are isolated indefinitely in a foreign jail run by aliens, and given nothing else to do but press levers which automatically administer unlimited quantities of drugs.

Enough! Time for a Brief Flight of Fancy:

In any case, what fool decided that the best way to study the effects of heroin, cocaine and amphetamines on humans was to give those substances to rats and monkeys? Surely animal testing is only necessary when willing humans are not available in sufficient numbers. Don't they realise how many thousands of humans in this country would be wildly enthusiastic about taking part in such trials? They'll sign any disclaimer you like, too. Let the monkeys go – just whisper it in any club in Manchester, Birmingham or Glasgow that there's free coke available for anyone who wants to help out with this study and they will be queuing around the block for a chance to take part. You wouldn't even have to pay them. Thousands of people whispering excitedly to each other: "What, all you have to do is press a lever? Shit, sometimes I've had to walk five miles and bang on eight doors before I got what I wanted – where do I sign?" No need to pay anybody. And when it's time for the amphetamine experiments they'll even clean your lab for you as well, from top to bottom. Clean out all the cages too, you can go home early.

In fact, human competition for a place on those trials would be fierce. You don't need to bother the animal kingdom at all, you could find out everything there is to know about the effects of heroin, cocaine and amphetamine on human behaviour in a single summer. There would be way too many candidates putting themselves forward.

Actually - just a thought - the pharmaceutical giants could be missing out on a massive promotional opportunity here. They should just put up posters:

> Calling all of Britain's heroin and cocaine enthusiasts:
> Somewhere out there, secretly placed in pharmacies
> across the land, there are fifty bottles of Night Nurse

with a Golden Ticket
to take part in our self-administration drug trials!
Will you be the lucky winner?

You watch that Night Nurse fly off the shelves. It's foul-tasting, but you never know! You want to see levers being pressed thousands of times for hours on end? Britain's finest could show the rats a thing or two. No need to be forcibly abusing rats and monkeys when there are so many humans that are more than happy to abuse themselves. And you're not even encouraging them, they were doing that anyway. They will be delighted to oblige, and you watch the incidences of shoplifting, theft from vehicles and burglary drop like a stone, too, now that they don't even have to pay the Dealer. Yes indeed, you'll find that they certainly don't need any encouragement to experiment the hell out of that stuff.

Experiments on nicotine though? No, then you'd have to pay 'em. And just watch their little faces fall when they find out they're on the nicotine trial, not any of the real drugs. See the enthusiasm just disappear, even though many of them are habitual smokers. You'll see it clearly written in their eyes: What, we bought all that fucking Night Nurse just for *this?*

N.B. I make no apologies for briefly making light of a serious subject – drug abuse – to make an equally serious point about the vast difference between real drugs and nicotine. Especially since the people who are likely to really appreciate the truth of the short passage above and laugh the loudest are the lifelong habitual drug-users themselves. In referring to them as "Britain's finest" I am neither approving nor disapproving, simply acknowledging the fact that many of them have become very experienced in the everyday applications of recreational and habitual drug use over time. It is just a factual observation, they inevitably develop expert knowledge. If anyone feels inclined to come over all offended by this sort of creative diversion then I would advise them to read tamer books, this one is meant to be hard-hitting. I'm trying to kill off a 1.2 billion-dollar-a-year international poison factory here, more or less single-handed. I can't be pussyfooting around.

CASE MYSTERIES 4: IF WE COULD TALK TO THE ANIMALS

Back to our serious analysis

So anyway, let's take a look at the claims for animal reactions to nicotine itself - rather than the real drugs, for which there seems to have been some genuine animal enthusiasm, perhaps not surprisingly.

It has been established that monkeys, dogs, rats and mice can all exhibit nicotine IVSA.

That sounds quite promising, doesn't it? Except for two points: why should these particular studies - which apparently manage to demonstrate nicotine IVSA - be automatically credited with "establishing" the phenomenon as some sort of accepted fact, but the other studies which fail to do so are dismissed as flawed studies? Because the writer of the article chose to interpret it that way, so that the reader is hopefully more likely to accept the suggestion that it is "established". Also, it is worth pointing out that *any* degree of evidence of nicotine IVSA, however tiny, could make the sentence quoted above technically true. Any measurable amount of lever-pressing, whatever the actual motivation for it, could warrant that generalisation without it telling us anything about addiction at all.

There is of course a nicotine *experience*. I know, I have experienced it myself many thousands of times. I can't say I was ever impressed with it, but I could easily recognise it were I to experience it again. (Actually I do revisit it: see *Rattus Humanus* in Section 7. It was horrid!) It may be a rather unexciting experience for the laboratory animal too, especially when compared with heroin or cocaine, but then they are not given a choice:

All these studies demonstrate that rats will self-administer solutions of pure nicotine in the absence of any other reward.

Well, exactly: "...in the absence of any other reward". I can't say I'm surprised that caged animals might resort to that, just as they sometimes resort to chewing at the bars. It doesn't mean they find it much of a rewarding experience, and indeed we will never know whether they enjoy doing that, or are just repeating it compulsively in the end simply because there is nothing else to do. Smokers commonly smoke lots of cigarettes when they have little to do, but hardly any when they are usefully occupied. That tells you nothing about nicotine. Lots of people eat excessively when they are bored. That says nothing about bodily needs, it is just a diversion, obviously. Why should other animal species be any different from us in this regard?

Why not Offer Them a Real Choice?

Where is the parallel with human choices? Ordinary smokers and drug users are not so limited in their behavioural options. What do you think would happen if we gave the laboratory animal a choice of three levers: one which gave them nicotine, one which gave them orange juice and one which just opened a door, let them out of the madhouse and returned them to their natural habitat? I think they'd have a quick drink of orange and fuck off, don't you? I very much doubt they'd be periodically popping back for a nicotine hit. Breaking in through a window, shoving the catheter back in. Looking needy.

Next, the experiments start to get a little more bizarre:

> Monkeys have pressed levers for nicotine at rates similar to those at which they pressed levers for cocaine. In these experiments, the nicotine or cocaine was paired (associated) with brief flashes of light, which in this model were functionally equivalent to the smell and taste stimuli associated with smoke inhalation.

What? How can flashes of light be "functionally equivalent" to taste and smell? And why is this confusing element useful at all? Surely the idea here is to focus on *nicotine,* in order to establish what that substance is doing. Why do we suddenly need to introduce lighting effects... what, are we going for *atmosphere* here?

What next for the monkeys? A mock-up of the inside of a club with a full sound-system, gyrating animatron monkey diva and Bacardi in the water-dispenser? In fact as long as we're going for realism now, why not give them matches or Zippo lighters to play with? Maybe they'll set fire to the scientists with a bit of luck. And no, that does not contradict my earlier criticism of animal liberation violence. If the monkeys do it, that is not terrorism. That's payback.

To be serious though, what idiot scientist decided that flashing lights, to a monkey, would relate in any way to smell and taste in the context of tobacco use in humans? I think they've been 'pressing a few levers' themselves, these scientists. I reckon they've been getting into some thoroughly inappropriate conditions, that's the only thing I can think of that could account for such a barmy proposal.

Both the nicotine and the light stimuli served as rewards for these animals, the latter by virtue of association with the nicotine.

Am I alone here in regarding that as an utterly pointless complication? Obviously the monkey could simply be playing with the flashing lights – in the absence of anything better to do – rather than aiming to dose himself with nicotine. It just confuses the picture, and there is no way to tell if the monkey is associating the light stimulus with the nicotine, or just playing with the light. And anyway, exactly how does it assist us to investigate the properties of nicotine to have the monkey associate the flashing light with the nicotine experience? It is about as relevant, in reality, as giving him cigarette cards to collect every time he presses the lever.

Nicotine IVSA has also been demonstrated in monkeys using simpler procedures without associated light stimuli, although rates and consistency of responding for the drug were less striking.

Oh, so it was the addition of the totally irrelevant flashing lights that made the other results "striking". This means that the effects of nicotine are less exciting than turning a light on and off. Yes, I'd agree with that actually. Now that I no longer have a smoking habit I'd rather play with switches than take nicotine, that makes perfect sense to me. Not sure I could say the same about free cocaine, especially if I was banged up in solitary confinement with nothing else to do… yeah, I'm with the monkeys on all these choices, in fact.

Dogs have also learned to press pedals to activate IV injections of nicotine. Up to several hundreds pedal presses were made to obtain a single injection of nicotine, indicating that its rewarding effect, although powerful, was less strong than that of cocaine.

This seems compelling on the face of it, does it not? Although cocaine was more impressive. Still, any smoker who has 'done coke' will hardly be surprised by that. No-one would dream of coughing up fifty quid for a gram of tobacco. There's no buzz, it wouldn't make that much difference to your Saturday night. But just allow me, if you will, to draw your attention to three points that might otherwise go completely unnoticed in the above quote:

a) Dogs have "learned to press pedals". Yes, dogs have learned to do all sorts of things, often just to amuse themselves. Exactly what the dog is pressing the pedal *for* remains an assumption.

b) Yet even if it *was* to repeat the nicotine experience initially – in the absence of anything else to do – the fact that the dog later continues to press the pedal "several hundred" times before a single further injection is given, can be read either of two ways. First, as the RCP conclude: "indicating that its rewarding effect, although powerful, was less strong than that of cocaine". Or second: that the dog, having learned to press the pedal often, is then happy to press it hundreds of times even in the absence of any reward. Perhaps it has simply become a conditioned activity that is continuing even in the absence of the original stimulus. Clearly it could be read either way, making it inconclusive, but that is not how the RCP are choosing to present the finding.

c) In the very next paragraph of the article, lever-pressing in rats is held to be convincing precisely because:

"The rate of lever pressing was related to the dose of nicotine, and the lever-pressing ceased if nicotine was no longer available."

You can't have it both ways, guys! Dogs continuing to press the lever in the absence of nicotine and rats ceasing to press the lever in the absence of nicotine cannot both strengthen the case that nicotine is significant - unless we are going to posit that rats are much quicker on the uptake than dogs. And really, what respectable scientific mind would not notice this glaring inconsistency in the interpretation of results? Setting Higher Medical Standards? I could set higher medical standards than that whilst bound, gagged and locked within a stout box. And when the RCP read this they will probably wish I was. Maybe they will even make tentative enquiries to see if they can arrange it, but it will be a bit late to rescue their tattered case by then.

Do you see how the established belief in the addictive attributes of nicotine in the minds of the medics and the scientists is affecting their objectivity throughout? They already believe nicotine is an addictive drug, and they are trying too hard to prove it! Or if you want to be really cynical, they know there is serious doubt and they are trying to prevent the public from catching on by creating 'evidence' of nicotine addiction.

Come off it, Hypnotist!

Why on earth would respectable scientists and medical authorities be involved in something like that? Well I'm not saying they are – respectable *or* involved - but some might suggest that a scientist whose livelihood depends upon carrying out research funded by drug companies may have more interest in producing results that might please their paymasters than results that will certainly frustrate them. And in the case of the medical authorities here in the U.K., they are already very deeply involved in the provision of smoking cessation services largely involving nicotine replacement products. In their article, the RCP do not mention who actually paid for this IVSA research, who instigated and funded these experiments, who collated and interpreted the results as they are presented here ie. in support of the notion that habitual tobacco smoking is drug addiction. In effect, the reader of the article is being assured that it is all sound and pretty conclusive – especially if they read it uncritically – when in fact it is full of inconsistencies and deeply flawed.

This particular review of the IVSA evidence has been prepared by the Royal College of Physicians and they are happy to display it to the whole world on their website, they are content to put their name to it - with all the flaws I am highlighting here - under the banner of Setting Higher Medical Standards. This should be ringing lots of alarm bells, because if I can pick so many holes in the case – and I am not even a scientist – then there is obviously at the very least a serious lack of intellectual objectivity in the matter of the IVSA tests.

If - as I strongly suspect - many of these experiments have been organised and funded by the drug companies who make nicotine replacement products, then they are not really a serious attempt to discover the truth about nicotine but an attempt to justify NRT as a treatment approach. That's not science, that's business. And indeed there would be nothing wrong with that provided everybody is aware of it and can therefore take into account, when considering the 'findings', exactly what the paymasters were aiming to find. Whoever pays the piper calls the tune.

To continue:

> Nicotine IVSA has also been reported in mice both with an 'acute' procedure in which stress may be a confounding factor, and in chronic IVSA experiments of the usual type.

a) Note: "has also been reported". UFOs have "been reported", it doesn't mean the report was convincing or significant. Clearly the evidence with the mice was unimpressive, or we would be given details. The attempt here is to throw in anything else that seems vaguely worth a mention in the hope that it will end up amounting to something 'collectively', as it were. Well I'm sorry, but even a mountain of faint evidence does not make a case more convincing. Quite the reverse, in fact.

b) No details are offered on the "acute" procedure that may have increased stress and amounted to a "confounding factor". Without details we cannot judge anything about the actual procedure for ourselves, so what is the reader to conclude from this vague assessment? Perhaps we should be reassured that there is an open mind at work here, some analytical rigour finally creeping in – if only for the space of eight words.

Next, a moment of jaw-dropping complacency:

> There is also some evidence for IV self-administration of pure solutions of nicotine in human subjects, but these studies do not seem to have been reported in full.

Do they not? And the RCP are content *to leave it at that?* This is the most bizarre statement in the whole article, since there are millions of people all over the world apparently self-administering nicotine every day. So to only be able to report that there was "some evidence", and to then have to admit that these studies "do not seem to have been reported in full" - well, this is just not good enough, is it? This is the only one of these barmy procedures that actually involves human responses. Surely the results should mirror the human smoking phenomenon if tobacco smoking actually was nicotine addiction. Make no mistake, if people are going to go to all the trouble and expense of doing scientific research there is no way they are not going to bother reporting the results... unless the people who paid for the research don't like the results. Can't the RCP investigate further, and tell us what happened in these studies? Why the lame shrug at the end of that sentence? Don't medical standards go any higher than that where nicotine is concerned?

Corrigall and Coen's "success"

The next section of the article is effectively presented as the best evidence that all this is not just a waste of time, and indeed seems more promising - at first:

In 1989, Corrigall and Coen succeeded in developing a rat model for nicotine IVSA. The rats learnt to press levers to obtain IV infusions of nicotine, but did not press an inactive (control) lever in the same test chamber. The rate of lever pressing was related to the dose of nicotine, and the lever pressing ceased if nicotine was no longer available. As in the experiments in monkeys and dogs mentioned above, the lever-pressing produced nicotine and no other substance. The nicotine served as a goal object (positive reinforcer) for these animals, much in the same way as other drugs of abuse and natural rewards.

These observations have been reproduced and extended in numerous published experiments from many different laboratories. All these studies demonstrate that rats will self-administer solutions of pure nicotine in the absence of any other reward.

So according to this evidence rats in lots of different studies have "learnt to press levers" that gave them shots of nicotine but not 'control' levers that didn't. The report doesn't actually state it but presumably the rats did press the control lever a few times to begin with, until it became obvious nothing at all resulted from doing that.

Otherwise we would have to wonder if the rats were psychic. Anyway it was the nicotine trigger they were mainly interested in, apparently. Aha, so nicotine must be an addictive drug after all then, mustn't it?

No. It merely shows that the rat - which is quite a clever little creature actually - soon figures out that if he presses lever 1, something happens: he gets a shot of nicotine. Exactly how the nicotine makes Ratty feel is something we can only guess at, but obviously he feels something. Apparently it doesn't hurt, or he wouldn't do it again but that is all we can safely conclude. When he presses lever 2 nothing happens, so he quickly loses interest in that. But again, the main problem with all this is the fact that this behaviour only becomes apparent:

"...in the absence of any other reward"

So this intelligent, lively creature is put into a situation where the only stimulation option is to press the lever that actually does something, and then we observe that it does that repeatedly. But this is hardly surprising, since the rats have nothing else with which to occupy themselves. This proves nothing useful at all. Office workers with nothing to do chew pencils, it does not mean graphite is addictive or has some particular 'habit-forming' property. Nor are the poor office workers becoming 'dependent' on graphite, no matter how many pencils they chew their way through.

The validity of the observation is supported by the finding that the plasma concentration of nicotine in rats during IVSA experiments can be close to that in heavy cigarette smokers who inhale.

This finding 'validates' nothing, in fact it is simply obvious that the rat ends up being full of nicotine. It would be truly astonishing to find otherwise, wouldn't it?

Leaving for Wonderland now – All Aboard!

Now it gets really amusing, and readers here in the U.K. who are old enough to remember the Autumn when train operators made the excuse that they were unable to clear leaves off the line - which had caused train delays - because they were "the wrong kind of leaves", may experience a little déjà vu here:

> Some studies have failed to show nicotine IVSA, but these used a strain of rat shown subsequently to be poor in performing this task...

"Poor in performing this task"? But it is not supposed to be a task! Surely the animals' self-administration behaviour is the inevitable result of the 'rewarding' properties of nicotine to begin with, and subsequently its 'addictive' properties! The rat is helpless to resist these compelling factors, is he not? He is a slave to the nicotine - this is exactly what the scientists are out to prove. So what is all this stuff about poor performers? It is only *skilled* rats that are prone to addiction, is it? Yeah, because we see an obvious human parallel there, don't we? It's only the high achievers who become smokers and smackheads, right? It's not just something any type of human can manage to do. Some people are not quite up to performing the task. Can't work a syringe, can't find the tobacconists, that sort of thing.

> ...strain differences in animal studies may reflect genetic factors that influence human use of tobacco.

So if the rat is not going to play the nicotine game, he's the wrong kind of rat, is he? Get lost, Dozy Rat - you can't be in our mainlining medical gang, you'll never be a true Self-Administrator! You can just be Sawdust Monitor, or something. Ooh, hey - maybe there's a *genetic* reason. Perhaps there is some correlation here between the human sissies who didn't want to try a cigarette, and the Wrong Kind of Rat. Let's test the Wrong Kind of Rat for 'scarediness'. Wooohoo, we're setting higher medical standards now!

Let's Get Serious, Shall We?

Ok, here's the real summary - forget the technical waffle they put at the end, this is the RCP's reluctant confession:

> It is, however, apparent in most experiments that nicotine is a weaker reinforcer than cocaine, its self-administration is acquired more slowly and maintained under a narrower range of conditions.

This despite the fact that there are about 12,000,000 smokers in the U.K. How many people use cocaine? And please don't anyone suggest that this enormous difference is accounted for by the prohibition of cocaine, there are far more regular users of cocaine now than there ever were before it was made illegal. Prohibition has simply made cocaine far more popular, just as it has done with all the other real drugs of abuse - and just as it did with alcohol, for the short period it was banned in the USA.

No, there are other reasons why nicotine is producing patchy and disappointing results here. We are often told that nicotine is supposed to be "more addictive than heroin" or "the most addictive drug in the world", mainly *because* tobacco smoking is so commonplace – forgive me for repeating it but the RCP admit that it is:

> ...apparent in most experiments that nicotine is a weaker reinforcer than cocaine, its self-administration is acquired more slowly and maintained under a narrower range of conditions.

That is a very different picture from the common myths about nicotine's legendary 'addictiveness'. The RCP are not sure how to interpret this, commenting:

> It is unclear whether this reflects on either the appropriateness of the animal procedures to model the richness of the human environment or on the importance of other reinforcers in human tobacco use.

I think that is the most inappropriate use of the word "appropriateness" I have ever encountered, but I think I have said enough about the ridiculousness of the animal procedures. I don't think it is unclear in any way. The whole of this article makes it obvious to any impartial, rational intelligence that the experiments are silly, cruel, inconclusive and certainly do not support any notion of nicotine as a highly addictive substance, even within the tendentious interpretation of the RCP article – where there seems to be a deliberate attempt to make the results seem more convincing than they actually were. The importance of "other reinforcers in human tobacco use" are in fact the entire reality. It never was a drug addiction, tobacco smoking is just a compulsive habit.

Case Mysteries 4: If We Could Talk to the Animals

The RCP are not entirely blind to the possible influence of other factors, as they tentatively suggest:

Non-pharmacological sources of reinforcement may be significant...

You think? Like the normal human automatic *impulse* to repeat the usual habit pattern, perhaps? Sometimes these are called cravings. And social influences, like what other people are doing? Traditional mental associations like the 'cigarette break' and the age-old link with alcohol. And beliefs, like *it's really hard to stop smoking*, or *it helps me deal with stress*. Copying what the cool people are doing, the influence of advertising and promotion, fashion, rebellion. The suggestion of addiction. Yes, I think that sort of thing may be significant... don't you?

...and recent studies provide indirect support for the presence of other psychoactive substances in tobacco in addition to the nicotine.

Oh my God, here we go again. Order some more patch-making machinery, we're putting new chemicals in the frame! Get a new batch of monkeys, breed some more rats – only make sure they're the lever-pressing strain, not those poor performers of really easy tasks – throw in some dogs and a beaver or two, we'll crack this problem if we have to poison half the animal kingdom... only don't bother testing the humans this time, they are a bit disappointing if the last lot were anything to go by...

One day we'll have a pill. The Holy Grail of smoking cessation: one day we will have a pill, and we'll make sure you have to take it for weeks or months on end, and we'll sell billions of them to half the adult population of the world, because they won't have a clue about the other reinforcers on human tobacco consumption, and we'll make vast fortunes that will make the poison gum and the poison patches seem like a drop in the ocean - and by the way, shoot that fucking hypnotist before anyone actually starts to pay him any attention - this is business, it's nothing personal you understand... make him an offer he can't refuse, I'm sure he's a reasonable man, every man has his price, money makes the world go around, the world go around, the world go around...

Meanwhile... in a sleepy laboratory somewhere in Berkshire... recent studies suggest... additional factors... poor in performing this task... the alpha4beta2 subtype are the most prevalent... may be significant... Higher Medical Standards, yes... rats... other species... zzzzz. Night night. Sleep tight. Don't let the monkeys bite.

<u>Could hypnotherapy have helped the animals stop Self-Administering?</u>

Not through any of the usual hypnotherapy procedures, no. But here's a wild and crazy idea: just disconnect the chronically-indwelling venous catheters and leave the cage doors open, and I'm sure any animals that are still alive will be happy to call it a day.

Section Six

Trance and Suggestion

i). What Really Happens in a Hypnotherapy Session

If you have never been to visit a hypnotherapist, nearly all of this section has been written with you in mind. If you have visited a hypnotherapist and got the success you were aiming for, you probably know most of this stuff already, but if you did not get success then reading this may help you to understand why.

If new clients came along to my office without the slightest idea what hypnosis was, that would be simply wonderful, but they don't. Instead, new clients have all sorts of vague notions about hypnosis which are nearly always wrong and are mainly assumptions drawn from watching stage hypnosis, but also picked up from the ignorant comments of other persons who know nothing about hypnosis either really, but imagine they do because they've seen stage hypnosis too.

As a result, new clients are expecting me to be dressed in black from head to foot, have piercing eyes and a cape, twirling my moustache and dangling a gold watch in front of their eyes. They are probably a bit surprised to discover that my appearance is perfectly ordinary, and all I do throughout the whole session is listen or talk. And in a perfectly ordinary way, too - none of this "Yoooou are feeeling sleeeeeeeepy!" sort of nonsense.

Now there may be hypnotherapists out there who do have twirly moustaches and capes and dangle watches and stuff, but I've never met one. There was one woman with a moustache, I remember, at some seminar I attended but it wasn't twirly and she didn't have a cape or piercing eyes, so you would never have guessed she was a hypnotist at all really. And although I have encountered the odd therapist who "taaaaalks liiiiike thaaaaaaat", most of us speak perfectly normally, whether we are addressing the conscious mind or the Subconscious.

I suppose I should have called this section "What Really Ought To Happen in a Hypnotherapy Session" because I am well aware that different hypnotherapists employ different methods, and there may be some who don't bother to do some of what I am describing here. Still, I regard all of these factors as important, so if you ever had a disappointing outcome from a hypnotherapy session it is worth asking yourself: "Did my therapist do all of this?"

A Warm Welcome

The first thing I do is to make people feel very welcome. It is important to appreciate that most new clients feel quite nervous and don't know what to expect, so getting them comfortable is a priority. Pleasant surroundings that immediately seem relaxing, private and secure play an important part in this, as does the demeanour of the therapist which should always be cheerful, warm and friendly.

An Easy, Comfortable Pace

Hypnotherapy can often achieve rapid results, but the process itself should be relaxed and leisurely. As I tell clients over the phone beforehand, all they really do during the session is relax in a comfy chair for a couple of hours. This reassures them that I do not require any efforts from them, so they can be looking forward to the experience.

Plenty of Time

I always set aside two hours for any session but I am aware that many therapists prefer hourly sessions. Anything less than an hour I would regard as rushed but I have to be careful here, because some therapists prefer rapid methods and can get good results, too. I have developed a more chatty style, over time. I started out doing one hour sessions, which gradually became ninety minutes and then two hours. This means I only do four sessions in a day - which often ends up being three, because on average about one in four sessions turn out to be no-shows, get cancelled or are postponed. But what it does mean is that those three or four people get my best attention and all my energy, which is much more difficult to achieve if seven or eight clients are coming along in one day.

The long session has three advantages for me. Firstly, it doesn't matter if the client is late. Even if they are half an hour late I can usually make the session work because I can always use rapid techniques anyway if need be. Sometimes people are travelling a long way to visit my office: from London, Glasgow, Swansea, or Oxford perhaps. I'm not trying to show off by the way, people really do travel these distances to see a therapist who has been recommended by someone they trust. I often say to them "Why not just find a local therapist?" but most of them would rather travel a long way than take a chance with a therapist that has not been recommended. Maybe they read Allen Carr's book:

Neither do I wish to appear to be knocking hypnotherapy; on the contrary, I use it as part of my own consultations. It is the power of suggestion and a powerful force that can be used for good or evil. Don't ever consult a hypnotherapist unless he or she has been personally recommended by someone you respect and trust."

(*Allen Carr's Easy Way to Stop Smoking,* Penguin 3rd edition, 1999)

What a ridiculous piece of scare-mongering! Don't ever accept ignorant suggestions about hypnotherapy from an ex-accountant who clearly knows less about hypnotherapy than I know about antique snuff-boxes. If you happen to pick the wrong therapist from the phone directory, the worst that will happen is nothing. There is no "powerful force" involved, hypnosis is just a form of communication. The power all lies within the client's Subconscious, the therapist has no power. The skill of the therapist is all about knowing what to say to that particular person's Subconscious as that precise moment – because if the therapist does not get that right, the client's Subconscious will probably ignore him.

The second advantage of the longer session is that I have plenty of time to let the client talk, and also to explain hypnotherapy properly in the first half of the session. Clearing the client's misunderstandings of hypnosis is essential – it must never be neglected – but also it is important that I get to hear a good deal from the client. I remember being advised during my earliest training in hypnotherapy: "Listen very carefully to the client, because the client will not only tell you what the problem is, but what the solution is as well." This is very often true, even though the client does not always realise it. I do not mean that in the obvious sense that the client says: "I'm too fat, and the solution is that I need to lose weight." It is all about how they express themselves, their thoughts, feelings and their personal priorities. The more I hear from them the more I know about these things and the more I can incorporate it into what I say later to their Subconscious. Then I will be 'speaking their language', as it were. It is easier for them to respond positively.

Thirdly, a longer session means we can often clear an issue in one go, which is how I personally prefer to work whenever possible. I love to do things in one session because it really makes an impact and the client is likely to enthuse about it later so it really helps to build a strong reputation. Obviously there are issues we cannot do this with, because some problems are never going to be a one-session thing, but when we can do it, not only does this impress people but it reassures them that although therapy isn't exactly cheap you can often expect rapid results. Also it convinces the client that this therapist, at least, isn't dragging the process out or stringing anyone along.

Sometimes people have privately suggested to me – partly in jest - that I am not acting in my own best interests by clearing issues in a single session. They assume I would benefit more financially from spinning things out for two or three sessions routinely, but what they do not realise is that if the process takes longer, hypnotherapy then appears (to the public) to be less dramatically successful *and* more expensive – where is the advantage in that for me? It would mean fewer referrals and not much of a reputation for rapid success. No, make people astonished and delighted, that gets the phone ringing off the wall. Don't forget that less than two per cent of the population have ever been to a hypnotherapist. There is a vast untapped market out there, so it is certainly not in the interests of therapists to "milk" that two per cent. Just impress them with excellent results and get them telling the other 98% all about it, that's the way to promote hypnotherapy and build a strong practice too.

The Whole session is Hypnotherapy

So the first hour seems to the client to be just a conversation but actually the pre-talk is full of useful 'waking suggestion' and the aim is to prepare the client very effectively for the trance part. Naturally the client thinks the trance part is the only really important bit but actually the whole session is hypnotherapy. Really talented and knowledgeable hypnotherapists will have done a good deal of the necessary work before the client even closes their eyes – if indeed there is any eye-closure during the session at all. Sometimes there isn't, but there will always be trance. If that puzzles you, read on! If you want to understand 'waking suggestion', there is a whole section on that in Section 15, Volume II.

Trance

As I am sure you will have gathered by now, trance is not what people think it is, and it is essential to explain this to the client *and make sure they really understand,* because otherwise they are likely to think they are not in trance at all, just like Allen Carr:

> "The whole session appeared to be a waste of time. The hypnotherapist tried to make me lift my arms and do various other things. Nothing appeared to be working properly. I didn't lose consciousness. I didn't go into a trance, or at least I didn't think I did, and yet after that session not only did I stop smoking but I actually enjoyed the process even during the withdrawal period."

Therapists allow this to happen too often – sometimes through their own ignorance or poor training - and although it doesn't necessarily blow the session, it can. In terms of accepting suggestions successfully whilst in trance, it doesn't matter what the conscious mind thinks about the hypnotherapy process. That is obvious both from Allen Carr's experience and cases like the Angry Satisfied Customer, but if negative thoughts trigger a negative mood on an emotional level, that certainly can interfere with the acceptance of suggestion. If a client is sitting there secretly brooding thus: "This is a waste of bloody time, I'm not even 'under', I can hear every word this fool is saying. I wish I hadn't bothered!", then the negative mood this creates can cause the *rejection* of positive suggestion at a Subconscious level. The mood there is quite different from: "Well, this isn't quite what I expected, but he seems to think he knows what he's doing, so we'll see what happens!" This person is more than happy to be pleasantly surprised, which is *accepting* of change. Some of you will have noticed that this can be a bit of a grey area: the Angry Satisfied Customer certainly seemed to be quite irritable, not just nonplussed like Allen Carr, yet that did not prevent him succeeding. Each client is different, and there is no way to judge what the outcome will be in cases like this until it becomes apparent later, it can easily go either way. What we can be sure of is this: any negativity in the mood or attitude of the client is not aiding success, so we seek to eliminate as much of it as we can.

The Thing That Surprises Everybody

Contrary to popular belief, you are awake throughout a hypnothearpy session and can hear everything as normal, because trance is a waking state. Being in hypnotic trance feels pleasant enough, but not strange. However 'deep' in trance a person is, they do not 'feel hypnotised' because there is no such thing. This is a surprise to everyone at first because they were expecting something new - something out of the ordinary - and trance is very ordinary, although a bit more comfortable than not being in trance because there is no mental tension created whilst in that state. If the client is not told about the ordinary nature of trance beforehand, then they are very likely to think they are not in trance at all, just like Allen Carr and countless others too.

Humans drift in and out of trances all the time, we just don't usually call them that. We certainly do not need a hypnotist to help us do that. Hypnotists *can* help us to do that provided we have no objection to it at the time but we certainly do not need their help to do that ordinarily. So it is not *hypnotising* someone that makes a difference, it is how they feel about what you say to them whilst they are in trance, that is what actually matters.

A Moment to Adjust:

Now, don't be surprised if your conscious mind is trying to tell you that hypnosis cannot possibly be that ordinary. The popular assumption is that 'hypnosis' or 'trance' is some *altered* state that is going to be different or unfamiliar. Most people have always been under the impression that trance is some strange state they've never been in, a zombie-like condition in which you have no control and don't know what is going on, and may not even remember afterwards what happened, a bit like taking Rohypnol. Fortunately that is not the case, and it would be very alarming if it were! That notion obviously comes from watching stage hypnosis and jumping to all sorts of conclusions which are in fact wrong.

Daydreaming is a trance. Sunbathing is also a deep trance state for people who enjoy that. Reading can be done in either trance or non-trance states (analytically or imaginatively). What we call "absent-mindedness" is simply trance - the conscious mind is not required at the time so it wanders off, and takes short-term memory with it. Temporarily.

We have lots of different words and expressions for trance states. We might say we were 'miles away', 'off in a dreamworld' or 'blown away' by something impressive. Words like fascinated, mesmerised, awestruck, dumbfounded, enchanted, magical, charming, entrancing - these all describe the process and experience of going into trance. It's just that people don't realise that because they assume hypnotic trance is something particular and different, some mysterious state they have never experienced. It is not.

Here is a classic example of a spontaneous trance state: Love at first sight - or infatuation if you prefer to be less romantic about it. Highly imaginative state, right? Everyone else can see you are suddenly wide open to suggestion about that particular person but you just think you are directly perceiving things as they are. It seems obvious to you that this wonderful person has magical qualities no-one else has, the only strange thing is that certain other people apparently cannot see it at all. Like your family for instance, or your best friend.

'Stardom' can elicit this response collectively, in other words amongst the public generally. A 'Superstar' has maximised this effect, but it is impossible to make it universal. No matter how popular a performer may become, no performer has ever been adored by everyone, because the performer – like the hypnotist – cannot *make* people go into trance, and without trance there is no adoration, because it is a work of imagination to assign 'super' status to anyone. As Oscar Wilde said: "Worship your heroes from afar - contact withers them."

So we have to be mesmerised to adore. Without trance there might be admiration, but that is a different thing. Of course it is not simply *being* mesmerised by a performance (ie. just being in trance) that makes the adoration occur, there has to be considerable appeal as well. We can be mesmerised by a truly awful performance too: that's what the early stages of X-Factor and Americal Idol are really all about, and zero adoration results, though we may be rivetted by the spectacle. Then suddenly, after freak upon freak has made us flinch and cringe, a vision appears with the voice of an angel, and our feelings change completely.

Quite why we have the ability to suddenly fall madly in love with a person we do not yet know is a bit of a mystery but it is certainly an imaginative process occuring within the Subconscious field, and it can completely overrule our skeptical, critical faculties. Later, we might snap out of it. Can hypnotherapy help a lovestruck individual to snap out of it? Yes! Ever fallen in love with someone you shouldn't have fallen in love with, as the old Buzzcocks song goes? Helping people to become once more unimpressed by a certain person is actually quite a fun process, and very liberating for the client. But be warned: that is usually not a one-session procedure. The Subconscious can be a bit clingy about that one at first.

People go into trance on the bus. Sometimes they stay in trance a bit too long because it is restful, and miss their stop. Then they snap out of it, hop off the bus and make their way back to their actual destination feeling somewhat sheepish. People go into trance whilst driving. Experienced drivers will drive in trance most of the time, especially on familiar routes. For habitual drivers it is easier, almost effortless in fact, and also the safest way to drive. Sometimes they will snap out of trance and realise they have gone the wrong way - or to be more accurate, the *usual* way, but today they had made a conscious decision to go a different way for some particular reason, it's just that their Subconscious didn't know. Your Subconscious mind is unaware of your conscious decisions, hence the notorious ineffectiveness of New Year's resolutions, promises to change and similar resolves.

Even when habitual drivers snap out of trance, it is still the Subconscious doing the actual driving because it is habitual. The conscious mind is merely making any new decisions about the destination, and perhaps the route. It is only novice and inexperienced drivers who are *driving consciously,* and that is why they find it stressful and difficult. They are also much more likely to make a mistake or overreact than a person driving in trance. An experienced driver who has dropped into trance is very unlikely to cause an accident unless: 1. they are also speeding 2. they are also drunk, or 3. they have a defective vehicle.

People often go into deep trance whilst sunbathing. Sometimes they stay in trance too long, because they are enjoying the total lack of stress and the warmth. So they get scorched, but they don't notice that until later.

People can go into trance watching television, listening to music, working out - especially on a running machine. Or in a theatre, if the performance is gripping... mesmerising... enchanting! We become fascinated, engrossed. Movie theatres are designed in such a way as to encourage you to drift into trance. They present you with an impressive focal point - the silver screen - then they darken everything else, so the rest of the world almost disappears. You are much more likely to get 'lost' in the action, and forget where you actually are some of the time. I remember being mortified once, when I was in my early teens, because I suddenly realised consciously that I had spoken out loud in a quiet cinema whilst watching the thriller *Puppet on a Chain* simply because I had completely forgotten where I was. I suppose I must have thought I was in my own living room at home. Deep trance!

Contrary to popular belief, hypnotic trance is not different from these states in any way. It simply has a specific purpose which is particular to therapy - or in the case of stage hypnosis, to entertainment. The common belief that trance is some sort of vulnerable or zombie state, in which people will follow instructions blindly or reveal secrets is utter rubbish, and those myths are entirely created by stage hypnosis, and also ignorant portrayals of hypnosis in movies and popular culture reflecting those same myths. In real hypnotic trance you know exactly what is happening at all times and usually feel very comfortable, but otherwise normal. You are completely in control of yourself and fully aware that you could open your eyes or stir yourself any time you choose.

Conscious Inattention in Trance

It is fairly common however for the conscious mind to wander off sometimes during the trance part of a hypnotherapy session, mainly because it gets bored and begins to entertain itself with other thoughts. The conscious mind is a bit of a grasshopper at any time and normally wanders all over the place in ordinary life, and it is the same in trance. Most of what I am saying to the Subconscious is information the conscious mind knew already, or heard me explain earlier in the session. The conscious mind does not like repetition, so it commonly drifts away for some parts of the session. This means the client will have no conscious recollection of that bit of the session because the conscious mind was paying no attention to it. It is exactly like the driving experience when the driver has no conscious memory of part of the journey. It doesn't mean *anything could have happened,* in fact it was precisely because there was nothing interesting going on that the conscious mind wandered off.

In some very deep states of mental relaxation, the conscious mind is more or less inactive in some people. This does not mean they are asleep, they are not. But provided nothing is bothering them, they certainly look asleep and the conscious mind is no longer bothering to record events as they happen, the 'short-term' memory faculty has become lazy to the point of inactivity. The Subconscious is still recording though, because Subconscious memory can be regarded as the 'black box flight recorder' of the human mind, it logs everything. This is quite different from conscious recall, which is ordinarily patchy. It is the same in trance, and can become even more so if we include deep relaxation as a part of the experience.

So not remembering parts of the trance experience on a conscious level is both common and ordinary, but not scary at all once you understand it. The therapist does not cause this or control it, and indeed has no idea when the client's conscious mind is paying attention or when it is wandering, so it is certainly not an opportunity for the therapist to do or suggest something that is not in the client's interests, as is often imagined by those who know nothing about it. Indeed, if a therapist did do something untoward the Subconscious would instantly bring that to the attention of the conscious mind anyway, and the client would snap out of trance instantly with full conscious awareness of the real situation. Your Subconscious mind is intelligent, and its number one priority is to protect you. It would instantly recognise any development that was not in your interests. Hypnotic trance is just like daydreaming, and you know how easily and quickly you can snap out of a daydream if something unexpected happens, regardless of how many "miles away" you were a moment before.

False Accusations against Therapists

So if you ever hear of a hypnotherapist being accused of taking advantage of somebody whilst they were in a trance, if the client's claim is that they were unable to prevent that *because they were in a trance* or just because of hypnotic suggestion, you will know that such a thing is literally impossible, and so whatever the truth is, it is certainly different from that. It is probably the fear of such a thing happening that causes some people to hesitate over using hypnotherapy, and there is no need for that caution at all. Accusations like that are thankfully very rare anyway, but it is not unheard of for some nutcase to drag a hapless therapist into court with a tale like that, just because they do not realise they will certainly be revealed as a liar - or at least a nutty fantasist - because such a thing is actually not possible and expert testimony will later establish that to the court's satisfaction. If the police and the prosecutors knew that simple fact in the first place, no case like that would ever go to court.

Abuse is possible of course, as is abuse of trust; but hypnotherapists are no different from doctors, dentists or indeed police officers in that respect. My point is that hypnotic trance makes zero difference, just as daydreaming would make zero difference. Simply being relaxed doesn't change that, obviously.

These rare cases in which somebody is trying to suggest that hypnosis could be 'used improperly' always get thrown out of court, or find in favour of the hypnotist once the experts have been called in to explain the reality. But mud sticks, and although this hardly ever happens anyway it must be truly awful to be accused of something like that, especially when you know for certain - as every hypnotherapist would of course - that levels of trance and relaxation are entirely controlled by the client, who is no more vulnerable in the therapist's chair than they would be whilst meditating, or doing yoga.

Irresponsible Reporting of False Accusations

Newspapers sometimes add to the impact of false accusations in the imagination of the general public because they often choose to cover court proceedings as if they are just another form of entertainment, and generally have no regard for truth unless it happens to serve their own circulation needs. Consequently the press will usually trumpet any dramatic accusations against a hypnotherapist on the front page - where anyone is likely to see it, even people who don't bother reading newspapers - and then later on when the therapist is cleared, that merits only a tiny paragraph on page seventeen where most people will certainly not see it. This sort of selective 'reporting' – which is the fault of editors really - is very irresponsible and has contributed to completely unnecessary fears about hypnosis. Not that the newspaper editors care of course, they love scaring people and don't give a damn about the truth anyway, they just want to sell papers. This infuriates therapists when it happens, but fortunately these accusations are rare.

Back to Reality

The truth about trance is that it is usually being misunderstood and also routinely confused with other things like relaxation, suggestibility and responsiveness - as if the nature or level of trance can be measured by those things. 'Depth of trance' is another concept which is frequently misunderstood, especially in scientific investigations into hypnosis in which it is regularly confused with 'depth' in relaxation - a quite different matter. There have been attempts in the past to standardise depths of trance or relaxation into various specific levels, and the theory has been that different things can be achieved in hypnotherapy at different levels of trance. My own view is that this seriously overestimates the significance of trance levels and is a distraction from the much more important matter of the *quality* of suggestion.

As this is really a brief summary of these realities for the layman, and not an academic thesis for the expert to consider I don't want to get too far into these points here, suffice to say that a good deal of the basic textbook 'facts' about levels of trance, and how that relates to the client's response to suggestion are actually rubbish. Attempts to standardise subjective human responses are always a rather silly project, and it is partly because the Subconscious endlessly subverts standardisation of its territory that science has usually abandoned these hopeless projects fairly early on. The ignorant assumption has been that these complications indicate the limits of the usefulness of hypnosis. It is more accurate to conclude that it is not the Subconscious that is the problem there, but the misconceived project of attempting to establish standardisation in a multi-dimensional and highly subjective field.

The Real Significance of Trance

The real significance of trance - from the point of view of doing useful hypnotherapy, not dumb experiments - is ridiculously simple, at least for the majority of work we do routinely. It comes down to this: when you are not in trance, your Subconscious mind is not really paying much attention to the world around you, it is leaving that responsibility to the conscious mind. So when I am talking to a person who is not in trance, I know that their conscious mind may be listening, but their Subconscious probably isn't. So if I want to get some important information across to their Subconscious mind for it to consider, that mental state is no good, the Subconscious is not listening. When they are in trance, it is.

Sorry if that sounds too simple for the academic mind (and it will! I know, I used to be an academic), but that is the reality. If you are a therapist who has been taught otherwise, I would not be surprised if you object to that statement and its simplicity, for I was taught otherwise as well. Experience has subsequently helped me to revise not only what I was taught but the many other observations written elsewhere, although I do not expect everyone in the field to agree with me on this. It now seems very clear to me that the level of trance – for *most* things that we do with hypnotherapy – is nowhere near as important as the acceptability of the suggestions at the moment they are presented to the client, and their general understanding of the proceedings, with the former being essential. I am so confident of this nowadays that I have not tested any client for trance level for years. If they are comfortable with the proceedings, comfortable with the prospect of the change, happy for those suggestions to be effective and the Subconscious has no objection of its own, then change is going to happen even if the level of trance is very light.

So it follows that if change does not happen - or does not happen at first - we need to look again at those factors to see which one was not 'green for go' on the day, and correct it somehow. It is not training that makes a therapist good at that, it is experience. And not just plenty of experience with hypnotherapy generally, but preferably in dealing with that particular issue. I am a great believer in therapists specialising in certain areas of the broad field of hypnotherapy.

So it is not surprising that scientists or medics who are not professional hypnotherapists but who are conducting general tests and experiments with hypnotic states and 'suggestibility' would be pretty clueless about the significance of such specialised experience. Not their fault, but it is easy to see how their own limitations in terms of practical experience and skill could be misconstrued as the limitations of hypnosis or hypnotherapy.

What is the Truth about Levels of Trance?

There *are* different levels of trance, and it is possible to 'test' in order to establish certain criteria, but how many levels there actually are seems easy enough to claim but impossible to prove. This means that some people may hold that there are really only four levels, whilst others claim that they can demonstrate that there are in fact seven, or three, or fourteen, or whatever. Some instructors declare such things to be important and if you accept that suggestion then it becomes important to you. But in reality, depth of trance is changing throughout a session anyway, just like levels of relaxation may change. So even if you establish via some testing procedure that at twenty minutes past two the client is apparently at level 3, that does not mean that he will still be at level 3 five minutes later when a crucial suggestion is presented.

Conscious Objections

Traditionally in hypnotherapy the aim of gaining depth of trance is based on the notion that the conscious mind may block suggestions if the trance is not deep enough, but in profound depths the conscious mind is no longer analysing what is being suggested to the Subconscious. This is a brief comment rather than an extended thesis, but I refute the traditional view on the grounds that it overestimates the significance of conscious opinion – as demonstrated in the case of The Angry Satisfied Customer – and implies that the pivotal judgement of the Subconscious can be confounded by the interference of the conscious mind - an idea the Subconscious would find most amusing, I'm sure. Conscious opinion and expectations are insignificant in hypnotherapy unless they adversely affect *mood,* and even that does not always block the change. In any case, this factor can easily be eliminated by proper instruction during the pre-talk. I have found this a much more reliable approach than attempting to get around conscious opinion simply via the highly-subjective phenomena of deep trance states.

A Simplification of "Depth" in Trance

Trance is really just a focused state of awareness in which the Subconscious is dominant and, for the time being, handling external reality as well as the internal world. The more a person's mental attention is focused upon a particular thing to the exclusion of other things, the "deeper" the trance. I already mentioned the cinema experience when I 'forgot' about my actual surroundings. Of course I was not in deep relaxation – I was watching a thriller, I was probably on the edge of my seat – and I did not have my eyes closed, obviously!

Similarly, I recall spending five hours in a video-editing suite one day all by myself, having just learned how to use the equipment. I was having great fun just editing video clips together. It only seemed like about two hours because I was totally focused upon the screens and the equipment, paying zero attention to the outside world – which was closed off anyway, just like in a photographic darkroom. I was working away rapidly the whole time, so it is obvious I was not in a state of relaxation and yet I seemed quite tireless.

Now obviously, the conscious mind was very much aware of the activity and may have had some minor involvement, but as editing is a creative business it is mainly the Subconscious imagination driving the process, and anyway the Subconscious can handle the complexity of the task much better than the conscious mind would. The conscious mind is really just along for the ride at a moment like that and the 'real world' of external reality is nowhere to be seen, so all the usual conscious concerns – like what time it is, where we have to be later, deadlines, financial matters, career, other people – have disappeared. Consequently I was in a state of bliss, just playing with the equipment and the pictures on the screen.

Is it any wonder people get carried away with hobbies they can really lose themselves in, like restoring a house or an old car? Spend far too much time surfing the 'net or playing video games? Playing fruit machines, or on-line gambling? It is only afterwards - when they snap out of trance and the conscious mind is back in the driving seat - that analytical processes reckon up the cost in lost time, broken marriages or gambling losses. The Subconscious was just having a ball, it doesn't have to concern itself with the reality of things like money, other people's opinions or arrangements to meet friends. That's the conscious mind's job, so it is the poor old conscious mind that now has to come up with a plausible explanation for the reckless or inconsiderate behaviour – or try to cover it up. The stress of that can end up being intolerable.

All this is easily fixed, you know. The Subconscious doesn't mean to cause a problem, it is simply unaware of those consequences. It is not the Subconscious that assesses the damage done, it just goes back to doing whatever it was doing before. It is the conscious mind that picks up the pieces and tries to make amends, and because the conscious mind has always been led to believe it controls all choices and behaviour, very often it dutifully shoulders responsibility for something it actually did not do and also could not easily prevent.

But the Subconscious can. It just needs a detailed explanation of what the problem is, and what needs to be changed to solve the problem and then it will change it. Hypnotherapy is essential if this change is going to be quick and easy, and it could become apparent in some cases that further hypnotherapy may be necessary if it is going to be permanent. A talented and experienced hypnotherapist with whom the client feels comfortable is also a necessary factor - as is a phone call, a booking and actually turning up for the appointment. Adopting the appropriate attitude towards the process before the trance bit begins is also a big help but the good news is that apart from that, the client does not need to do anything else to achieve complete success. Which is a lot better than gambling or drinking away your business, your marriage and then hanging yourself.

Back to Inductions

Since I became really comfortable with conducting hypnotherapy sessions, I found myself drifting away from induction procedures (formally 'hypnotising' people), testing for level or bothering with 'convincers' and my success has only become more consistent. This may be partly an advantage of confidence, but it also reflects a deliberate move away from the traditional features of hypnosis generally, many of which are unnecessary and sometimes unhelpful. Some hypnotherapists will have been taught to use these approaches though, so I had better explain them. It is not that they do not work – they usually do – but not everyone responds to them positively and for some clients they involve too much mystery, which makes them feel dubious and suspicious.

'Hypnotising' People

I suppose new clients generally assume that the moment when I 'hypnotise them' is the crucial event of the session! A moment of tension: Will he be able to do it? Will it work? How will he attempt to achieve this mysterious transformation, and will I resist, or be unable to enter the hypnotic state? Will the session end right now, in embarrassing failure and frustration?

Sometimes I forget, nowadays, that clients may actually be feeling like that because they don't always show it. If they act as if they haven't a care in the world regarding such matters I just assume they don't. I certainly haven't, and if they have been listening to my detailed explanations and genuinely taken it all in – as most do, actually – then all this stuff becomes pretty irrelevant. Having said that, some people just nod and smile in all the right places and assure me they completely understand everything I have explained - and then turn out later to be very surprised that they didn't go to sleep! Surprised they could hear everything as normal, and felt they could open their eyes any time they wanted to, feeling relaxed but otherwise normal. Just like I told them, in fact.

The truth is that although I explain the realities of hypnosis to everyone in considerable detail quite a few clients still hold on to their original misunderstandings of hypnosis, almost as if they do not believe me. This is simply because they are so familiar with the old fantasy notion of hypnosis that they may not find it easy at first to adjust to this new concept, which is after all less dramatic than the imaginary one.

I suppose these days I no longer *induce* hypnosis. I *introduce* it, as it really is. I explain it, and invite the client to use the state to allow me to get the message across to their Subconscious mind. It takes a while to explain it all in detail, hence the two hour session. But I have found that this achieves universal acceptance – of *trance* that is, not necessarily suggestion - which is not true of any other method of attaining the state of hypnosis. It also proves that the common idea that some people cannot adopt the hypnotic state is not true.

The way that idea is usually expressed – that some people cannot *be hypnotised* - actually reveals the problem for that sort of client - they have a problem with the idea of being hypnotised by someone else, and it is easily removed by proper explanations. The only exceptions to that are people who are literally too stupid to understand the explanations, or are not listening anyway as in the case of The Cartoon Man.

N.B. When I say "too stupid" I am talking about people who are so slow on the uptake they could easily be outwitted by the dumbest person you ever met. Ordinary ignorance or poor education do not cause any problem at all, so even people with no faith in their intellect need not worry. I've had plenty of success with folk like that, and indeed I've only met about three or four people so far who were genuinely too thick to understand what I was saying to them. That is three or four people out of thousands, so it's pretty rare.

There is one further exception: the kind of person who is so awkward, difficult to get on with and contrary there is no way to work with them at all, and my attitude towards individuals of that sort is very straightforward indeed. These two exceptions – Lonely Brain Cell and Impossibly Awkward - are so rarely encountered in hypnotherapy that they just do not matter at all.

So having developed an approach to the trance state that is successful with just about every client, I naturally dropped all other methods over time. These methods of attaining trance states are called inductions, and hypnotherapists are trained to use various types of hypnotic induction to 'help' their client into hypnosis. You will probably encounter methods like this if you visit a hypnotherapist, so if I explain it here it should help you to understand what it is all about and respond positively.

Just before the Induction

For the trance part of the session, very often the client will be seated comfortably in a recliner of some sort or on a sofa. Actually hypnotic procedures are just as easy to do whatever kind of chair is used - or even standing up, as evidenced by stage hypnosis - but for therapy, the standard procedure is the recliner because we want the client to feel comfortable. A few therapists work with the client lying down, but this is not the norm. Some clients might feel awkward with that as it is a bit undignified, and there are other associations with that physical position inappropriate to the therapy scenario. Has the therapist considered that? And if they haven't, what else might they be failing to take into account in terms of the client's feelings and expectations?

The Physical Element

The temperature and general cosiness of the room should be well-managed and adjusted to the client's preference. Simply being too cold can adversely affect the mood of some people, whereas others hate being too warm. Even something as basic as needing to go to the toilet can get in the way of a positive response during the trance part of the session. Feelings matter very much in hypnotherapy, and it is important to consult the client on this, as personal feelings can vary greatly.

After I have asked the client if they have any questions, just before the trance part of the session, I pointedly ask if they are *comfortable, physically*. This will prompt anyone who needs to relieve themselves to ask if we have a toilet they might use. Many people can be quite shy about these things and need that sort of prompt. Not everyone is hesitant about such matters, but it is up to the therapist to anticipate this sort of thing and make sure it doesn't cause a problem. It is easy to avoid.

The Auditory Elements

It helps if there is minimal background noise during the trance part of the session – not because it is a problem but because the new client will *assume* it is a problem, so once again it can affect their mood. If background noises cannot be eliminated, they can still be made a non-issue by explaining why it is not a problem. In other words the irritation normally triggered by background sounds can be eliminated by the effective use of reassuring suggestion. This can be entirely successful even if the noises are quite loud, surprisingly enough. Put simply, the Subconscious does not care about background sound. It is the conscious mind that thinks it is a distraction, because the conscious mind can only really focus on one thing at a time. Once the conscious mind has been reassured that noises do not bother the Subconscious, it becomes far less bothered about them too. (This is a classic example of 'waking' suggestion: if the client accepts the suggestion, they will not then be bothered by background sound simply because I have just explained why it will not affect the outcome, which is the only thing that they were really concerned about.)

Music of a relaxing nature is often used by hypnotherapists although it is not essential. It has no particular significance but it can enhance the ambience and make the whole experience more pleasant. However, this should be checked with the client to make sure that particular client finds that sort of recording enjoyable. Also the volume level needs to be right for that client and they need to be able to hear the therapist clearly enough over the top of it. Listening comfort and all that entails must be attended to and nothing should be assumed.

Actually all these things can be managed with a catch-all suggestion: "If anything is bothering or worrying you at any time, do let me know straight away and we can take care of it immediately. Please don't feel you should just put up with anything that is getting on your nerves!"

Hypnotic Inductions, or 'being hypnotised'

The presentation of hypnosis *as if it were something somebody does to you* can be practised in any number of ways. There is the dramatic, such as the Stage Hypnotist prefers. These are sometimes called shock inductions. Earlier I explained how the conscious mind is usually 'in the driving seat' when we are dealing with other people, but if something unexpected suddenly happens, the Subconscious leaps into the driving seat, unceremoniously shoving the conscious mind out of the way. It is an instant state of alarm, which is sometimes triggered in ordinary life too - this is what we are referring to if we say that something "made us jump". That jolt was your Subconscious grabbing the controls, and triggering the release of some chemicals which might be handy, such as adrenaline. Immediately the Subconscious is paying full attention to your surroundings. This is a defence mechanism which helps us cope with the unexpected because the Subconscious can handle several things happening at once, which the conscious mind finds too confusing. If it turns out there's nothing to worry about really, the Subconscious soon hands back control to the conscious mind, but until then you are actually in 'waking' (ie. eyes open) hypnosis. This is also why being 'in shock' has a certain dream-like quality to it. It is another trance state.

A Useful Aside

Because of this fact, if a person you are with is in shock you should be very careful to say only positive things to them – and say as many soothing, reassuring things as you can. Often people get this very wrong without realising it, saying things like: "You need to understand that you've been in a serious accident", or "Of course you feel woozy, you've lost a lot of blood!" Everything you say can function as a very influencial suggestion, as the imaginative Subconscious mind assesses the situation. "Help is on the way", "You're going to be okay" or "I'll stay with you, everything's going to be alright" is more what the Subconscious needs to hear. Believe me, it makes a difference.

Back to Inductions

So the Stage Hypnotist knows that a sudden slap on the shoulder or the forehead, a shove, a shout, a sudden jerk or even a snap of the fingers right in front of the face - all these will cause the Subconscious to sit up and take notice, and relieve the conscious mind of command. If this is accompanied by an instant suggestion like "Sleep!" then as long as that person already knows what is implied by this - not sleep proper, but the state of relaxation associated with hypnotic trance - then the person will very likely choose that state as preferable to being shoved or shouted at, and immediately drop into a nice comfortable state of relaxation. This decision is made in a fraction of a second, and the conscious mind is not involved. Of course the person concerned has to be already comfortable with the general situation (the stage show or demonstration) or the relaxation bit will not happen, or will be only partially or temporarily accepted.

Now, let me reiterate that I am talking about Stage Hypnosis here, or public demonstrations which are nothing to do with therapy. Some hypnotherapists will be aware of how to do shock inductions like this too, but will rarely have a use for them in therapy because clients are more comfortable with a less abrupt aproach. There are gentler inductions that are more appropriate for hypnotherapy.

Inductions in Therapy

The first induction every hypnotherapist is taught is the one known as the progressive relaxation induction, and there are hypnotherapists who simply stick with that for years. It goes something like this:

"Now I want you to focus on your toes, and just relax your toes... just your toes... really relax them now, let all the tension go from those toes.."

...and very gradually working up the body, section by section, until eventually you reach the top of your head. That is assuming the top of your head is still there, you haven't blown your brains out because of the excruciating boredom of this induction. For some strange reason this induction is probably the most commonly used, especially amongst beginners and people who don't really do hypnotherapy in any advanced form but use the basic ABC stuff as part of a yoga class or pre-natal relaxation classes, something like that. Purely as a relaxation method it is fine, especially if you are new to such things. But it is still bloody boring and long-winded.

Real experts in hypnotherapy are unlikely ever to use this induction. Personally I hate it because it is slow, dull, and rarely achieves a quality state for advanced hypnotherapy. I don't use formal inductions anymore anyway, but even when I did I never bothered with that one. So if your therapist is using that induction they may not be very expert. This does not necessarily mean the therapy will not be effective, but if it isn't, this may be one indicator that your therapist is no great master of the art.

There are thousands of inductions, all variations on a theme which is really quite simple. Trance is all about getting information to the Subconscious. If you are not in trance then only the conscious mind will get a chance to consider the information, and that's not hypnotherapy. The trouble is, if the induction process seems *mysterious* to the client in any way, it can create the false impression in the client's mind that:

1. What the therapist is doing is nonsense
2. That it doesn't seem to be working properly
3. That the therapist is 'trying' to 'put' the client into a trance
4. That this might be a tricky process in itself.

This is why it is important to enlighten the client as to the true nature of hypnosis or they end up like Allen Carr who - even though he was successful – was left with the impression that his success had nothing to do with the hypnotherapist:

"The whole session appeared to be a waste of time. The hypnotherapist tried to make me lift my arms and do various other things. Nothing appeared to be working properly. I didn't lose consciousness. I didn't go into a trance, or at least I didn't think I did, and yet after that session not only did I stop smoking but I actually enjoyed the process even during the withdrawal period."

But does it matter what he believed, as long as he was successful? Yes, of course it does! How many people have subsequently read his books or been on his courses? His misunderstanding has gone a very long way! Sure, he has helped a lot of people nevertheless because it is only a partial misunderstanding - most of what he says *about smoking* is quite true. But if his hypnotherapist had explained the whole thing properly in the first place, Allen Carr would have understood his own quitting experience completely from the beginning. Then hypnotherapy and the Subconscious could have got the credit they rightfully deserved, instead of Allen Carr being hailed worldwide as some sort of genius for what *his hypnotherapy session* actually achieved. But obviously his therapist didn't explain it effectively enough, hence the cluelessness of his statements above and the confusion and inconsistencies in Mr Carr's later work, especially regarding the role of nicotine.

Testing and Convincers

Some inductions involve testing, both for trance states and depth of trance, and that's why Allen Carr's therapist suggested lifting his arm up in the air and "various other things". This sort of test can also function as a 'convincer', which I mentioned earlier without explaining, so I am going to explain it here. A convincer is a demonstration or test which is aimed at convincing the client that they are in hypnosis, as the new client will commonly doubt this.

'Involuntary' Muscular Response as a Convincer

The Subconscious controls the body. The conscious mind is sometimes allowed to control it too of course, but only on licence. So when the Subconscious is in the driving seat directing your behaviour (trance) it may choose to operate an action that can astonish the conscious mind, because the client may recognise that they had no conscious intention of doing that. Actually there are many common intances of this, such as when a ball is flying towards you but you don't see it until the last second, yet catch it 'instinctively'; or when you knock something off a table but catch it before it hits the floor. Notice how delighted and astonished your conscious mind is when that happens?

The success of these reactions is not infallible because the Subconcious often isn't paying much attention to external events, but the fact that both those events would probably 'make you jump' indicates that the Subconscious had half a sleepy eye on your surroundings and leapt into action with a swiftness and accuracy that can amaze the conscious mind, for conscious mental processing is not that fast. Conversely, if you didn't 'jump' and the ball just smacked you in the face then the Subconscious didn't see it coming, even if the conscious mind did see it in the final second or two. Conscious reactions are slower.

So – in theory - if the client has adopted a trance state and the Subconscious then chooses to respond positively to the therapist's suggestion by lifting the arm, the therapist is supposed to know immediately that the client is in trance and that their Subconscious is also choosing to co-operate - even with a pointless suggestion like lifting an arm, so meaningful suggestions should hopefully be accepted also. At the same time the client's conscious mind should be convinced that something unusual is apparently happening, so they would be reassured that this 'hypnosis' thing is working, and the therapist now *knows* that the client has realised that. Right?

Not necessarily, which is why I never bother with any of this. There may be several things wrong with that technique in practice. First of all, the therapist does not know if the client is complying by a conscious decision or a Subconscious one unless they register obvious conscious amazement, which does not usually happen at the time. Secondly the client is often unsure whether they are responding 'on purpose' or automatically anyway, so they can be left feeling confused and uncertain, which is a long way from convinced. Confusion and uncertainty can allow doubt to creep in, and this can affect mood in the wrong direction. The very pointlessness of the task can make the client feel doubtful about the validity of the whole procedure. They may be too polite to actually say "What on earth is the point of this supposed to be?" but if they are thinking it, that in itself can also be taking matters in the wrong direction.

Further: even if the person does not lift their arm, it does not mean they are not in trance, they may well be. The pointlessness of the task is something the Subconscious can easily recognise too, so there is very little Subconscious motivation to respond to a request like that. The silly idea that a person in trance is 'more suggestible' and will blindly obey instructions has led many a novice hypnotist to assume the client is not in trance, when really the Subconscious is just choosing to ignore the daft suggestion. It doesn't do what it is told, it does what it likes.

Allen Carr thought he wasn't in trance, but the end results prove he was. If he had not been, his smoking habit would have been unchanged at the end, he would never have developed 'EasyWay' and become a multi-millionaire and he certainly would never have allowed some form of hypnotherapy in his clinics, which wouldn't have existed anyway. His Subconscious evidently wasn't interested in waving his arms about pointlessly, but it was interested in shutting down his smoking habit because that seemed like a good idea. Just because it didn't respond to a stupid suggestion doesn't mean it cannot recognise a decent suggestion when it finally hears one. The Subconscious mind is intelligent.

If you go and see a hypnotherapist, any simple tests of this nature that may be involved are not really important in any way, so whatever your personal response or lack of response, please don't think that means there is a problem because it doesn't - as Allen Carr's case proves. In fact the best attitude to take to this sort of test is that it is an unimportant detail of minor curiosity, but what really matters is *how you feel about the issue you are there to address.*

The risk a therapist takes with any test procedure is that the client may well assume that the test is crucial, and if there is a lack of response the client might be worrying about that from then on, generating negativity that certainly will not help the outcome and may even scupper the session. Allen Carr wrongly assumed that when the therapist tried to get him to lift his arms he was 'trying to hypnotise him', an assumption which most new clients would probably make. That is why I prefer to just explain everything. Techniques can be much quicker but can also backfire, and often contribute to the perpetuation of mystery and misunderstanding in hypnotherapy, which is a damn nuisance to therapists and certainly not something to which we should be contributing.

So if your hypnotherapist seems to be using some sort of professional technique but isn't explaining it, the best attitude to take is that it is probably of no importance to the outcome of the session - whether it is apparently 'working' or not, just like in Allen Carr's case. However if your therapist seems to be displaying any frustration or uncertainty, that might well indicate that you have picked someone who is not expert in these matters and may be of little help. If it seems so, try someone else.

Rapport

For hypnotherapy to be successful, you need reasonably good rapport between therapist and client, and that means that the therapist should be easy to get along with. Clients may be awkward sometimes but therapists should never be, so if your therapist is ever bad tempered, tells you off for being late or betrays frustration because you had to cancel a session or anything like that, forget it, you should not attempt to work with that person. Partly because they are not very professional but also because that kind of thing breaks rapport, and generates Subconscious resentment that makes progress unlikely. This is particularly true of hypnotherapy because of the central role of the Subconscious, the emotional part of the mind.

So lots of things matter and may have a bearing on outcomes, but testing isn't one of them and neither is depth of trance, certainly for the majority of issues hypnotherapists normally deal with. New clients are always surprised to find that trance - although quite pleasant - is not dramatic or mysterious at all and isn't even a new experience really, but something with which they were already familiar. In fact trance doesn't make much of an impression at all as an experience, however 'deep' into trance the client may go. What often does make an impression is:

Relaxation

Trance and relaxation are separate things but they are often confused with each other, and even some hypnotherapists seem to be unclear about the distinction, so we shouldn't be surprised that non-hypnotists are too. In the practice of hypnotherapy we often put trance and relaxation together simply because they make a nice combination, for as well as eliminating mental and physical stress the relaxation element also encourages a pleasant mood in the client. This is the function of relaxing music too, and of course the minimizing of background disturbance.

As I have mentioned many times, the emotional mood of the client is quite a significant factor in the process of accepting change. It is not the deciding factor, but it can have a key bearing on response so we aim to get the mood as happy and carefree as we can. That is the main function of the relaxation aspect of the session. In explaining this to the client though, it is best not to give them the impression that relaxation is all-important or some clients will immediately start to panic about whether they will be able to relax enough, and obviously panic and relaxation have opposing trajectories. This concern can easily be avoided by reassuring the client thus, both before and very soon after going into trance:

"People often assume that you have to be in some deep state of relaxation for all this to be effective... not at all! Relaxation is an optional extra, we just throw it in to make you feel good really, it's all about being comfortable. How much people relax varies enormously from one person to another and honestly doesn't matter, so feel free to relax just as much as you please. There is certainly no mystery to it, it's only relaxation."

Suggestions like this can be enormously reassuring, in fact for anyone who is new to hypnotherapy this is a very welcome suggestion and they are virtually certain to accept it immediately, with relief. Acceptance of the suggestion that it doesn't matter enables deeper relaxation simply because it takes the pressure off completely. Easy!

Sometimes I don't even mention relaxation at all. For example, if a client is in pain and has come to learn hypnotic pain-relief techniques, there is no point telling them to relax - they're in pain! They'll relax later when they are no longer experiencing that discomfort, and then without any specific suggestion from me. Or if someone is very tired when they arrive, I just leave relaxation suggestions out of it and put forward a few basic suggestions about 'getting comfortable' instead. It is actually possible to send someone off to sleep by going on and on about relaxing when they are already unusually tired.

The 'Sleep' Thing

After the session is over it is quite common for some clients to come to the conclusion that they actually fell asleep at some point during the trance part of a session. It is surprisingly rare for clients to fall asleep for real, in fact I would guess that out of the thousands of hypnotherapy sessions I have conducted, only around twenty or thirty clients have actually drifted from relaxation into a proper sleep state, and those cases were usually elderly people during late afternoon sessions. One memorable exception was a young hod-carrier, who had spent the entire day running up and down ladders with a hod full of bricks, so I guess that counts as unusually tired.

It is *very* common, though, for people to *think* they fell asleep and it comes back to the fact that the conscious mind wanders off. If you are driving a vehicle and your conscious mind goes walkabout, when it returns to what you are actually doing you may have no conscious recollection of the last bit of driving, but you know you didn't fall asleep because your eyes are open and you are still on the road. If the same thing happens during the trance part of a hypnotherapy session, not only will you have no conscious recollection of what the therapist was saying before your conscious attention drifted back, but you also have your eyes closed and are in a dozy state of relaxation. Of course some clients will assume that they must have dropped off for a while. Actually the conscious mind just wandered off, but it is difficult for the client to detect the difference.

Does it matter? Well, I prefer people to know the truth, and not be under the wrong impression. If the client thinks they fell asleep but didn't really, that will not make any difference to the outcome. But if they did not get an ideal response anyway for some *other* reason, they are very likely to assume this was because they 'fell asleep' and it can be quite difficult for a therapist to persuade them otherwise. This can lead to them feeling afraid of 'falling asleep again' in a subsequent session, and that can be a nuisance because being *afraid* of anything at all can be a negative enough emotion to thwart success again next time, even if the true stumbling block is detected and removed. Again, detailed explanations are the best way to prevent this.

Does it matter if they genuinely *do* fall asleep? Well it rather depends upon exactly when that happened. If it was five minutes before the end of the session, then probably not. But if it was five minutes into the trance process - as in the case of the hod-carrier, actually - then yes, which is why I woke him up. Unfortunately he fell asleep again and again, and in the end we had to abandon that session and do the trance bit on a different day, but we got there in the end. It is apparent that ordinary hypnotherapy proceedings will have no effect upon a genuinely sleeping client, but any therapy that took place before they actually fell asleep can have its full effect.

Hypnosleep

There is such a thing as attaching the therapeutic process to sleep – sometimes called 'Hypnosleep' – but that is quite another level and I am going to leave the details of that out of this explanation because so few clients ever truly fall asleep in a session, it would be something the average hypnotherapist would have no practical knowledge of anyway. If you're curious though, read *Hypnotherapy* by Dave Elman. In fact I would recommend that book for anyone who is serious about understanding hypnosis. It's a bit dated, but it is still a milestone in the development of the hypnotherapy profession.

Relaxation is a fascinating phenomenon in itself. Since it is really just the opposite of stress - the antidote to stress, in fact - it should not be surprising that it is a universally appreciated experience. In other words, everyone enjoys it. Deep trance is unremarkable as an experience, but deep relaxation is something else. Most people do not know it, but we are all capable of reaching states of relaxation so deep and so wonderful that you feel like you could stay there forever - a state of bliss that is quite beyond normal experience and marvellously enjoyable. The vast majority of people need guidance to get there, especially at first, but we can also learn how to get ourselves into this deeper level any time we choose.

The Euphoric State

At the deepest level of relaxation there is a euphoric state in which there is no experience of bodily discomfort whatsoever, and a top to toe experience of pure joy that just goes on and on. For hours, if you like. This state was 'discovered' in a modern sense by English surgeon James Esdaile in the middle of the nineteenth century, and although it usually took him an hour or two to get his patients that deep, once they were in that state he was able to perform major surgery and they experienced no discomfort. They were awake and could hear perfectly well during the proceedings, and also would have been able to rouse themselves if they wished - they just preferred not to, obviously! This was before chemical anaesthesia was developed. (See *Hypnotherapy v Science,* Section 17 Volume II.) Faster techniques are now used to reach those depths in minutes if required. This state has in the past been termed "The Coma State", which is very misleading because it has nothing to do with coma at all. Anyone in the euphoric state is absolutely safe and can return to normal any time they like.

For ordinary therapeutic purposes the euphoric state is no use for changework, because euphoria is a state of bliss in which the person hasn't got a care in the world. Great for surgery, but no use for hypnotherapists ordinarily because we may need interaction or motivation from the client. If the client is so happy that they don't care at all about what the therapist is saying, then the therapist's suggestions are obviously going to be ignored. But it is nice to know - when you drift into whatever state of relaxation suits you best - that although you cannot get all the way down into the euphoric depths by yourself, the deeper you go, the better you feel because you are simply getting nearer to that euphoric state.

The Fear of being 'Stuck' in Hypnosis

As a hypnotherapist I find the fear of becoming 'stuck' in trance very amusing because it is exactly like suggesting somebody could become 'stuck' in a daydream, or literally unable to stop sunbathing. You may as well be afraid your head will fall off - except for the fact that it is at least technically possible for that to happen if conditions were right. The conditions would need to involve a guillotine or something similar, but it is possible. Being stuck in trance is not, but there is a reason for that idea getting about in the first place. It has to do with the euphoria state.

In the past, when deep states of relaxation and trance phenomena were not well understood by anyone, hypnosis demonstrations were already being staged in many parts of the world. The vast majority of people taking part in these shows would never go into the euphoria state, because this level of relaxation is profound and it usually takes some time and a series of particular procedures to achieve it. There are however a tiny number of people who are lucky enough to be able to drop into the euphoria state easily, and just occasionally one of these types would find themselves taking part in a hypnosis demonstration.

Even today, most stage hypnotists are not really experts in the field of hypnosis. Up until the last century *nobody* was, so it is not surprising that when a stage hypnotist was confronted with a person who did not just go into trance and relaxation - in which state they might be comfortable with playing silly games for half an hour - but dropped right down into the euphoria state, the hypnotist didn't know what to do. Here was a person who was enjoying a trance experience in which they felt so good they completely ignored everything, including instructions to come out of it. The hypnotist would have had no idea that was the real state of affairs, and as this is outside the usual range of reactions he begins to panic and lose his composure.

Imagine being a spectator watching that show. Here were people doing all sorts of crazy things which you didn't understand anyway, and now some poor soul has apparently gone into a trance so deep that even the hypnotist cannot get them out of it. Oh my God! What's going to happen now? Of course the hypnotist was likely to panic: this is ruining the show, people are getting alarmed. Quick, get this zombie off the stage! So the person in the euphoric state is wheeled off - without a care in the world, actually - and the hypnotist tries to continue as if nothing happened. But nobody is about to forget that something apparently went wrong, there. It looks for all the world as if that person got stuck in trance, and since the hypnotist has been acting as if he is controlling all these people, the fact that even the 'expert' didn't seem to know what to do makes everyone afraid.

Like I said earlier, humans can be afraid of something as simple as a camera or a cigarette lighter if they have never seen one before and don't understand what it is or how it works. This is the reason for many fears about hypnosis and the real origin of specific fears about being 'stuck' in trance or losing control, and it is all so unnecessary. Those people weren't stuck in anything, they were just having such a fantastic time they could not be bothered about the hypnotist or his show and were not about to return to dull old normality anytime soon – and could you blame them?

Finally someone figured out the way to get the person to exit the euphoria state of their own volition. Like most ideal solutions, it turned out to be very simple: the hypnotist only has to tell the person that if they don't rouse themselves on the count of three, he will make sure they never get to experience this wonderful feeling ever again. They will open their eyes on cue. Having experienced that wonderful feeling once, no-one wants to take a chance on losing it forever.

Back to the Office

None of this extraordinary experience is likely to be going on in a hypnotherapy session. In fact, it often seems like there is nothing really happening at all. The client may feel quite relaxed but not dramatically so, it is simply pleasant. During the trance part of the session, as the client you often don't have anything to do and it doesn't even matter whether you pay attention or not on a conscious level. Your Subconscious takes it all in, weighs it in the balance and does what it likes - taking into account how you apparently feel about whatever this hypnotist fellow has been woffling on about. It is useful to know that if you are looking forward with enthusiasm to the change - already welcoming those helpful suggestions with enthusiasm - then that helps. But apart from that, you don't really need to do a thing.

All of the changes take place at a Subconscious level, so of course you don't notice that happening because it is SUB-conscious. You only know what your conscious mind is doing, which is nothing much really so it usually seems like nothing significant is happening. Don't let this throw you, it is normal. It is also a very good idea for the therapist to tell you this beforehand, so you don't start worrying about the fact that nothing is apparently happening.

Sometimes there is more interaction than that, there can be conversation back and forth with the client – but it still seems like ordinary conversation to the client, although it might resemble the sort of lazy conversation between two people on sunbeds because of the relaxation. The only real difference from everyday conversation is that when a person is not in trance, the Subconscious is unlikely to be taking any notice of that conversation. When you are in trance the Subconscious is taking it all in, but in terms of the client's experience there is barely any noticeable difference. It is the *results* that are different - often dramatically so, because the Subconscious can do all sorts of things the conscious mind cannot do and maybe didn't even know were possible.

<u>Secrets, Lost Information and Personal Matters</u>

Sometimes – especially in movies – hypnosis is conducted like an interview, involving questions which it seems as if the person in trance must answer, or must answer truthfully... as if the Subconscious will just automatically produce any information it has 'upon request', as it were. This is part of the mythology of hypnosis, and the idea scares some people for obvious reasons. Fortunately it is absolute rubbish - and indeed if it really was possible to do that, of course there would be no such thing as interrogation or torture, because information could be easily accessed through hypnosis. In reality hypnosis cannot be used as if it were a truth drug, because the Subconscious does not do what it is told, it does what it likes - and is able to lie effortlessly, make stuff up or withold information whenever it chooses. I'm not saying that this is fortunate in the sense that interrogation and torture then still have an application in human conflicts, but at least it means that no-one needs to fear revealing any secrets in hypnosis.

Is it Over Already?

At the end of the session when you open your eyes – if indeed your eyes were closed at all – you may feel a bit dreamy or dozy for a little while, but this is just the state of relaxation continuing temporarily. It is nice to be relaxed. Some clients only relax a little, but those who relax deeply may be surprised to find that although they knew they were not asleep, the process of opening their eyes again feels a bit like waking up. This is really because trance with relaxation is sort of a halfway-house between waking and sleeping, but it is certainly on the waking side.

Do we ever conduct hypnotherapy sessions without eye closure? Certainly. We *could* do it all the time, but to some extent we have to work within the expectations of the client. Most people have no idea you can be hypnotised with your eyes wide open. They expect to have their eyes shut, so let's not confuse them too much - they already have to adjust to the surprising fact that they are not asleep and feel fairly normal really, apart from the pleasant relaxation. Let's not make this experience so far from their original concept of hypnosis that they cannot respond!

However there are a few people who seem to be afraid to close their eyes, even after I have explained everything. If they cling to this fear, the best thing to do is ask them to pick a spot on the wall and just gaze in that direction - letting their eyes go out of focus whenever that seems more comfortable. This produces the same focussed state of awareness that eye-closure does. At the end of the session they may still have their eyes open, or they may have closed them anyway somewhere along the way – it makes no difference, their Subconscious will have got it all anyway.

If it was a smoking session, cravings are gone and no willpower will be required after that. The successful client simply does not feel any urge to smoke and has now been returned to non-smoking normality. As part of the same session weight-gain and over-eating are prevented, removing a major worry for a lot of people.

In short, the habit has been eliminated, and the client has achieved this total success without doing a thing themselves, apart from:

a) Turn up for the session, with a genuine preference for change.

b) Adopt a positive attitude to the process, welcoming the change.

If total success is not the immediate outcome, it simply means that more time is needed on that issue because there is a conflict somewhere, which is bound to be the case for some people. This should be regarded as quite normal for that individual case – as normal as any other outcome of a single session - and is certainly not a 'failure' (See Section 14, Volume II). However, if another session with that same therapist were to bring no joy, my advice would be to try a different hypnotherapist. Success with smoking these days should normally be one session or two, providing of course there are no other major issues attached to the problem that need to be cleared. Even if there are, many things like that can be cleared in session two provided the therapist has been properly trained, is talented and most of all an experienced smoking cessation expert.

ii). The Role Of Suggestion: How and why we respond

We hear a lot about the 'Power of Suggestion', but this phrase is misleading. There is no power in a suggestion itself. If there were, then each suggestion would have the same effect upon everyone. Allow me to demonstrate:

> I suggest you take all the money from your savings account in used ten pound notes, come over to my office, lay all three of them down on my desk and then leave, having no memory later of doing any such thing! (Gerry Kein, Omni Hypnosis)

I am quite confident that you would find that suggestion completely unappealing whatever state of mind you happened to be in. Even if you were in deepest trance imaginable, there is nothing in that suggestion that could possibly motivate any part of your mind to act upon that, is there? Without the motivation to accept a suggestion it is ignored, which is why the stage hypnotist first has to find a few people with some inclination to entertain others or just be the centre of attention for a bit, because there is nothing appealing about the suggestion to bark like a chicken (or whatever) if you hate the limelight and have no desire to make people smile.

There is no power in a suggestion. It is how you feel about taking it up, that is what motivates a response. The idea that someone may feel more inclined to respond to the suggestion to hand over their savings simply because they were in a trance is laughable. Being in trance does not make you 'more suggestible', as has often been stated: suggestions are still accepted or rejected in trance on the basis of their appeal. Just as your conscious mind would have no desire to comply with that suggestion, your Subconscious would not either. The Subconscious has its own agenda, and if there is no advantage in responding to that suggestion according to the Subconscious mind's agenda then it will ignore the suggestion, just as the conscious mind would.

In Stage Hypnosis each participant has been carefully selected from the audience, not randomly selected. In fact the majority of them have selected themselves, although they may not realise that. Their emotional attitude to the proceedings has already been established: these are the people who are happy to play the game. They may all have their own reasons for being happy to play the game at that moment, but by far the most common one is simply that they like being the centre of attention. The stage hypnotist plays the game with that person's Subconscious mind, which is dominated by their imagination. Their conscious mind may be a bit surprised by some of the silly games the Subconscious is happy to play and therefore be a bit confused afterwards, but the notion that the *hypnotist* was in control is an illusion, created by the stage hypnotist himself. The conscious mind may become aware that *it* was not actively controlling those responses, so it might accept the suggestion that the hypnotist was in control, because it doesn't realise that the Subconscious mind exists. The same is true of the conscious minds of the audience.

So contrary to popular belief, being in trance does not make you 'more suggestible', as if you would simply obey instructions. It just shifts the agenda from a conscious to a Subconscious one and also brings the imagination into play, which is crucial because the imagination can conceive of experiences beyond any previous real experience, as we all know from dreams in which we are flying, fighting monsters or falling off cliffs. To the Subconscious, everything is potentially possible, and certainly anything is imaginable.

Here is the real difference trance makes:

When you are not in trance:

Only the conscious mind is considering the incoming suggestion. So if it is a suggestion the conscious mind likes the sound of, and the conscious mind is *able* to respond in the manner suggested then the person might well respond, under the direction of the conscious mind. If it is a suggestion the conscious mind likes the sound of but it is not within the gift of the conscious mind to create the response (such as shutting down cravings) then there will be no response. And of course, if the conscious mind does not find the suggestion appealing in the first place there will be no response in any case.

When you are in trance:

The Subconscious is then *also* considering the suggestion. The Subconscious is able to do all sorts of things the conscious mind cannot do, which broadens the scope of possible outcomes. If it is a suggestion the Subconscious likes the sound of - or at the very least, has no objection to - it may respond, provided it is capable of creating that response of course. If it has any objection at all though, it is likely to hesitate, partially respond or not respond at all. There is nothing the hypnotist can do about that, except to present the suggestion again for reconsideration, add some other incentive or change tack.

When I present a suggestion to the Subconscious mind of a client, I am not telling it what to do, I am *putting forward an idea for consideration*. Of course it is possible to make it sound like a command, which is what the stage hypnotists often do - "When I snap my fingers you will believe you are James Bond: on a dangerous mission to photograph Goldfinger's secret plans!" - but it remains an idea, nothing but a suggestion in reality. The Subconscious will consider it. Then it will do what it likes, because it is entirely independent. So if a hypnotist wants to create the illusion that he is controlling the Subconscious mind of another human being he has to use all kinds of selection procedures, distractions and social pressures to stack the deck in his favour beforehand, preferably without the audience noticing any of that, or this house of cards will come tumbling down. And as every stage hypnotist knows it can easily come tumbling down at any moment whatever he does, because the central suggestion aimed at the audience - that the hypnotist is controlling people - is false in the first place. And even if he is very good at what he does, not everyone in the audience will believe it anyway, will they?

The Agenda of the Conscious Mind

Your conscious mind's real responsibility is to deal with the world around you and other people, so it is concerned with how you see yourself in relation to the rest of the world and what you want from it, and also may well be concerned about what other people think. Work, money, social identity, politics, ambition, sporting achievements, social or business aims and aspirations, material possessions, image, appearances, reputation and the impact we have on others and the world in general - these are the sort of matters the conscious mind tends to regard as important. It may also be idly interested in any other curiousity that crops up from time to time, which might be worthy of a few moments of conscious attention, but usually not for very long.

The Agenda of the Subconscious Mind

The Subconscious *can* become engaged with some of the things listed above. For example it is apparent that some people become deeply involved in sport on a Subconscious level as well as a conscious level - in other words, they can become emotionally involved in it. But the main Subconscious agenda is roughly the same in everyone and can be summarised thus. Your Subconscious mind cares about: your survival, safety, emotional security, health, well-being and happiness on a daily basis, usually in that order of priority. If you later have children, it then also cares about their survival, safety etc. with the same set of priorities. The Subconscious mind is the emotional centre and is creative, so its way of handling these issues will tend to be emotional and imaginative rather than necessarily logical. Since the Imagination knows no bounds, this gives us endless scope for dreaming up all kinds of problems our children have or might have one day, regarding their survival, safety, health, security, well-being and happiness on a daily basis... matters about which we will then feel very emotional. Oh yes.

Cultural variations apply, in the sense that cultural differences inhibit some drives whilst bringing others to the fore, but as a general indication this gives you a pretty clear outline of the primary concerns of the human Subconscious mind. In addition, whenever there is a switch to the Subconscious agenda emotional issues become more influencial, and spontaneity and impulsiveness become more likely. Primal drives hold more sway, such as physical pleasures like eating, drinking and sexual activity. There may be cravings for excitement, for some, or alternatively comfort.

Once the Subconscious is in the driving seat there is likely to be very much less concern with what other people think, varying degrees of impulsiveness (or 'recklessness' as the conscious mind might see it) can be a common feature of Subconscious-driven behaviour... but not *necessarily*. In a normal individual their general sense of fun will be enlivened, as will general excitability. Past emotional issues that have not been resolved may also resurface, nostalgia is more likely, as is musing over future dreams. Imaginative time-travel is effortless in trance, with a dreamlike quality to it.

If on the other hand the Subconscious chooses to stay in the present, instant gratification is very much the order of the day. It is the conscious mind that sometimes defers pleasure or relaxation to a later time. "I want some chocolate and I want it now!" is more in the spirit of the Subconscious. I don't mean to suggest that the Subconscious is just impulsive, wild and undisciplined - but it is goal-driven, and although the conscious mind gets lots of advice and guidance from an early age about the risks and dangers of this or that, which usually makes the conscious mind more hesitant over risky things, nobody ever talks to the Subconscious about anything like that, which means it can sometimes make decisions that seem rash and impulsive. (Nobody, that is, except myself and my professional colleagues. You'd be amazed what a difference it makes.)

Here is just one simple example: the Subconscious learns early on in life, through multiple social experiences, that chocolate is apparently special because we can't always have it, we can only win it by being good or we might have to wait for a special occasion. It is therefore regarded as a reward, or a treat. Later in life the conscious mind learns from the world around us, through education – to which the Subconscious is not paying attention because there is no *real* chocolate involved – that chocolate is rubbish from a nutritional point of view. It is fattening and damages health if eaten regularly. So the conscious mind resolves to eat less, or give it up. But all eating behaviour is driven by the Subconscious, which knows nothing of all this so it keeps on reacting to chocolate as if it is simply wonderful, triggering repeat impulses to buy and consume it. However, when we explain the reality to the Subconscious through the hypnotherapy process it will usually cease to do that. No impulse = no conflict = no willpower required + no chocolate required either. If the issue ever returns it is not a problem, we just do it again. Sometimes the Subconscious needs reminding, just like the conscious mind. On the opposing side, meanwhile, there is a tremendous amount of suggestion in the form of advertising and promotion, shamelessly trying to push all your emotional buttons with regard to your early childhood impression of chocolate, and sugary things generally. (I like to explain advertising to the client's Subconscious, which makes it far less effective from then on.)

So we see that the agenda of the Subconscious differs markedly from that of the conscious mind. These are brief summaries of course, but I have listed all the main points. After that it gets highly individual, so it is silly to map it further but if you need another beam of light to shine upon this, just look at the differences between what a person cares about when they are sober and how that typically changes when they are engaged in drinking alcohol.

There are many trance states, and inebriation is one of them. People drink alcohol to go into trance, they just do not realise that. It takes more mental energy for the conscious mind to dominate - to keep it in the driving seat, governing our behaviour - than it does to drop into trance, and let the Subconscious take over. Alcohol is a central nervous system depressant, which does not simply mean it makes you depressed, as some people assume - otherwise it would not be so popular at weddings and funerals, obviously – but when alcohol gets into the bloodstream, it becomes even more of an effort to operate analytical processing (conscious thinking). So we drop into trance very readily, almost as soon as alcohol's effects become noticeable in fact. We certainly don't need to be *drunk* for that to happen.

Immediately, everyday concerns fade, money worries disappear from the agenda and this can be quite a relief of course, leading some people to seek 'comfort' in alcohol, often with pretty uncomfortable results in the end. These immediate effects are temporary changes, but very noticeable. Emotional issues come to the fore and people may become impulsive, giddy, unreasonable perhaps. Alcohol temporarily creates an unnatural imbalance of power and influence within the mind. The Subconscious tends to be dominant anyway if it is strongly motivated, but with alcohol in the system the Subconscious is given free rein in a way which is not normally the case. Usually Subconscious drives are being tempered by the more cautious influence of the conscious mind through the application of analytical processes which can predict likely consequences. Typically it would seek to oppose or inhibit risky choices, but now the conscious mind is drugged and dopey, barely able to think beyond the moment as it occurs.

This can feel good - liberated, living in the moment, devil-may-care, hang the expense, who cares what anyone else thinks, fuck you mate! Don't stop me now I'm having such a good time - I'm a freebird - bollocks to the rat race, I'm going to ring my boss right now and tell him what I think of him... wow, who's that girl, she's gorgeous! I'm going to ask her out. Eh? So what, I was going to get divorced anyway. Anyone fancy a curry? Oi! Who you looking at? Hey! Where's my drink?

Someone suggests going to a club in a different town: "Yeah! That's a great idea - let's grab that taxi, I'll pay!" It's one o'clock in the morning, and you have to be at work by 9am, but so what? You only live once!

Without the Subconscious mind getting all enthusiastic about these things you would never get excited about anything. Consequently you would never get the gig, the wheels, the girl, you would never see the world, start a business empire, have a hit record, win the match, have a good social life, try a few illicit substances, dance until dawn on a beach.

Without the conscious mind sometimes inhibiting these drives and getting all cautious about the possible ramifications of such impulses, you would be forever waking up in a skip, a police cell or a hospital bed, jobless, spouseless, penniless, thinking "Oh God I did it again". The trick is to get the balance right. Hypnotherapy helps enormously.

You can easily see from all this what kind of advertising suggestions are likely to appeal to the conscious mind, such as:

"14% Tax-free interest – Guaranteed!"

...and what might be more likely to appeal to the Subconscious:

"This time next week, you could be in Bali! Don't you deserve a break?"

Now, just because those suggestions may well be appealing to either side of the mind does not mean the person *will* respond. But if they did, it wouldn't be very surprising, would it?

Section Seven

Why Nicotine is not even a Drug

What is a Drug?

Can any chemical be called a drug? Only if it has a use. Tobacco smokers are certainly smoking tobacco – but are they *using nicotine?*

Just because many smokers nowadays have come to believe that they are 'using nicotine' does not mean that is what they are really doing. Here is an interesting historical fact. According to the Royal College of Physicians:

"The early growth in popularity of smoking tobacco was largely due to its supposed healing properties."

Yes, healing properties! And physicians were involved in making these claims at the time. In 1571, a Spanish doctor called Nicolas Monardes wrote a book on the medicinal properties of various plants, in which he claimed that tobacco could cure 36 health problems, including toothache, worms, lockjaw and cancer.

Surely everyone would now find such claims laughable, especially the idea that smoking could cure cancer. But here is an even greater surprise: tobacco smoking is genuinely credited with helping to prevent endometrial cancer. And also Parkinson's disease. But before you all go rushing off to the tobacconist, the list of horrible diseases smoking causes is much longer, so any notion that tobacco might be generally beneficial was abandoned by the medical profession long ago. Quite a few medical people still smoke themselves, but they certainly don't recomend that you should do it.

But this is yet another example of just how surprising and convoluted the tobacco story can be. If you stood on a street corner and asked a hundred passers-by if they thought the Royal College of Physicians - right now in the 21st Century - credited tobacco with helping to prevent certain diseases including one form of cancer, do you think you would find one person who would find that believable?

The RCP do not mention specifically whether *nicotine* is supposed to have any role in reducing the incidence of endometrial cancer or Parkinson's disease, or whether that effect is due to one of the other 4000 or so chemicals in tobacco smoke. But if we are going to call something like nicotine a *drug* - if we are going to dignify it with that name - surely that particular substance alone would have to prove to produce either a useful effect or a pleasant effect. To be described as a drug it has to have a practical use, so if it is not pleasurable or medicinal it is not a drug, merely a chemical compound. There are only two types of drug: medicinal drugs and recreational drugs.

Medicinal Drugs: are only truly *drugs* if they directly bring about a useful effect that cures or eases a medical condition. Many thousands of concoctions and compounds have been tried out over the centuries to see if they would do that, and I think it is fair to say that the majority were abandoned at some point as it became apparent that they did not truly prove useful, or no more useful than a placebo. Or else they proved to have side-effects that were just as severe, or worse than the presenting condition.

Nicotine is a compound that has been known to medical science for quite some time, and yet has never had any modern *medical* application, because all the effects of nicotine are toxic. No-one is going to benefit from a temporary increase in their heart-rate. No-one needs their blood pressure intermittently raised, an increased risk of thrombosis or restrictions to blood circulation in the extremities. So therefore nicotine would never be prescribed to treat a medical condition, in order to *make someone better*. It has only ever been prescribed as a stop smoking aid, in accordance with the theory that the smoker 'needs nicotine' – a theory which is wrong anyway. In fact it is a theory I successfully disprove just about every working day of my life, to the delight of my clients and their loved ones. In short, nicotine is only a poison because all its effects are entirely toxic, it doesn't do anything that is *useful* at all. So it is not a medicinal drug.

Recreational Drugs: are used principally for pleasure and their use in this way is officially discouraged by the medical profession, politicians, the police and just about anybody in authority. Since most of *them* use alcohol, the most widely-used recreational drug in the world - and some of them use other substances too - there are lots of contradictions and mixed messages in the debates that rage around recreational drug use. Or 'abuse', if you are a hardliner. But one thing is for sure, all over the world people have been using interesting substances to alter their feelings and perceptions for thousands of years, often just for fun. Some of these practices became ritual, or just habitual and they can often cause serious damage in the long run. Or even immediately - it is all a bit unpredictable so the *results* are not always fun, but pleasure or gratification is certainly the aim.

Now, some smokers are genuinely under the impression that they enjoy smoking tobacco but even this is an illusion in reality, as I explain in detail elsewhere in the book. This illusion is partly just the effect of a colossal amount of suggestion (eg. advertising), but also partly a result of the fact that smoking is being closely associated in the mind with other things that really are a pleasure, such as: taking a break, relaxing, socialising, drinking alcohol, or taking other recreational drugs like cannabis, cocaine or amphetamine. In describing those last three as a pleasure I am not recommending them, you understand. But their recreational use isn't rare so there is clearly enough enthusiasm about them in some quarters, at least, to create a sizeable international trade in those substances.

The global trade in tobacco is absolutely gigantic - far greater than all recreational drugs put together, of course. And yet nicotine itself isn't any fun at all. Try chewing the nicotine gum. Try sticking a patch on. Or if you have never smoked, try inhaling tobacco fumes, and then write down on a piece of paper precisely how much you 'enjoyed' that.

Stick that piece of paper on the fridge, read it every day and you'll never smoke again. That's how great nicotine is.

Nicotine is an oily, colourless compound which is very toxic indeed. It is of absolutely no use to humans. Nicotine has no useful effects, so it is certainly not medicinal and it doesn't have a pleasant effect, as we notice the first time we try to breathe the smoke in. It causes nausea and faintness, which could never be described as a high - at least, not by anyone who had ever taken any real recreational drugs. The mere fact that we can become accustomed to that nausea and later tolerate it quite easily is no more significant than the fact that sword-swallowers learn to tolerate cold steel in their upper digestive tract, or that a human can learn to regurgitate a live goldfish. That doesn't make it pleasant, useful or a good idea, just an example of how extraordinary human behaviour can become, if we are determined to override our natural resistance to such invasive procedures. Like the sword and the goldfish, the principle intention when most of us first start smoking is *display*: the main aim is to impress.

Sometimes humans, particularly young ones are impressed with out-of-the-ordinary behaviour, especially if it appears fearless. So anything that appears difficult, or looks as if it might hurt, can influence the young impressionable mind, and the mind of a sheltered or naive person. The imagination kicks in, Subconsciously of course: "Hey, if that impresses *me,* maybe if I do that too it will impress other people!"

Look at tattoos: there is a fine example of what I am talking about. Acquiring tattoos and learning to smoke are strategies adopted with the onlooker in mind, and the onlooker is supposed to be impressed. Smokers may well deny this, and some people with tattoos may also object to what I just stated, but it is important to realise that one of the onlookers – the key onlooker, really – is themselves. It is narcississtic, like so much human style and performance. Humans are animals, and animals are competitive. We have to have one eye on the competition, and the other eye on ourselves: how are we doing, how do we look, is it working, what does everybody think of us, how are they reacting, do we need to change anything, what else might work... what else is new? Wow, look what he's doing! That certainly got my attention – maybe I should do that! Martial arts are another good example of this, albeit a much more complex example with regard to levels of skill and discipline. In terms of the visual impact upon the new observer though, it is very similar to the other examples and many more.

Right from the beginning, tobacco smoking is not drug-taking. People take drugs – whether they are legal or not – to change the way they feel. If they continue taking those drugs, it is because they like the way it makes them feel. Ask any smoker how they felt the first time they inhaled tobacco smoke and they will either say they don't remember, or that it made them feel dizzy and sick. From this we can safely surmise that it made all of us feel dizzy and sick, it is just that some people have forgotten that – and really, why should they want to remember it?

So when we tried the second cigarette, it was certainly not because we enjoyed the effects of the first one. No, it was for the same reason as we tried the first one: to join in with our friends, to break the rules, to be all grown up, to try to impress someone else, or just ourselves. The actual effects of the carbon monoxide, the nicotine and all the other poisons in the smoke were just what you had to put up with if you were going to learn how to smoke. Smoking is at first a performance - an adopted attitude, and a way of posing with a theatrical prop. It is all about style and appearances. It has nothing to do with nicotine at all, and when you were thirteen you knew that. There are millions of smokers alive even today who had never heard of nicotine when they started smoking tobacco.

Try to find a parallel: any cocaine users who had never heard of cocaine when they first started using it? Never heard of alcohol? Never heard of heroin? Of course not, the drug was the whole point! So people carry on with those substances simply because they like the way it makes them feel right from the beginning. But when we persisted with the attempt to learn how to smoke, it was in spite of how the smoke made us feel, not because of it. And that is not drug taking.

N.B. With real drugs there can be nausea in a few cases too at first, in fact with heroin and morphine it is fairly common. The difference is that with those drugs the nausea passes and the high continues for much longer, whereas with tobacco there is no high, only nausea, and all new smokers experience it, not just some.

It is not long before tobacco smoking becomes a habit, because it is not long before anything becomes a habit. Then it just repeats automatically. **Compulsive habits are entirely caused by repetition and regularity, and then the Subconscious simply continues them for no other reason than they were already part of the usual routine.** The continuance of the behaviour, then, has nothing to do with the contents of the smoke at all, except in the sense that the smoker may come to believe it does, so that belief then becomes one of the notions potentially supporting the habit. Even if we remove that belief at conscious and Subconscious levels with hypnotherapy, the habit would continue anyway without it, if that were the limit of our intervention - proving that beliefs are not essential in the persistence of compulsive habits, just as we can clearly see from the closely-related habit of nail-biting.

Looking through the Wrong End of the Telescope

When nicotine was first *wrongly* identified as the apparent cause of compulsive tobacco use, you can bet that medical science went looking for a drug already believing a drug to be there. Not having an accurate, detailed model of the Compulsive Habit available to them, or an accurate understanding of the Subconscious mind, scientists started with the fact that people are apparently 'unable' to stop smoking, and then assumed that this must be because of something in the smoke. With a theoretical model of drug addiction already in existence, the simple fact that people evidently found the behaviour difficult to stop led to a simple conclusion. Conveniently forgetting that there are many other things people apparently can't stop doing once they get started which don't involve drugs at all, the search was on for the Thing that 'must' be there: a chemical culprit, a drug.

I suspect that one of the main reasons they picked on nicotine is simply because it has a measurable effect on the body. Lots of other things in the smoke have effects on the body too but they're not so easily measurable, and scientists love to measure things so that they can produce figures – data - without which, nobody in the scientific world can speak at all. But just because you can measure the effect a chemical has upon the body doesn't make it a drug, and it certainly doesn't mean it is addictive. Not only that, it doesn't even mean that the measurable effect of nicotine is the real reason anyone smokes. And indeed it's not, although many smokers currently believe it is. The main reason they believe that is because they've been told to believe it. Thousands of times.

You see, the scientists keep being very unscientific. For example, a recent piece of research (circa 2002) that received widespread press coverage in the UK was reported as indicating that young smokers:

"...became addicted to tobacco more quickly than was previously thought."

How did they discover this? By asking them! That isn't science, it is arbitrary subjective comment from youthful people who are very likely to misrepresent their behaviour (i.e. show off or exaggerate) at that age anyway. Also, all that the questioners are truly discovering - at best - is at what point people *feel compelled to do it,* without ever considering that this factor can commonly trigger repetitive behaviour without any drug being involved - as evidenced by nail-biting, chocolate eating, gambling etc.

It also ignores the factors which are most crucial of all when young smokers begin smoking, i.e. the main reasons for starting, which are certainly not the effects of nicotine. These are as follows: what the new smoker imagines it makes them look like (older, tougher, more daring, less like a kid), the fact they're not supposed to be doing it (rebellion, devilment) and the security of joining in and being accepted by the group. How soon do these factors become compelling? Well, when they're a few years older and are likely to be honest about it, you could ask them. In the meantime just cast your mind back to when you were an adolescent. If you can bear to, that is.

In the report mentioned above the self-conscious, self-dramatising, subjective opinion of young smokers was then given a completely unnecessary gloss with the addition of a bit of 'scientific' speculation:

"Scientists believe this may be because of the effect of nicotine acting more powerfully on the young, still developing brain."

I see. And now they've decided that, I'm sure they'll waste lots of money trying to prove it is true, instead of trying to prove it isn't, which would be far more scientific.

The actual effects of nicotine are as follows: it makes the heart beat faster than it should, it causes constriction of outer blood vessels drawing blood toward the centre of the body, away from the skin and the extremities, which is why it is bad for the skin and bad for circulation generally. The combined effect of these two things raises blood pressure. Blood fat-levels are also raised, and the risk of blood clots is increased. None of these effects are either useful or pleasant.

Everyone who has ever tried smoking tobacco knows that from the first time we attempt to inhale tobacco smoke it is blindingly obvious that the effects are not useful or pleasant. Virtually every smoker says the same thing: it made them cough, choke, perhaps even retch, and when the nicotine and carbon monoxide got into the system, feelings of clamminess, nausea, faintness and dizziness were the actual experience. Nothing in tobacco, and nothing in tobacco smoke is remotely of any use to a human being. But none of that matters at all, because the actual effects of the smoke were never the reason we were doing it anyway.

If you ask a drug-user when they first started using drugs, will they begin by telling you when they learned how to smoke tobacco? No of course not, they will tell you when they first started taking real drugs. It would never occur to them to talk of tobacco in that way. They might begin by talking about alcohol though, if that was the first substance they used to change the way they feel.

When a person starts smoking – at whatever age – they certainly do not think they are taking a stimulant drug. Not only that, no-one experiences it as a stimulant either. If anything the smoker feels exhausted or queasy as they grind out that cigarette-end. They don't feel vibrant and energised, as they might if they took amphetamine or cocaine. They don't even experience the sort of up-tempo boost that the caffeine in a decent cup of coffee can produce. In fact many habitual smokers are under the impression that tobacco *relaxes* them. They are surprised and confused when first told that nicotine actually stimulates the heart and raises blood pressure, because they didn't know that, so it obviously forms no part of the new smoker's motivation.

So if we are supposed to believe that smoking tobacco is drug-taking, doesn't it seem a bit odd that most of the people who are doing it are astonished to find out what this 'drug' actually does because they always thought it was doing something totally different? In fact they may even believe it does different things at different times. Sometimes it seems relaxing. Sometimes it seems to aid concentration - yet relaxation and the mental effort of concentration are polar opposites. Sometimes it seems to the smoker that tobacco can ease suffering, be it physical or emotional. There are times when it appears to alleviate boredom, enhance social life, boost confidence. Another peculiar aspect of this 'drug' is that it apparently rounds off a meal in excellent fashion.

But when you open a packet of cigarettes they all look the same. As you take them out one by one, they're all blank: you don't find one with *Concentration* helpfully etched onto the side of it... or *Stress Relief* or *The One After The Meal*. How does each cigarette know what is required of it, at that particular moment in your day?

The answer is: it doesn't. But you do. And of course the effect required by you is produced by you, entirely. All nicotine can possibly do is make your heart beat too fast, raise your blood pressure, raise blood fat levels, make you feel a bit dizzy and restrict the circulation of blood to the skin and the extremities. And it will do exactly that every time, whether it is coming from a cigarette, a patch, a wad of gum, a nasal spray, a lozenge or by chewing tobacco leaf.

Not only is this not pleasant in any way, it is of no use to any living person. In fact it is dangerous. It doesn't matter how you felt beforehand or what the circumstances, no normal person needs their heart artificially accelerated and their blood pressure raised. And although other stimulants also have those effects, that's not why people take them. People take stimulants like cocaine, amphetamine or ecstasy because of the powerful highs involved, not for the dangerous side-effects. There is no such thing as a Nicotine High, there is only the vague nausea that goes with breathing smoke in and out, and that is why the habitual drug-user would never refer to their first cigarette as the occasion of their first drug experience.

This is also the reason nobody abuses the Nicotine Replacement products. There are lots of people out there who enjoy taking all manner of recreational drugs simply for the experience, just to change the way they feel for a while. And they'll try all kinds of things, whether legal or illegal, natural or synthetic. But no-one 'abuses' the nicotine patches, the gum, the inhalator or the lozenge. The only people who ever try them are people who are already smoking habitually and are attempting to quit. And they usually don't try them for very long because they don't like them. Which seems very peculiar doesn't it, since they are supposed to be 'nicotine addicts' already? Why don't the vast majority of them prefer this nice, clean, 'clinical' and slightly safer form of their regular poison?

Despite the fact that many people who enjoy taking drugs will notoriously abuse virtually anything from poppers to cough medicine and whatever else they can get access to, they never bother with nicotine replacement products at all. Why not? Because there is no drug experience, no enjoyment or satisfaction to be had out of it, at all. There is no *enthusiasm* for these products, despite the daft medical assumption that it is the effects of nicotine that smokers are 'enjoying'. Even drug-takers who also happen to have a smoking habit don't waste time trying to get a kick out of the patches because there's no pleasure there at all, no buzz, no nice feeling. Nobody abuses these things because there's no enjoyment to be had - nicotine is just a poison and it makes you feel poisoned, until you get so accustomed to it that you barely notice. It did that from the beginning; right from the moment you first bravely breathed it in, and it made you want to puke.

If nicotine was a drug, the following statements would be commonplace:

"Hey, you look kind of bored – try some of this excellent nicotine gum, it alleviates boredom and also gives you something to do with your mouth."

"You know, you seem stressed – let me stick a nicotine patch on your arm, that'll calm you down. I'm wearing three, that's why I'm so serene."

"Darling, what a splendid meal! Now pass me the nicotine nasal spray, that'll round it off to perfection."

Never happens! It isn't a drug! It's a poison! And no-one likes it! The only reason it has ever been *called* a drug, is to try to make it fit this recent drug addiction theory, which it doesn't. The world has been hypnotised from the 1980s onwards, by the endlessly-repeated suggestion that smokers are nicotine addicts. The drug companies have got everyone believing this poison is a medication.

When I snap my fingers, wake up and smell the smoke. Millions of pounds of taxpayers' money are blazing away.

The Nicotine Experience

Now don't get me wrong, I know there is a nicotine *experience* – or at least, a tobacco-smoking experience. I have experienced it myself many times. But let's not get confused between the actual effects of inhaling the smoke, and all of the other things the smoker may be experiencing at that moment - because of the situation, their usual habits, their mood, their expectations, their personality, recent life-events, their current beliefs about smoking and also the action of any other toxins that may be in their system like alcohol, cocaine or cannabis. Even having a hangover can dramatically change your experience of the effects of tobacco smoke, as every smoking drinker knows.

Hypnotherapy can change it so completely you will never feel inclined to smoke again. This is simply a return to normal, in fact.

When people are smoking tobacco, it is not possible to know how much of that experience is caused by nicotine itself, or by a combination of nicotine, carbon monoxide and any one of the many other toxins in the smoke. Smokers often mention noticing a light-headed or dizzy feeling, especially when alcohol is already in the system, or after a period of abstinence from smoking. This is partly caused by carbon monoxide causing a rapid drop in oxygen levels in the brain. Does this make carbon monoxide a *drug?*

Obviously not, it remains nothing but a poison. So who decided that *nicotine* was a drug? Here is a job for a really dogged researcher! So far I have been unable to locate the moment in history when some fool decided that nicotine was a drug, and not just one of the many poisons in the smoke. If nicotine is a drug, then sugar is a drug. Oxygen is a drug. Any substance that has an effect on you that can be measured qualifies as a drug on that basis, whether the 'user' knows what it actually does or not.

Of course real drugs can often be regarded as poisons too, since there will be a level of concentration that would cause damage or even death. But it is the *intended effect* that is the key in understanding the difference.

When scientists are trying to understand addiction, one of the markers they regard as significant is the continued use of the substance *in spite of obvious detrimental effects;* which they then mistakenly assume means that the drug has taken control of the behaviour, because the user's logical mind can recognise the problem but not prevent the behaviour. However, once you understand that all habitual behaviour is controlled by the Subconscious, and that the conscious recognition of the damage it is doing *is not perceived* by the Subconscious - and also that the Subconscious has more clout if there is a conflict - then you can easily understand all compulsive habitual behaviour. It also becomes obvious why this is perplexing and frustrating to the conscious mind, which has previously been misled to believe it controls all choices and behaviour. This leads to *an illusion of powerlessness* in the conscious mind, combined with simple unawareness in the Subconscious that there is a problem.

All that is needed to correct and resolve this is to explain the situation effectively to the Subconscious and resolve any other associated conflicts there might be, so that the habitual behaviour can be changed by the Subconscious. The only way to do this is through effective hypnotherapy. When I say effective hypnotherapy, I do not mean some guy on a CD reading from a script while you lie on your bed wondering why the guy's voice is so irritating, and why you don't feel any different and you want a cigarette. Real therapy cannot be mass-produced, sorry. Poisons can, but not therapy, not healing. That's a human thing.

A Little Harmless Retro-Speculation

Sometime during the the last century when the medical profession was on a roll, the kind of people who aim to eliminate all suffering, damage and disease decided to tackle the problem of tobacco smoking – with the best will in the world, people were dying in considerable numbers and the habit was rife. They looked at smoking behaviour and thought: "Hm, here is something people can't stop doing once they get started... Oooh, that reminds us of addictions!" And off they went up that track. Not surprisingly, because medical training typically gets people thinking in terms of either surgery or drugs as an intervention. Since they could not cut the problem out with a knife, they found themselves seeking a chemical solution, and off they went looking at all the chemicals involved to identify an "addictive" chemical culprit.

What they failed to notice right from the start – or perhaps ignored - is that there are lots of things people can't stop doing once they get started which don't involve drugs at all: nail-biting, compulsive gambling, chocoholics and shopaholics are obvious examples, as indeed the tobacco companies have sometimes pointed out, but nobody wanted to listen to them. All the 'obsessive compulsive disorders' too, where behaviour becomes repetitive and driven - all characterised by *a powerful urge* to do whatever it is, which won't leave you alone or give you any peace of mind until you do it.

Everybody Guessed Wrong - even the Tobacco Companies!

Here is a quote from the website of the medical 'anti-smoking' group ASH (Action on Smoking and Health):

"Tobacco industry documents dating from the 1960s have shown that tobacco companies recognised that the main reason that people continued smoking is nicotine addiction. A lawyer acting for Brown and Williamson said: "Nicotine is addictive. We are, then, in the business of selling nicotine, an addictive drug." Publicly, however, tobacco companies denied that nicotine was addictive, because such an admission would have undermined their stance that smoking is a matter of personal choice. ...In March 1997, Liggett Group, the smallest of the five major US tobacco companies, became the first to admit that smoking is addictive as part of a deal to settle legal claims against the company. More recently the tobacco companies have tried to cast doubt over the meaning of addiction by comparing smoking with other common pursuits such as shopping or eating chocolate."

Scientists have been looking for a drug in chocolate for years, convinced there must be a chemical compound in the stuff which causes compulsive chocolate-eating in so-called 'chocoholics'. There isn't - and there isn't an addictive element in fingernails either, to cause the seemingly unbreakable habit there. It is the *behaviour* that is compulsive, the product or object is irrelevant. Tobacco, chocolate or salted peanuts are no more habit-forming in themselves than fingernails. *The brain forms habits,* and it can form them just as easily without a product (nail-biting, finger-picking, hair-twisting, whistling) as with one (tobacco, slot machines, chocolate etc.)

Smoking is compulsive behaviour: just like nail-biting, compulsive gambling, compulsive shopping, compulsive skin-picking, or habitual chocolate-eating. It is automatic behaviour directed by the dominant part of the mind - the Subconscious. It is the same kind of automatic mental process which directs the obsessive-compulsive disorders, resulting in endless hand-washing or checking routines and rituals. The conscious mind is not involved in the operation of these behaviour patterns, so it cannot cause them to cease. But the Subconscious can. So if we aim to change these things, that's the part of the mind we need to talk to. Hypnotherapy is the only way to do that quickly, effortlessly and safely.

All the compulsive habits listed above are notoriously difficult to stop just with willpower – i.e. conscious efforts alone – but really rather easy to sort out with hypnotherapy because those behaviours are not really outside that person's control at all, merely outside their conscious control. Their Subconscious is controlling them fine, it just doesn't know about the conscious decision to change them. In practice, during therapy there may also be some *resistance* to changing them as well, but it's all up for negotiation with the Subconscious mind. Changes may be accepted immediately, or it might be after a bit of negotiation; other issues may have some bearing on that. We commonly need to deal with these additional matters along the way. But just as often there is no resistance anyway, the Subconscious is perfectly happy to change it right away. The only reason it had not changed it before is because it had never been consulted on the matter before. How long the habit had been operating before that is absolutely irrelevant.

"Old habits die hard", that is what we are taught to believe. But this is true only if you try to change them with a conscious decision followed by a conscious effort - willpower – which is exactly what most people *are* trying to do when they seek to change these things. This makes virtually no impression on the Subconscious, which doesn't have any idea about the thoughts and intentions that are going on in the conscious mind. But if you explain it all to the Subconscious mind, that part of the mind can change it all at the drop of a hat with no apparent effort at all. It's just that most people don't know that because it is not something they have experienced themselves, and they are more familiar with the idea that habits are hard to break. Now add the fact that their conscious mind doesn't really believe in their Subconscious mind anyway at first. Except maybe in theory. Is *your* conscious mind struggling to believe all this?

<u>To Summarise</u>

If you ask a heroin addict what heroin does, they will have no difficulty in enlightening you. It would be the same with cocaine users, of course they know what it does. Ask any smoker what nicotine does and you will find that they haven't got a clue – or even if they do know, it will then be impossible for them to claim that the actual effects of nicotine are the real motivation for their smoking behaviour.

When you are young and fit you don't ordinarily notice how fast your heart is beating. So if it beats a bit faster, you genuinely don't notice that. You certainly don't know what your blood pressure is, even if it is dangerously high. So the so-called "stimulant" effects of nicotine as described in the BMA's Medical Dictionary are not noticed by the smoker, so that cannot form any part of their motivation. The idea that smokers smoke cigarettes in order to make their heart race and their blood pressure go up is frankly ridiculous. And as for "reducing fatigue, increasing alertness and improving concentration", well this is just mythical, isn't it? When I smoked tobacco I just felt tired most of the time. Just look at people sitting there, puffing miserably away on the old coffin nails: do they look bright and alert, full of energy? Any sign that they've been taking powerful stimulant drugs, at all?

You can smoke tobacco at any time of day and it doesn't affect your behaviour. You cannot do that with alcohol or any other recreational drugs, because that would influence your behaviour. Tobacco smoking is not drug-taking because it doesn't alter your perceptions or judgement, which alcohol and all other recreational drugs do. This is where there is a clear difference between smoking and drinking, which some people mistakenly regard as being linked. Most habitual smokers will smoke from one end of the day to the other. They don't *drink* from one end of the day to the other, because it would disastrously affect their lives. No, drinking is drug-taking - people do that *to change the way they feel,* and it does. Smoking does not, so you can smoke at any time of day and life continues just as it would if you had not. Unless you suddenly have one of those heart attacks or strokes that nicotine is so adept at dealing out to smokers without the slightest warning. *Then* your life continues quite differently. If it continues at all.

<u>The Drug That Never Was... an Offence Either</u>

Law enforcement officers in many countries now will test a driver's blood after an accident to see if there is any alcohol, because everyone knows that alcohol can affect their perceptions and therefore their driving ability. Likewise if they find opiates in the blood, if they find cocaine, amphetamines, cannabis, they will prosecute the driver for driving while their faculties are impaired. Not all these substances make you dopey: cocaine and amphetamines both reduce fatigue, improve alertness and aid concentration - just like the BMA suggest nicotine does. So if your airline pilot or your school bus driver has been doing coke or speed, they should be okay to handle that journey, right? No! Of course not, because we all naturally feel that *normal perceptions* - totally unimpaired by any drug - are what everyone on the road and in the skies has a right to expect from the person in control of any vehicle.

So if you see your pilot taking nicotine just before the flight you can have him arrested, right? He wasn't just smoking a cigarette in that airport lounge, he was putting everyone's lives in danger by taking a stimulant drug to reduce his fatigue so he could be more alert and concentrate better. Oh my God I've just realised, this is a nine-hour flight! He can't smoke on the plane and nicotine levels start falling after just twenty minutes. What is going to happen to his concentration and alertness then? What sort of distracted and dozy state will he be in when he tries to land this plane, nine hours after his last fix? Quick, anyone got any patches? We've got to get some nicotine replacement to the pilot, or we're all going to die!

See how ridiculous this nicotine nonsense is? In the RCP article about the IVSA animal testing I critiqued in Case Mysteries 4, attempts were continually made throughout the article to get the reader to accept the suggestion that nicotine was a drug which caused the same kind of dependence and changes to normal behaviour as cocaine and heroin, even though it obviously doesn't. But if those scientists who conducted the tests and the medical people who reviewed that evidence really believed it was all true, why were they not calling for drivers with nicotine in their system to be banned from the roads? Let me just remind you of certain statements that were included in the introduction to the IVSA section of their article entitled *Nicotine Addiction in Britain:*

This drug-seeking and drug-taking behaviour can dominate the animals' behavioural repertoire to the detriment of normal behaviour, just as in cases of serious drug abuse in humans.

It has been established that monkeys, dogs, rats and mice can all exhibit nicotine IVSA. Monkeys have pressed levers for nicotine at rates similar to those at which they pressed levers for cocaine.

These statements turn out to be extremely misleading when properly analysed in the context of the actual details of the tests, as I point out in my critique. But if the Royal College of Physicians truly believed that nicotine affected humans and animals to the detriment of normal behaviour, as claimed - *resembling cocaine and heroin* - why is smoking while driving still acceptable? It surely cannot be that the authorities are just turning a blind eye because there are too many smokers to prosecute them all - if smokers are going to be busted for smoking in a bar now, why not behind the wheel?

I'll tell you exactly why: because everybody knows, really, that tobacco smoking is not drug taking. Deep down everybody knows it, it's just that people had kind of forgotten, and hadn't quite recognised consciously that they *knew* all this stuff about addiction was hyperbole, just as it is with chocolate and computer games. Somehow we let the simple fact that compulsive habits are hard to break with willpower confuse us into accepting this bogus portrayal of nicotine as a 'drug of addiction'. But the moment someone seriously suggests that drivers should be prosecuted for driving under the influence of nicotine, this ridiculous exaggeration comes crashing down amid howls of laughter. It is every bit as silly as suggesting that the smoking driver is "impaired by the drug carbon monoxide", and that is exactly why no-one has ever suggested it. It is true that there are calls for smoking to be illegal when driving, but that is because lighting up or handling the cigarette may momentarily distract the driver, not because the effects of nicotine might – and that's the giveaway, right there. That very fact proves my point exactly: what fucking drug? There is no drug involved.

The End of the Debate

So there we have it. There are lots of chemicals in tobacco smoke, but none of them can be classified as drugs. Nicotine Replacement Therapy is entirely based on a myth. It is at best a placebo and at worst... nothing but a poison fraudulently posing as a medication. Nobody needs nicotine because cravings are signals produced by the brain and are related to patterns of habitual and communal behaviour, not high or low levels of nicotine in the blood. No-one needs nicotine 'replacing', in fact it's the last thing they need.

What they really need - if they just want to get rid of their smoking habit easily, quickly and without ongoing internal conflicts - is hypnotherapy. The useless poison nicotine, far from being an addictive drug turns out to be the most extraordinary case of mistaken identity in medical history. It is the biggest medical mistake of the 20th Century.

It truly is THE DRUG THAT NEVER WAS.

The Inhalation of Smoke

Breathing smoke in and out is something that humans have done for a long time. Many 'primitive' cultures feature some sort of smoking behaviour in one form or another. But that doesn't make it natural or a good idea. Humankind has always been full of ideas – some great, some not so great – but purposely filling our lungs with smoke has to be a contender for The Dumbest Idea in History.

Now there are lots of substances that are smokeable, and as one smoking material goes out of fashion another may take its place. I'm not going to get into any moral debate about that because it would lead us into a discussion around whether or not people should take drugs. I have no moral position on that as a therapist because it is a health issue - and anyway, this book is about tobacco smoking. There is no drug involved.

If indigenous people somewhere in the rainforest are smoking some strange and wonderful herbal preparation as part of a mystical ritual, I reckon that's up to them. I still think - though it's none of my business of course - that from the point of view of their lungs, certainly it would be better to make space cakes out of it, or brew it up in a pot and drink it, but smoking is quicker, I understand that. It is also more dramatic. And from the point of view of spiritual significance, more in line with the notion of some ephemeral essence flowing in and out of us: bringing visions, ecstasy, hallucinations and a thumping headache.

If at the same time someone on a council estate in Dudley is smoking heroin, again I hesitate to comment. I don't live there, maybe I'd feel inclined to smoke heroin if I did, I don't know. What they are doing is putting the health of their lungs later in their list of priorities, some way behind getting the narcotic into their system rapidly. That's their issue, this book is not about whether they should or shouldn't do that.

It's about smoking tobacco. Which is quite different.

The Inhalation of Smoke

Let's be simply factual: all smoking is unnecessary, unnatural and damages the lungs. Our lungs are the only method we have of getting the oxygen we need, every moment of every day to sustain our lives. To damage them in any way is completely stupid, unless you genuinely do not care whether you live or die. But when people are taking drugs *you can at least see the point*. It then becomes a judgement call, and everyone has to make those choices for themselves. They may live to regret their choice later but hey, that's personal responsibility for you.

So why is tobacco different? Because contrary to what many people in the world currently believe there is no drug or pleasure involved in reality, it is an illusion. Also, because this is by far the biggest cause of preventable human illness and death in history. In fact, the misunderstanding of the tobacco story constitutes the most catastrophic error in human history. I can think of no other blunder that even comes close in terms of the loss of life, the suffering and the grief.

It is all for nothing. An empty puff of smoke. There is no high, no benefit. No pay off except the relief of a craving, which is unconnected to the smoke anyway, just an impulse to repeat the established habitual behaviour. This is the only 'vice' with no reward at all, and worse consequences than most other vices have, yet it has often been regarded as the most permissable and 'ordinary' of vices. This is mainly *because* it is not a drug, so it does not change anyone's behaviour. It does not cause loss of control, lewd or offensive behaviour, dangerous driving or prompt anyone to commit crime. It is only anti-social in the sense that it gradually poisons whole sections of the populace to death, but so slowly that the shadow it casts over those people is almost imperceptible until the very end. Some smoking is even referred to as 'social smoking', which is a mad expression. It is a bit like describing two emphysemic patients seated together wearing oxygen masks as an example of "social breathing".

Literally Insane

So the inhalation of smoke is always damaging but sometimes it does at least have a point, i.e. when there is a drug involved, such as cannabis or heroin. That does not make it a good idea, but it does make it purposeful. By contrast, the inhalation of tobacco smoke is both damaging and pointless, which I think defines it as insane behaviour. As indeed we would all instantly recognise if we had never previously seen anyone do it, and then first witnessed a demonstration when we were around the age of 35, at which point on life's journey we are not so impressionable as we were at 13. If we saw a vagrant doing it perhaps, whilst begging in an underpass. We would think "What on earth is that old loony doing, breathing in s*moke?*" Probably we would be quite alarmed - what other insanity might the wretch be capable of, if he thought nothing of inhaling hot fumes?

The mad craze of tobacco smoking had already become established, dear reader, before you stepped up for this particular ride on Life's Rollercoaster. Just imagine - if you can - what you would think of it today if it were a completely unprecedented suggestion.

Rattus Humanus, *or* Go On Then, Give Us a Go of That Patch

Recently someone I knew was trying to stop smoking with the use of patches. Of course I don't go preaching about hypnotherapy to ordinary people around me, as in my experience that tends to put people off, if anything. It's like when someone says: "Oh, you *must* go and see that film!" I don't know about you, but that always makes me feel a general disinclination to do any such thing. So I didn't offer any professional advice they hadn't sought.

It struck me, though, that here I was writing a book about nicotine and yet I hadn't personally experienced the effects of nicotine in a very long time, and suddenly I was curious. Also, although I had used the nicotine gum quite a bit during various attempts to quit in 1990 and 1991, I think I only ever tried a patch once, and no longer have much memory of the impression it made, if any. Of course I was a smoker then, and so I was accustomed to nicotine being present in my system, along with lots of other toxins contained in tobacco smoke. I couldn't help wondering now what the nicotine experience would be like for a person who was not. Someone just like that was standing close by at that very moment. Right next to me, in fact. Closer, even. Yup, it was me.

Now I could have simply tried a cigarette, but nothing seemed more disgusting than that idea, and anyway, as a former habitual smoker – and more especially, as a hypnotherapist – I knew that if I did that, the old habit could be kicked off again by accident. Easy enough to fix, but surely better to avoid. In addition, that would be an experience of cigarette smoke, which includes all sorts of chemicals in addition to nicotine. What would nicotine feel like all by itself, to a person who had not smoked, or taken nicotine in any form, for many years? Naturally I had no reason to fear becoming 'addicted to nicotine', because I knew that idea was mythical.

So in the end curiosity got the better of me and I asked if I could try one, for research purposes only, and after looking at me as if I was nuts (which I am used to) my friend handed over a nicotine patch. I fetched a pen and some paper upon which to make notes of the experience, and immediately noted down that it was a NiQuitin CQ 21mg 24-hour patch. I didn't intend to leave it on for 24 hours, but I did aim to leave it on for most of the day, just to monitor the experience. As it turned out, it didn't quite happen that way.

This was at 10.15 on a Sunday morning, April 22th 2007. We were planning to take the kids to the park at about eleven, which I was looking forward to because it was a nice day. This is an exact transcript of the notes I made at the time.

10.15am. Stuck patch on inside upper left arm.

10.20am. Tingling in both hands, mild tightening feeling in the throat.

10.25am Feel nauseous, patch burning skin a bit.

10.30am. Feel like blood pressure is up, not a pleasant feeling. Tense. Uncomfortable, want to take it off actually. More nauseous, feel a bit ill. Patch really burning. Bowels upset a bit.

10.35am Head fuzzy. Feel rather sick. Got that feeling like I don't know where to put myself. Feel really uncomfortable and irritable now.

10.37am. Took patch off. Don't feel safe. Big red mark on arm. Hands/wrists aching. Feel sick and faint, balance and even speech abnormal. Wrists and hands quite red. Bowels churning. Feel rotten, very definitely ill. Poisoned. Really want to feel normal again, regret trying this.

10.50am. Still feel just as rotten, but feeling of real alarm that made me take it off now subsiding. Just feel ill.

The patch was only in contact with my skin for 22 minutes. Before I began the experiment I felt fine – healthy and in good spirits. Now I felt absolutely terrible, really unwell and although I don't usually scare easy, actually afraid to leave the patch on any longer. But here's the thing - according to the BMA, nicotine:

"stimulates the central nervous system, thereby reducing fatigue, increasing alertness, and improving concentration."

So, did nicotine make me feel more alert, able to concentrate better, as the BMA described? Well, by the time I took the patch off I was anxious, irritable and no longer able or willing to hold a normal conversation - so I would have to say no, it certainly did not. Well, why not? If that is what nicotine does, that is what it does. I would have noticed. It just made me feel poisoned, and actually it did remind me of the first cigarette I ever tried, when I was eight. My pal Ian Coates stole a single Embassy No.1 from his mum, and we hid at the bottom of his garden and smoked it. It left me feeling pretty much like the experience I described above, but with a foul taste in my mouth as well. It was years before I tried one again, and even then it wasn't because I liked it the first time. It was just because I wasn't allowed to, and because smoking makes you look grown-up and cool, despite being twelve and pimply with awful hair and silly clothes. And feeling very queasy, if not actually vomiting.

At eleven o'clock, we all left for the park. Sure enough I felt very queasy, delicate and anxious I might suddenly need the toilet – that IBS feeling. I really didn't want to go out at all now, I felt more like going for a lie down, which I only ever feel inclined to do if I am quite ill. Of course some fool might suggest that the dose was too high for a non-smoker, or that I was irresponsible to try that without medical advice, as if that were the reason it made me ill. But that's ridiculous: none of us took medical advice before we tried our first cigarette, did we? And very few kids start with a low-nicotine cigarette, certainly not my generation anyway, or the previous one. So it was, in fact, an experiment that roughly replicated most initial, real smoking experiences but this time focussing entirely on nicotine itself, and guess what? Nicotine just makes you feel ill, because it is nothing but a poison. I'm not saying you can't get used to it – boxers get used to being slammed in the face, and I'm sure that stimulates the central nervous system too, but that don't make it medicinal, baby.

In my younger, wilder days I tried just about every drug there was, and really hammered some of them too, so I know a thing or two about drug effects. Some drugs are less pleasant than others and technically, you could class them all as poisons in a sense, but here's the thing: drug taking is pleasure-seeking, thrill-seeking if you like. All recreational drugs have to have a 'buzz' - or to put it another way, cause sensations that are supposed to be broadly preferable to, or more fun than normality at least temporarily. But it was blindingly obvious to me there was no buzz in my nicotine experiment – and I was really searching, too. I was even making notes. Read them through again, see if you can find anything that might pass for recreation.

On reflection, I would say that the only 'substance of abuse' that has effects remotely resembling that – and it is still not a close resemblance - is amyl nitrate, sometimes called poppers or liquid gold. As recreational drug effects go, amyl nitrate is a truly lousy experience which really just messes with your heart rate and blood pressure for a few minutes and usually leaves you wishing you hadn't bothered. (I'm not suggesting habitual smokers experience effects like amyl nitrate, of course. They barely notice any effect at all, I'm only remarking that nicotine hits you slightly like that if you haven't been poisoned by it at all for a long time. Your head goes funny, you don't feel normal and you don't quite feel well, that's the similarity in a nutshell.) Amyl nitrate is a very cheap and nasty rush that most habitual drug users would never bother with, but have probably tried at some time, which tells you all you need to know about its lack of appeal. But even with that, there is at least something resembling a high, even though it only lasts a couple of minutes, and the nausea is just a side-effect that comes after, rather like the nausea and sickness that follows solvent abuse. Also, all of the effects of amyl nitrate usually wear off within five minutes, so you don't even have to put up with any of it for long.

My nicotine experience did not quickly disappear. It ruined my trip to the park: I just stood by feeling dreadful whilst the kids and the dog raced around enjoying themselves. I found it difficult to make the effort to hold a normal conversation with my wife - which makes the claim for alertness and improved concentration obviously doubtful - and although I was no longer making notes, I did make a note of the time as very gradually the nausea began to fade at around 12.40, a little over two hours after I took the patch off. By about 12.50 I felt almost normal again, but very tired despite the fact I hadn't been exerting myself in any way.

Just occasionally during the writing of this book, I have momentarily wondered if I may have gone just a little too far in declaring emphatically that nicotine is not a drug at all. I always knew that some people would find the idea hard to believe, because they had already been brainwashed with the idea that it was - but I never worried about that, I only wondered once or twice about whether I might be slightly overstating the case. My nicotine experiment put paid to that. This is supposed to be the most addictive drug in the world? What ridiculous nonsense, it isn't a drug at all!

I bet if you took a bunch of young teenagers – say about 12 to 14 years of age, about the age many of them first try smoking - and got them to sign up for an experiment in which you stuck 21mg 24-hour-patches on them every day for a month, just like the one I tried, all of them would drop out of the experiment within 48 hours. This would certainly be the case if they had no idea what the substance was, so that attitude played no part in their subjective experience. People do experience substances in different ways to some extent, but I doubt if any of those young people would be prepared to carry on with NRT for even a week. The idea that you could create an addict that way is absolutely laughable.

Doctors would probably advise that such an experiment would be unthinkable anyway, and that it would be dangerous to allow a twelve-year-old to try a nicotine patch at all, let alone a high-strength patch like the one I used. If I tried to organise a public trial like that, I would be confident that some media-savvy doctor would immediately step in and try to prevent it 'on medical grounds'. But you have to ask yourself why that should be, if it is safer than an ordinary cigarette? The same doctor would scarcely glance at a twelve-year-old walking down the road with a cigarette, that is commonplace enough. No need to slam on the brakes and intervene in a professional capacity, no – that's really just a part of growing up, something he probably did himself. He may also think nothing of prescribing that same 21mg patch, which I'm sure he would regard as dangerous to the 12-year-old, to the boy's mother or grandfather, and assume he is helping them.

He is not. A poison is a poison, and all it can do is poison people. It makes no difference how old you are. That's all it did to me, not only when I was eight but all the time I was smoking, all the time I was trying to end the habit with the nasty gum seventeen years ago, and during the short, horrible experience of my recent nicotine experiment. I have experimented with many chemicals over the last few decades, and I have to say that even the roughest drugs you could find traded on the streets are nothing like as unpleasant as that nicotine patch was, although I wouldn't recommend them either. All drugs make you ill in the end, if you take them for long enough, but nicotine makes you ill right from the beginning, and without a high to compensate. One or two of the recreational drugs – heroin particularly springs to mind – can make some people nauseous at first, but that's not all it does, obviously. That is a side-effect which only affects some people anyway. And at least everybody is fully aware that heroin is a drug, and might be harmful.

Nicotine is not even a drug at all, but it is being called a drug, and as a result of that catastrophic medical error, this nasty little poison is also able to pose as a 'medication', and the fact that the British taxpayer has to pay for all the hundreds of millions of doses dished out by that dozy leviathan known as the NHS means that the drug companies have pulled off a bigger hustle in the UK than the conman who sold Tower Bridge to a Texan.

The FDA have a hell of a lot to answer for in all this, but they're not the only ones. These Poison Products are now raking in billions, and they are not only fake medicines, they are fucking dangerous. It is obvious - not only from my little experiment which served as a shocking reminder of what nicotine is actually like, but also from anyone's first smoking experience *and* many a smoker's difficulty tolerating NRT products – that there is no such thing as *therapeutic nicotine*. It is as ridiculous a notion as therapeutic cyanide or therapeutic carbon monoxide. The drug companies are just poisoning people. Millions of them. And the fact that those people were already poisoning themselves with something else is no excuse – at least cigarettes aren't posing as a medicine.

Still have doubts? Wait until you have read Section Nine.

Section Eight

How we Shut Down Cravings in Therapy

Question: When is a Need not a Need?

Answer: When it is Only an Impulse!

Remember when the actor Michael Douglas received treatment for his "addiction to sex"? Who did not smile at this? Hollywood actors, just like other famous people, have been notoriously promiscuous before, no-one ever called it an addiction. We now commonly hear of people 'addicted' to shopping, 'addicted' to playing computer games. Watching violent movies, or exercising. The word is being used journalistically to comment negatively upon the behaviour, not accurately understand it. It is sensational, because the word 'addiction' in the popular imagination is like a cell-door slamming shut: now you're caught! You are hooked, helpless - and what's more you've brought it on yourself, you *deserve* to be a wretch. Isn't this the implication of the word 'addict', the stigma? It is more of a judgement than anything else: this is your punishment for indulging yourself. And of course it can sound like an excuse as well, which rather seemed the case with Michael Douglas.

It is all nonsense. What we are talking about here is repetitive compulsive behaviour, not addiction. There's a difference! By that other definition, we're all 'addicted' to eating, drinking and breathing. Certainly we don't feel like stopping, but we are not addicted. We are responding to compulsive urges to do those things, urges that originate from the brain. Whether we call them urges, impulses or cravings may depend upon the context and our immediate suppositions about these motivational feelings, but they are not coming from the conscious mind. In fact they are usually misunderstood by the conscious mind.

Cravings or compulsive urges are signals sent by the Subconscious mind prompting a certain behaviour or reaction. The exact aim of the signal may be any one of these three things: to spur us to act immediately, to remind the conscious mind that it is an appropriate moment to do something we regularly do, or else to suggest that it might be useful or gratifying to do that, according to presently-held beliefs and expectations. (N.B. I refer to Subconscious beliefs. The conscious mind may hold beliefs that are not the same.)

What has caused all the confusion about cravings is that although these signals are fired off by the Subconscious mind and are entirely controlled by the brain, they are directed via the body. The Subconscious mind is sometimes prompting us directly to act without thought, and sometimes using the body as a signalling system to get an idea across to the conscious mind. The signals are actually *mimicking bodily needs*, so we feel them in the body, they are like a pang. Hunger is one, thirst is another. The signal to light up cigarettes is just another example, as is the urge to buy a chocolate bar if you are a 'chocoholic', and there are many more.

The Stomach Doesn't Speak

I remember recently seeing a psychologist on television telling the TV audience that a hunger pang is "the body telling you it needs food". Either she was dumbing-down for the TV audience to a patronising degree, or else she didn't know what she was talking about. It is the Subconscious mind that is sending the message, not the body. The aim is to *suggest* to the conscious mind that there is a 'bodily need', when actually there may be no real need at all.

For example: in the case of ordinary thirst there appears to be an obvious connection to bodily requirements, but the urge to order a last drink at the bar when time is called after an evening of liquid indulgence has obviously got nothing to do with bodily requirements. Dehydration due to alcohol has not yet occured, so the impulse is certainly not 'thirst'. The body isn't short of liquid, yet it is often an overwhelming impulse. Just like the 'temptation' to order something from the sweet trolley after a hearty meal - clearly there is no bodily need there whatsoever, but the urge can be very compelling - easily powerful enough to overturn conscious resolutions. What would the psychologist call that: "The body telling you it's a greedy bastard"? There is a pleasure-seeking principle in the mind driving that impulse, it has nothing to do with the body. The body could well do without it actually, as the conscious mind knows perfectly well, but nobody has talked to the Subconscious about that. The body may be the apparent locus of the *urge* - the physical experience of the impulse to respond - but the signal originates from the Subconscious mind. And whether the signal happens to be linked to real bodily requirements or not, the signal itself is not need at all, but a *prompt*.

How do I know? I worked it out logically, from my observations of the results of hypnotherapy. The body is not intelligent in any *conversational* sense, and therefore cannot respond to suggestion. So if these signals originated from the *body*, hypnotherapy to remove cravings would have zero effect. The Subconscious on the other hand is intelligent, and is usually happy to respond to suggestions to change anything, as long as it is not inconvenient and will be useful – often responding perfectly to requests presented in very specific, particular detail too. So when the cravings disappear, just because we asked the Subconscious to shut them down, that proves that the Subconscious intelligently responded to the useful information and changed the sensations it was previously directing in the physical body. The Subconscious controls the body in every last detail, and can change anything about the operation of the system if it chooses to. It's just that most people - including psychologists, apparently - don't know that.

So let's go back in time and look at the development of tobacco smoking behaviour to see exactly where cravings really came into play.

The Three Stages of Tobacco Smoking

Stage One: Before the Cravings: Experimentation

Very early sampling of tobacco, from about the age of eight upwards is really only occasional experimentation and does not usually start the habit off. Regular smoking rarely begins this early, and these flirtations with tobacco are more devilment and curiosity than anything else.

Some children are strongly attracted to things that are forbidden: the more they are not supposed to do it, the more appealing it seems. They may well persuade a friend or sibling to join them in exploring this forbidden experience as well, but neither of them are likely to find tobacco attractive on any other basis at that age, so once their curiosity has been satisfied smoking tends to be neglected again for some time.

This particular inclination to try tobacco is not always restricted to very young children. Curiosity is a factor that can lead to experimentation at almost any age. Even devilment can suddenly break out in the most submissive of souls, well into their twenties or thirties, if they suddenly decide, perhaps, that they have always allowed their strict upbringing to hold them back and prevent them living life to the full. From that sheltered perspective, lighting up a cigarette for the first time can seem almost like a declaration of independence, a joyous rejection of miserable oppression. A moment so emotionally powerful, in fact, that it almost obliterates the revolting experience of trying to inhale smoke for the first time - as well as installing a thrilling 'anchor' (attached emotion) to the act of smoking that serves as a strong inclination to light another one before long.

It is ironic and sad that such moments serve, in fact, to throw off one yoke only to attach oneself to another even more oppressive one - sometimes for life.

Stage Two: "I'm Not a Kid Anymore!" Tobacco as Contraband

From the age of ten upwards, children gain greater access to tobacco on a regular basis and are also likely to have some money on a regular basis too. It is between ten and sixteen that most people try tobacco for the first time, and it is highly significant that they are not supposed to be doing it. During these years tobacco is contraband, illegal for minors to purchase, and also an illicit possession. History demonstrates beyond doubt that if you want to make something very popular you only have to ban it, and the very prohibition of tobacco for minors provides one of the most powerful inclinations to pick it up. As contraband, it has a significance during these years in a person's life that completely vanishes the moment it becomes legal – but by then the damage is usually done because the habit is established.

In any case, the 'illicit' taint never disappears entirely from tobacco even for adult smokers. There remain lots of places where they are not allowed to do it and there are always some people who forbid it or disapprove. Smoking is often sneakily done - and sneakily shared too, in a conspiratorial way – not just behind the bike sheds at school but often by much older people who are supposed to have quit, or perhaps are just being banished to 'Smoker's Corner' by the non-smoking majority. To smokers themselves, Smoker's Corner can be anything from a haven to a humiliation depending upon how each smoker chooses to look at it, but there is often a certain camaraderie about it. As there usually will be, when humans are united by a common vice. Whilst being judged by the virtuous, we naturally relate better to those who are similarly flawed, judged or misunderstood.

Since tobacco has long been taxed, it has also traditionally been smuggled in order to evade those taxes and this lends it a dark glamour on another level. Black market trading of anything adds the thrill of risk, and the satisfaction of defying authority as well as 'saving' money. For many people this illicit, devious aspect to the trading of tobacco recurs often, from their earliest purchase - some shopkeepers used to sell single cigarettes to minors - to the more recent enthusiasm in the UK for importing large quantities of tobacco and alcohol upon return from foreign trips, and sometimes selling it on. Then there are the 'Booze Cruises', where Brits would nip across the English Channel to France on a ferry, to fill a van with booze and baccy. This last practice I'm sure on some Subconscious level appealed to the imagination, recalling tales of smugglers landing boatloads of barrels on a Cornish beach by moonlight, avoiding the Customs Men ...and even though it is now legal to make these ferry trips, it retains the satisfaction of evading UK tax.

All this creates a recurrent inclination to keep stocking up with large quantities of tobacco in advance – and therefore to keep smoking - because it seems 'canny' or clever. It also reinforces an inclination to regard smoking as some sort of demonstration of independence - a petty rebellion from the start, that never really loses its pettiness nor its unruly message: "I'm not a kid anymore, you can't tell me what to do!" Many smokers will readily admit that in certain circumstances, the very act of lighting up is really just the smoker demonstrating to the world that the world cannot stop them.

Hidden Significance in: Purchase, Possession, Use and Sharing

During adolescence particularly, the purchase, possession, use and sharing of tobacco can be socially significant. A number of important statements are being made, generally to one another but also sometimes directed outwardly at the rest of the world.

<u>Purchase:</u> In adolescence buying tobacco becomes a dare, an opportunity to prove your mettle before your peers. It takes nerve to look a retailer right in the eye and ask for cigarettes when you are obviously too young to buy them. It is also an adrenalin rush, because there is a real risk being taken: not so much a fear of the law, but of the humiliation of being turned down and having to troop shamefacedly out of the shop again in front of your friends. But it can be worth the risk - if you succeed you are a cool dude and your status within the group is strengthened.

For minors, purchase can also be achieved by an illicit route if the tobacco is bought on the black market. Alternatively purchase can be avoided altogether by stealing tobacco and even selling it on. If you think about it, the first few cigarettes smoked by minors will almost certainly have been stolen, often from their parents. So in fact there is a similarity here between obtaining cigarettes and obtaining drugs: before you can smoke, first you have to "score". At the very beginning it is an achievement just to get hold of the contraband, which lends cigarettes a thrill value and significance which creates further inclination to get involved with the whole smoking pantomime. It's a challenge!

<u>Possession:</u> Possession is also a dare, but on a different level. It functions as a *hidden* defiance, a covert rebellion which might be

discovered at any moment. There may be a risk of censure or punishment, interrogation concerning how the contraband was obtained and who should be held responsible. And this brings into the picture a key element in all this for illicit young smokers, the question of trust.

From the age of ten onwards, we are beginning to liberate ourselves from family bonds and begin to negotiate the minefield of wider social relationships. Many will drift away from the control (and security) of parental and school authority, and seek to form new bonds within the peer group. In adolescence we tend to communicate less and less with adults at home or at school, and begin concealing all sorts of things: true likes and dislikes, plans, sexual explorations and contraband of all kinds. It becomes uncool to be on good terms with parents and teachers, and for the next few years the 'coolest' individuals may appear to be the ones with least regard for the values of parents and teachers.

It is a dangerous time for all sorts of reasons, and therefore (it has to be said) rather an exciting time too. Risks are being run, but this also creates strong bonds because information is held by each that could get the other into trouble, and possession of tobacco can function as a demonstration of trust - especially if it is discovered. Once caught in possession of illicit tobacco (and really, what kid hasn't been?) there arises a perfect opportunity to protect a friend, or drop them in it to protect the self. Whose is it? Where did it come from? Who actually bought it? Parents and teachers often miss the true significance of this little melodrama because they are thinking in terms of rules. Young people don't mind much what rules they've broken and they certainly do not worry, at that stage, that tobacco could kill them decades later, but they care very much what their friends think of them.

<u>Use:</u> The actual use of tobacco in early adolescence has significance only in terms of the *drama* of it. Physically it is completely useless, as the ordinary young smoker knows perfectly well at the time. Very few kids will ever smoke alone, unless they are practising how to do it. The main point is to be seen doing it, and for the message that conveys to

be the right message. Virtually every adult smoker will readily acknowledge that the first time they breathed in tobacco smoke they found it a revolting experience and it made them feel ill. So it must be recognised clearly that the inclinations to smoke that get people started have absolutely nothing to do with the way it makes you feel, and therefore nothing to do with nicotine at all.

This clearly separates tobacco smoking from all forms of drug use. People start smoking for reasons *other than* the way tobacco makes them feel and continue doing it in spite of the effects of nicotine, not because of them. Smoking has a meaning - or a series of meanings - and the early inclinations to adopt smoking behaviour are really related to these. These meanings are clearly compelling enough in many people to overcome the natural *disinclination* to inhale a cloud of toxic gases, which is exactly what tobacco smoke is. Also important enough at the time to allow new smokers to tolerate the nausea that the poison nicotine causes them to experience, as well as the effects of carbon monoxide and other poisons in the smoke, for long enough for the whole sorry business to accidentally become habitual. Some people drop it before that of course, but it is truly astonishing how many of us did not.

<u>Sharing:</u> The sharing of tobacco as a bonding ritual is something virtually all smokers are aware of, and easily able to use - even with a complete stranger - as a focus or trigger for small talk, or in the case of males, to comfortably avoid small talk. But we all started out sharing cigarettes, and those early experiences of passing a cigarette back and forth are quite an intimate bonding experience, since we were actually passing the soggy, smouldering thing from one mouth to another.

Later, sharing is more likely to involve giving away whole cigarettes rather than passing one back and forth, so cigarettes then also become a currency: something you advance one day, then call the debt back in due course. This currency circulates only among smokers and consequently the trading of comments and conversation too will often exclude non-smokers. In any youthful peer group, the 'coolest' individuals are likely to be the least obedient where authority is concerned, and also the toughest and most daring. They are highly likely to be smokers too, largely because of that. Other adolescents who are not that influencial - and not that tough - usually wish they were, and may feel uncomfortable about being excluded from that social group or marginalised by it. If you are going to join it, or attempt to join it, you have to mirror the behaviour of the movers and shakers within the group, and this is the real 'appeal' of tobacco at this point in a person's life.

None of this has anything to do with nicotine, the contents of the smoke or the direct effect of inhaling it. It's just that taking up smoking kills several birds with one stone. We hope it will make us look older, tougher, less like a kid and more like the cool guys, which may lead to us being accepted by them, which is of course safer than not being accepted.

These matters are very important at the time. Years later, these buttons can be pushed again at any time, in any smoker, and tobacco used to defuse a tense moment, advance a favour, reconcile, or just find a level of recognition.

It is true that just occasionally in therapy we encounter new 'reasons' for starting smoking that we do not usually hear. Some of these are surprising and amusing, like the slightly-built Asian gentleman who explained that his wife bullied him into smoking cigarettes during the 1970s because other men were doing it: "Be a man!" she said, "Start smoking!" Nowadays this seems incredible, even mad - but she may have been uncomfortable about other women's opinions of her man, and concerned to make him appear more macho. A couple of decades later, she exercised the woman's prerogative of changing her mind, and began to nag him to stop again.

Then there are the unusual reasons for starting that break your heart, like the chain-smoking woman in her late sixties who told me that she started when she was six, smoking rolled-up newspaper that she lit from the coal fire when she was alone. She had heard someone say it was relaxing and made you feel better, and she hoped it would help.

She was being sexually and physically abused by her father, a violent drunken bully who terrorised the whole family.

Even in the above cases, it is noticeable that the smoking behaviour starts *as a response to suggestion*, and that suggestion comes from others. In fact this is always the case, but for most smokers the circumstances were more ordinary and familiar to the majority.

Stage Three: Something's Changed

Let us put aside all the social factors now, and look at what changed physically in the course of becoming an habitual smoker. The first time we attempt to inhale smoke, it is because we made a conscious decision to try it. The instant it hits the airways, the Subconscious identifies that this is not air but smoke, and violently objects - using the reflexes of coughing, choking and retching to reject the smoke and dissuade us from attempting that again. This is unpleasant of course, but we know that if we persist, we too can probably learn to casually breathe smoke in and out as if it was no big deal, because we have seen other people overcome this obstacle fairly easily.

If we persist in trying to inhale smoke, it is not long before the Subconscious mind – which is intelligent of course – comes to the conclusion that the daft little conscious mind is going to keep trying to perform this stunt anyway, no matter how much resistance the Subconscious kicks up, so it drops the objection since it is simply being ignored. Then it adjusts the reflexes so that this particular type of smoke can be tolerated from that point onwards. Any other type of smoke would still trigger the coughing reflex if inhaled. This is why cigarette smokers would struggle to smoke a pipe, or their first cigar; it is not quite the same thing and they would have to get used to that also if they wanted to develop the ability to do it comfortably, i.e. without Subconscious objection.

The Voluntary Phase

So off we go, we have learned how to breathe smoke in and out without coughing. Another rite of passage and another string to our bow. But we do not have a problem yet because we don't have a habit yet, that takes a little longer to develop. At the beginning – and many smokers will remember this – there is a voluntary period, during which we can take it or leave it. We don't actually like the smoke or the way it leaves us feeling queasy and faint, we are just doing it for all those other reasons really but the fact that we can freely take it or leave it lulls us into a false sense of security at first, because we think it will always be that way. We assume we will be easily able to drop it at any time, and during this phase we could. But it doesn't last long.

In truth the length of time for which smoking remains voluntary will vary from one person to another, depending upon their other routines at that time. In school years it might last for weeks or even months, depending upon how regularly smoking episodes occur. Sporadic smoking episodes are the norm at first, so stopping and starting is both commonplace and quite easy during this phase. This unfortunately adds to the false sense of security amongst these smokers, and they may be particularly puzzled later, when it eventually becomes a habit, as to why they now find it hard to stop because they always found it easy enough to stop and start before. As a contrasting example, anyone who started smoking shortly after starting a new job because their colleagues were regular smokers will find that they quickly fall into regular daily habit too, because the smoking patterns in work situations are likely to be more regimented than they ever are at school.

In just a few cases, a regular habit never develops because no pattern is ever established for the Subconscious to repeat. Smoking will remain voluntary for as long as this remains the case.

The First Inclinations to Smoke are Not Cravings

Question: What prompts a person to smoke the first cigarette, what is their motivation? Obviously not anything in the smoke because they have not consumed any yet. So it isn't nicotine. And it follows that if it is not any need for nicotine which motivates them to smoke the first cigarette - which it cannot be, obviously - then we should certainly not assume it must be any need or desire for nicotine which motivates them to smoke the second, or the sixth, or the seventeenth, or the thirty-third. Why can't it be the same motivation that caused them to smoke the first one? In fact it is very likely to be exactly that. Why should they need new, extra reasons?

Later on, the whole process becomes habit-driven and that is when the reminder signal (craving) comes into the picture, but cravings are absent from the initial stages of getting accustomed to tobacco. There may be any number of reasons for adopting the smoking behaviour in the first place, and obviously nicotine itself is not one of them, otherwise schoolkids would be sneaking nicotine gum, patches and lozenges into school along with the cigs, because those could be used *during* lessons, and without the giveaway smell, too. But you would never hear a teacher saying: "Turn out your pockets, sonny – and you'd better take your shirt off too, so I can check you for patches..."

No, that is never going to happen. Neither will there ever be a bunch of kids behind the bike sheds passing around a box of nicotine patches or a nasal spray. The possession of tobacco has rebellious significance for schoolchildren, as does the act of smoking – but what fourteen-year-old wants to be seen wearing patches? What kind of devil-may-care performance is that? Nicotine itself is of no significance whatsoever to the teenager because even when they do smoke cigarettes they are not 'taking nicotine', they are acting out the smoking behaviour and its associated performances – with attitude of course – exactly as they have seen others do for years. It later becomes a Compulsive Habit by the same automatic learning process by which anything else becomes a Compulsive Habit. There is no drug involved.

During the voluntary phase there are no cravings, although there may well be inclinations to light up a cigarette sometimes. There may also be disinclinations. The smoke is very unpleasant but we gradually get used to it, and slowly begin to feel more comfortable with the new activity because we know that we are in conscious control of it, we could drop it if we chose. During this time there may be days when we don't smoke at all, and we would not worry about running out of cigarettes, it doesn't matter. We have no sense of 'needing a ready supply' at this point. However, this phase does not last long, because all we are really doing at this time is making conscious decisions about when, where and why we smoke. There is no clear pattern at first, but gradually a pattern emerges and eventually we have made all those decisions, and we are just repeating and repeating the same behaviour in the same situations.

The brain notices this. It is very good at spotting patterns. At some point it arrives at this conclusion: "We don't need the conscious mind involved in this anymore - there is nothing to think about, is there? We've got all the information now, there is nothing new developing anymore. It's the same routine every day... we can do this on autopilot." So the Subconscious takes over direction of the smoking behaviour for us because it has become predictable. In fact everything that we learn to do and then repeat regularly will go through this process of *becoming second nature.*

This does not mean that all behaviour that becomes second nature will become a Compulsive Habit, of course not. But it does mean that the behaviour can then be effortlessly directed by the Subconscious without conscious thinking being necessary, whether it is noticeably compulsive or not.

Now your conscious mind does not realise it at the time, but it just lost control of that behaviour to the Subconscious. The conscious mind doesn't understand that because it thinks it controls everything, thanks to the way we were educated in the first place – as if the Subconscious does not exist. Your conscious mind is still able to direct voluntary smoking behaviour *as well* – in other words you can still light up a cigarette according to a conscious whim. You can always do that, you could at the start. But once you have drifted past this point of it being taken over by the Subconscious, becoming second nature, conscious decisions or conscious efforts to stop it or change it usually have little or no effect, or only temporary effect. This is because the Subconscious does not know about the new conscious decision, and conscious efforts (willpower) can only repress the behaviour temporarily.

N.B. Recognition of the initial *voluntary* phase of smoking has virtually disappeared in recent years due to the relentlessly determined promotion of the idea of 'nicotine addiction'. Yet once mentioned, nearly all smokers remember it – giving the lie to the mythical concept of "one cigarette and you are hooked".

Most smokers and ex-smokers will remember, if they think back to their earliest smoking experiences, having the same packet of cigarettes for days on end, without actually smoking at all on some of those days - when it was all about opportunity and secrecy, and hiding cigarettes away. When it wasn't so easy to buy them, so the ones you already had were hoarded like precious contraband. And of course sometimes you did not have any at all – were you climbing the walls, beset by desperate cravings? No, it was no big deal.

Having said that, I do remember kids at school *pretending* they were "gasping" for a cigarette, but this was only because they had heard adults talking like that and thought it sounded suitably dramatic. Young people love being dramatic, teenagers especially. The whole smoking business is copying anyway: monkey see monkey do. Monkey hear monkey repeat. Gasping for a smoke? Of course you are son – you must have smoked at least ten cigarettes in the last four days. You must be in a state of terrible deprivation! Couldn't wait to get out of that maths lesson this afternoon, could you, and get round the back of the gym for your second cigarette of the day. It's been hours since you had one while waiting for the bus to school.

In fact I think I knew that adolescent 'gasping for a smoke' performance was bullshit even when I was thirteen. I certainly never felt like that, and I'd been smoking cigarettes on and off since I was eight. I didn't enjoy the smoke in any respect, I was only doing it because I wasn't allowed to and because it was all part of the act – trying to look older and tougher than I actually was.

Voluntary Phase Ends: Now it becomes a Compulsive Habit

Habit because it fits the pattern you have programmed in through repetition on a daily basis, which is why it must become a regular routine before the voluntary phase is concluded.

Compulsive because what the Subconscious now very helpfully does, is to wait until one of those situations arises where you would usually reach for a cigarette, and then send you a nudge: *Time for a cigarette! Isn't it? Nudge!* That is a craving. It is a signal from the Subconscious mind to remind you when to light cigarettes so you never have to think about it again for the rest of your life. It is supposed to be for your convenience, ironically. Indeed it *is* convenient, until you make a new conscious decision to change the behaviour.

'Social' Smokers

A minority of smokers develop habits that are not daily, but a response to certain circumstances. They may not have developed a regular pattern of smoking in the usual sense, yet they exhibit predictable smoking behaviour on special occasions or perhaps on a Saturday night out. Their Subconscious is responding to the circumstances in which they have smoked before, but ignoring other situations where they have not. Contrary to the assumptions of regular daily smokers, these so-called "social smokers" are not strong-willed or 'controlling' their smoking behaviour, they simply have no urge to reach for tobacco at any other time. It is still a compulsive habit, and it could yet develop into more frequent smoking quite easily at any time. Or it may not.

Craving? Impulse? Urge? Temptation? It is really just a Prompt

Cravings have been the cause of all the confusion and the misinformation about smoking because they have wrongly been identified as withdrawal symptoms – which they are not – and linked to nicotine, which they have nothing to do with at all, except in the sense that most smokers may *believe* they are linked, which would account for the mild placebo effect of NRT *and* the slightly-raised placebo effect of NRT products in scientific trials compared to control placebos which do not contain nicotine. Since any smoker may recognise the presence of nicotine in any product, their belief that nicotine is the thing they require may soothe their agitation at the thought of being 'deprived', obviously. This may not relieve their tensions indefinitely, but it is likely to be more effective than a product that seemed to have no nicotine-presence – unless of course an even more reassuring suggestion was attached to that one.

In reality we are all very familiar with cravings. We get lots of cravings, they are not all about tobacco. They are signals from the Subconscious mind to the conscious mind, usually reminding us when to do something but they can also be suggesting that it 'might be nice' or it 'might be useful' to carry out the habitual behaviour now, based upon current Subconscious beliefs and expectations. The main cause of the misunderstanding about cravings is that although they originate from the Subconscious mind, and are controlled by it, they are *experienced* in the body, causing a conscious impression that they are genuine bodily needs. They are not, but it can be a very convincing impression.

Cravings Are Annoying

The most unwelcome attribute of cravings is that they are irritating. Actually that is what makes craving signals so effective: they need to be unsettling and difficult to ignore, because the signal has to *distract* us from what we were focusing on consciously – just long enough to realise what we should do next – and also *prompt* us to do something other than what we were already doing. So the signal has to have the same quality as someone tapping you on the shoulder - it's annoying, but it gets your attention.

Any craving signal can be very difficult to ignore, and may wind you up progressively if you try not to respond. If at any point you do respond, the prompting nudge immediately ceases - relief! But if you don't, the signals get more insistent and persist for longer... eventually making you feel distracted, irritable and tense. You start to become snappy and unreasonable.

How We Shut Down Cravings

It is easy to see why smokers so readily accept the notion that this indicates a desperate need for a fix, but really it is simply what results from trying to ignore irritating reminder signals. The longer you actually put up with this before you finally respond, the greater the relief when the irritation stops. This creates the illusion that the event of 'lighting a cigarette' brings peace, relaxation and a feeling of relief. In reality the cigarette did no such thing, it was just that you finally responded to the reminder signal, so it shut off and that is why peace of mind returned.

If you turn a key to shut off an alarm, it is not the action of turning the key that brings peace, but it can certainly seem that way. It is the fact of the alarm no longer irritating. The same thing happens if you cut the power, the key isn't even needed. (Scratch that last suggestion, if you have criminal tendencies. I was hoping it would serve as a useful metaphor for the Subconscious shutting down the craving signals in hypnotherapy. The 'key' is the cigarette, that really isn't needed... ok, lousy metaphor. Of course we don't want to suggest that the cigarette is the 'key' in any respect, as peace returns. Anyway, The Subconscious Has The Power, that's the point. And let that be a warning to all of us, about the off-hand use of metaphor: it can turn out to be the sort of mixed message that blows up right in your face. Never be tempted to just risk it, without thinking it all through careful beforehand. I'll recover, and carry on just as if that never happened, but you might not be so lucky. Think on.)

Now although smokers often tend to interpret that prompting signal as a *desire to smoke,* actually it is not. It is a compulsive urge to light up – or to begin rolling up, in the case of handrolling smokers and habitual cannabis users. For the ordinary cigarette smoker the impulse peters out as soon as they light up, which can sometimes leave them wondering what they are smoking it for. But since it is already paid for, and lit... their general assumption is that they 'might as well' smoke it. Some people put the cigarette out half-way through, but they cannot help feeling they are 'wasting' half of it - as if it would be making better use of it to inhale more of the smoke!

The word "craving" is wrong really because it implies need, and this is actually a prompting signal, not a true need. But it *feels like a need*, and that is what has caused the misinterpretation. So it is common to hear people say "I need a drink", "I need a cigarette" or "I need something to eat now", because the signals are annoying and distracting. They disturb our peace of mind, and we naturally feel that we 'need' to act out the usual habitual behaviour in order to restore that peace of mind.

Still we do not have to respond, we are not robots. However, the habitual smoker quickly learns that if they go ahead and light a cigarette, the irritating signal will go away and stop irritating them. It has done its job, it is just a signal. But if they do not respond – for whatever reason – they will get another signal. And if they keep ignoring them, the signals will first come more frequently and then get more annoying. The lack of response is noted by the Subconscious, which assumes the conscious mind hasn't noticed so it sends a stronger signal. Apparently the conscious mind needs MORE DISTRACTION! It must be busy or something.

So the Subconscious will keep on doing that automatically, and with increasing intensity until it drives you up the wall.

Resistance is Useless!

Well, not quite useless - I just like that expression because when I was kid I enjoyed watching old movies about World War II in which German officers frequently say: "Resistance is useless!"

With regard to the idea that smokers should be able to quit by toughing it out simply by an effort of conscious will, we might more commonly remark that "Old habits die hard". But for a realistic impression of just how useless conscious resistance to cravings would normally be, see: *The Willpower Myth* in Section 12, Volume II. There's a clue in the title.

Who Needs a Cloud of Poisonous Gases?

So it is not a need in reality – what you are really up against when you try to quit smoking the hard way is an automatic reminder system controlled by the Subconscious mind. It is reminding you about all sorts of things throughout the day, it isn't only directing the smoking habit. Craving signals can be vague – such as hunger - or they can be highly specific: a person can get a craving for a biscuit, for example. A *chocolate* one... and if there isn't a chocolate one, those plain ones just won't do at all! Now that is very specific, as signals go. And obviously the body never *needs* a chocolate biscuit.

Actually this is a very important point. Where's that TV psychologist - can we just get this quite clear? The overwhelming impulse to go against the conscious mind's resolutions and eat something like that is *not* an example of "the body telling you it needs a chocolate biscuit". This is the Subconscious mind simply suggesting to the conscious mind: "Wouldn't we rather be eating a chocolate biscuit right now?" It doesn't put it into words, but images, memories and feelings.

This is a mental process, and it has nothing to do with the contents of the biscuit or the effect upon the body of consuming that. And you may have noticed – those of you who ever signed up to some diet programme that did not include chocolate biscuits – if you were normally partial to a biscuit, those signals came along anyway, did they not? That is because it was your conscious mind that decided to go on a diet, your Subconscious signed up to nothing. It is completely unaware of this new restriction or the reasons for it. But it quickly notices the change in the usual routine. "Hey, what happened to chocolate biscuits all of a sudden?" thinks the Subconscious, and starts prompting the conscious mind with tempting distraction signals aimed at locating the object of desire. "Daft little conscious mind," thinks the Subconscious, " it gets all wrapped up in that work stuff, and worrying about money or what other people think – fancy forgetting all about chocolate biscuits for *days!* Good thing I'm here to remind it. Life isn't all about work, now is it?"

I'm being playful of course. The Subconscious probably does not muse about it in that way, it simply pursues its own aims. It does not concern itself with resolves and reasonings of the conscious mind at all, because it knows nothing of them. These are separate mental departments just doing their own thing.

The Imagination is brought into play of course, in the Subconscious' pursuit of its aim: daydreams of chocolate, fantasies, memories and even recall of taste causing salivation. This sort of 'longing' process can also happen to some degree in people who are using willpower to try not to smoke - although it is likely to be a bit less sensual because the experience of smoke is not actually pleasant in any way. Nevertheless, the Imagination is powerful enough to make it seem so, and of course link it to memories of good times to make you feel as if you are really missing something. It can bring emotions into play too: feelings of desolation, deprivation and yearnings. Your Subconscious certainly knows how to motivate you, and the poor little conscious mind really has its work cut out trying to resist all this pressure. Physical sensations can be created in the body, too. Smokers who have tried to quit with willpower alone sometimes report feeling tightness or similar sensations in the chest, anxiety feelings, or a strange 'lump in the throat' experience. Not all smokers have feelings like this when they try not to smoke, but they are common enough.

Why should the Subconscious go to such lengths to pursue something it originally tried to reject? Because now the aim is different. When we first attempt to inhale smoke the Subconscious aim is simply to protect the body using reflexes. To overrule that, we had to make repeated conscious efforts to inhale, which is hardly the fault of the Subconscious. Having forced the Subconscious to abandon that position, a different section of that mental department later adopted a new aim, of helping us to repeat a now-predictable action without us having to think consciously about it. Unaware of any subsequent conscious decisions to stop smoking, it pursues its current aim – to repeat the smoking activity at the appropriate moments – with everything in its arsenal. So if it aims to do that by creating the impression that you are really missing something, it can do that very convincingly.

In reality though "smoke inhalation" is something for which people are treated in hospital. If you were rescued from a house fire, you may well be carted off for life-saving treatment for smoke inhalation, with an oxygen mask strapped to your face. The truly bizarre fact is, some of the dedicated medical staff who treat you might later go on a break and nip around the back of the hospital to engage in a bit of mindless smoke inhalation themselves.

I wonder: if any of them are *bogus* doctors, do they have to *pretend* to feel awkward about the contradiction?

<u>So Cravings really have nothing to do with Need at all, then?</u>

No. But when the Subconscious creates an illusion it can be very convincing. Remember those dreams that can bring people to orgasm, or make them wake up screaming? Look at phobias. Look at phantom limb pain - the experience of real pain in a limb which is no longer there. Don't underestimate the Subconscious mind's ability to convince you of something which is not actually real at all. Look at the differing religions, with their millions of devotees: can't all be right, can they? Yet many of them utterly believe that they are, right down to their very soul. Even to the point of blowing themselves up on a crowded train, apparently.

How deluded do you have to be to feel the 'need' to do that, eh?

No more deluded than to lay down your life for 'King and Country', despite the fact 'the Royals' were originally German anyway, which really confuses the issue in the First World War particularly, if you think about it in any depth. And here's a rather amusing historical fact: centuries ago many European commoners believed that their illnesses could be cured by "The Royal Touch". If they could only get the ruling monarch to touch them, they would be healed. The challenging bit was to figure out how to get the monarch to go anywhere near them.

<u>Yet it can Work!</u>

Providing the *belief* is real enough, we now know that the effect can be real enough, but the monarch's role is only symbolic in reality. The King's touch is only truly significant in the imagination of the commoner. It is the notion that the monarch has Divine Right to rule – is chosen by God – and therefore it is indirectly a Divine Touch, that is what makes it more significant than being touched by the Mayor or the doctor. Exactly the same thing happens with faith healing, but the hypnotherapist would argue that it is the Subconscious that does the healing, not Jesus or the Holy Spirit. Yet when the healer claims that the follower was healed *by their faith,* of course he is right. Also it has to be something the Subconscious can actually fix, or it doesn't work. Unless it is a real miracle, I suppose. Some of these faith healers are bogus, of course – but so are some doctors. Doesn't mean they all are, does it? Unless you don't believe in doctors.

Even today thousands of people believe they will be healed if they are blessed by the Pope, for exactly the same reason: God's representative on Earth. The fact that he was once Hitler's little representative on a much more local basis does not trouble them because Christians have this wonderful notion of forgiveness, which means you do have the right to make mistakes as long as you are sorry later and do something to make up for it. And I suppose going so far as to become Pope is making up for it in style. In terms of the outfit, that is definitely an upgrade from the uniform of the Hitler Youth. They didn't have robes, did they? That would have been contrary to the ideology. And they weren't big on forgiveness either. Or loving their neighbour. In fact they were more likely to get their neighbour arrested by the Gestapo.

Some people honestly believe that if they don't touch the light switch thirty two times before they open the door, they cannot leave the room. Or that if you possess an ornament in the shape of an elephant it is unlucky. Or if you open an umbrella indoors. If someone puts shoes on the table. If the fridge is facing the dishwasher there is a 'need' to change that, because the energies are not properly balanced. Or something. Humans are imaginative creatures, and the imagination sometimes doesn't know when to stop. Left to itself, that is. That's why I keep going off on these little historical and mildly philosophical diversions. But look! Here we are back at the point:

No 'Need' to Light Up at all

Just to get rid of this idea of 'need' completely – because this is a real red herring in the matter of tobacco smoking, which has led to the addiction theory and also added to the myth of the "addictive personality" - here is another example of a reminder signal you will probably recognise. Not all these signals are about *consuming things,* you see:

If you decide you are going out for the day, and you lock up the house because there is no-one else in... then you suddenly realise, just as you pass through the gate, that you don't remember locking the back door... What do you do? Do you carry on with your journey regardless, or do you go back and check?

Almost every time, you will go back and check – even if you are late, and it is really inconvenient, because even though you know that you probably did lock it, you don't want this reminder signal bothering you all day long because it will ruin your peace of mind. So you trudge back and take a look: yep, sure enough it's locked. That clears it, and you will not be troubled by the reminder again that day.

So we get many of these familiar prompts and signals from the Subconscious throughout the day: so that we don't have to think consciously about every little thing we do regularly, we get a little *nudge* when it's time to take care of that, or just to make sure we haven't forgotten it. These signals are meant to be useful, they can be annoying and they can easily become attached to something which *later on* turns out to be terribly dangerous: like tobacco, like alcohol or gambling. These things are often called addictions – they are not, they are compulsive habits. And although they are notoriously hard to break with willpower, they are really rather easy to change with hypnotherapy especially if there are no complications. This is because the problematic behaviour is not outside that person's control at all, only outside their *conscious* control. Their Subconscious is controlling it fine, and has no idea they want to change it.

Or why. You see, everything you ever learned about why it is not a good idea to smoke, gamble, take drugs or drink too much *you learned from the outside world,* either in conversation with other people, via the media or through a process of education. The Subconscious ordinarily pays scant attention to such things, it has stuff to do. Under ordinary circumstances it trusts the conscious mind to deal with The World Out There, so all that important information was absorbed by the conscious mind, not the Subconscious. All the conscious mind can do with that information is worry about it. And make the occasional big conscious effort to change the habitual behaviour, which usually makes little long-term difference. Or try to ignore it completely by focusing on other matters, which it does most of the time – out of necessity really, we don't want to drive ourselves mad with fear by worrying about the consequences of smoking every minute of the day. Besides, the conscious mind tends to reason that it probably won't happen anyway... because so far, it hasn't... let's not dwell on the 'logic' of that one for too long.

This is why the *trance* part of a hypnotherapy session must – this is an absolute necessity - include plenty of information that the conscious mind knows already about the damage smoke can do to the body. Details like that should never be included in the pre-talk, because that is just patronising. The conscious mind would normally feel insulted by yet another lecture on the dangers of smoking. But the Subconscious needs some stark facts so that it can get the priorities right immediately.

It is also a very good idea to explain the necessity for this beforehand to the conscious mind. Remember that during the trance part of the session the conscious mind never really lets go of the idea that the therapist is still talking to *it*. The whole idea of the Subconscious is vaguely mythical to the conscious mind, and so it helps if the client has been advised beforehand that almost everything the therapist says during the trance part of the session is information the conscious mind already knows. Therefore the client should not be surprised if there are occasionally conscious thoughts along the lines of "I know all this, I've said all this to myself many times. I don't see what difference this is going to make!" That is just the conscious mind not realising that the therapist is actually talking to the Subconscious, and that part of the mind does *not* already know this, or not much of it anyway.

This way we can avoid creating a state of annoyance and resentment during the trance section. No-one likes to be patronised, and we want to get the mood right. The more the client understands hypnotherapy, the easier it is to get the mood and the response correct.

The Craving is the Key: but not the whole story

Shutting down the craving signals is the thing that makes hypnotherapy the only truly effortless way to stop smoking. But if we simply did that, and did not attend to all the other factors in play: the habit pattern and its relation to other daily routines, the beliefs and myths that support the habit and, crucially, the way the smoker feels about tobacco, hypnotherapy and the prospect of stopping smoking – permanent cessation would not be the usual outcome. It is highly likely that any scientific trials of hypnotherapy that achieved poor results were not attending to these matters. In other words it was lousy therapy conducted by people whose understanding of the art of hypnotherapy was primitive, or even wrong.

For the Subconscious, shutting down cravings is as easy as blinking and it already switches them off regularly anyway. Every night when you go to sleep, for a start - you don't need tobacco but you do need your sleep, the Subconscious isn't going to wake you up over it. But that's not all. The fact is, it shuts them down many times during the day too. Just consider now:

When Cravings Shut Down Simply For Your Convenience

Smoking has long been banned in certain places and most smokers have adjusted to this easily. When the smoker goes somewhere where they know they can't smoke, because nobody can – provided they *accept* that restriction because they need to be there anyway (i.e. they do not choose to resent it), then the reminder signal will not bother them while they are there – even if they are in that situation for hours.

So when smokers are travelling on aeroplanes, trains or buses, most of them find they are not bothered by the restriction and only get the reminder signal when they get off, or when they realise they will soon be getting off. Likewise when they enter cinemas or hospitals – all enclosed public places are now smoke-free in many countries – the majority of smokers are able to comfortably adjust. What is actually happening is this: as they walk into the restricted situation, the Subconscious mind registers that there is *no smoking opportunity here*, so the reminder system is shut down. If an opportunity presents itself, or as soon as they leave the situation of course the reminder signal kicks in again, but it will not usually bother them while they are there.

The Storm before the Calm

The arguments in many countries recently about banning smoking in public places can become quite a heated debate at times. Non-smokers are concerned about their health, and people who believe they are nicotine addicts or even believe they are smoking out of choice are concerned about their "freedom" to smoke.

In reality, this is all nonsense. We had the same fuss about crash helmets being made compulsory, and seatbelt laws being introduced. I can remember seeing big demonstrations by motorbikers on television, vowing to defy the law and claiming that biking would never be the same again. When wearing seatbelts in cars was made compulsory people claimed they would defy that too. Critics predicted it could never be policed, or that the courts would be jammed with thousands of ordinary people rebelling and protesting - willing to go to jail for the noble right to go flying through the windscreen in the event of a collision. A few weeks later everybody calmed down and got used to the idea, realising the obvious sense in organising things so that unnecessary harm is averted.

People just don't like being told what to do, that's all it is. They were not already *in the habit* of wearing seatbelts or crash helmets. It's not about freedom, it is all about what you are used to. Cigarettes got banned on buses, smokers moaned and boycotted the buses for two days then calmed down and got over it, and their habits adjusted in next to no time. As soon as the Subconscious catches on that the bus is no longer a smoking opportunity, which doesn't take long at all (about a week for most people, if they use the bus every day) then it no longer sends the reminder signals while they are on the bus. Easy.

Nothing More Than Feelings

How the smoker *chooses to feel* about this new situation can be quite significant though. Most smokers are actually quite laid-back about these things - once they get used to the idea - and although they may moan amongst themselves for a week or two, they soon get bored with that and simply adjust. Then it never really bothers them again, just like the crash helmets and the seatbelts in fact. Yet there will always be a few uptight, irritable and resentful smokers who will nurse and cultivate their resentment for ages, boycott restricted places and struggle to cope with the ones they cannot avoid, join the pro-smoking lobby and look for every little bit of evidence that smokers are being discriminated against - as if 'The Smoker' were a species, and the whole world was against them.

Actually *those* individuals already thought the whole world was against them, or they were against it, or at least any part of it that did not agree with them. To defend smoking in the name of freedom is laughable because habitual smokers are not *choosing* to smoke, not since it became a compulsive habit anyway. Smoking is no longer something they *do* but something they cannot help doing, just like nail-biting. They just prefer to tell themselves that they are choosing to smoke, when in reality they are smoking whether they choose to or not.

If you know a person like this, challenge them. Say to them: "OK, you say you are choosing to smoke, simply because you want to. That implies you could just as easily choose not to, so just to *prove* that, choose not to for a couple of months and then we will actually take you and all this stuff about freedom seriously."

whine on about their "freedom to smoke" sound like some Broadmoor Prison Hospital saying "Oh no, I'm not in prison! I'm not really locked up because I am a dangerous nutcase, no, I just like it here. I could leave anytime I want to, but I *enjoy* Broadmoor, there's so many interesting people to talk to. I may choose to stay here forever, I haven't quite decided yet."

Smokers are no different from anyone else, nobody likes being told what to do. Motorbikers didn't like being told to wear helmets when they were used to pleasing themselves, but how many bikers complain now? Nobody liked being threatened with a fine if they didn't have a seat belt on, but they soon got over it. Now it is just an automatic thing, you just belt up without giving it a second thought. Drivers don't pause to think: "Dammit, what about my freedom?" It was the same with smoking on buses and trains - how many smokers are bothered about that now? It will be the same in all the other public places once everyone has got used to the idea.

Tobacco smoking has had its day. It has been steadily going out of fashion for half a century, and if compulsive habits and hypnotherapy had been properly understood by the public during all that time, it would be gone already. Tobacco smoke is not just a threat to the smoker, but everyone in the room. This isn't about freedom, it is simply a matter of safety like the other examples I listed. Nobody likes being told what to do, but as soon as everybody has got used to the idea, most people are really not bothered at all. That shouldn't take more than a week or two.

Never mind all that: How does *therapy* get rid of the cravings?

With ridiculous ease, actually. First we explain all the details to that part of the mind – not the conscious mind, which usually doesn't believe any of this - and then we simply ask the Subconscious mind if it would kindly shut down the reminder signals – just as it does at night, and in lots of other ordinary situations - but this time permanently. The Subconscious mind is usually quite happy to do that. If you remember, your Subconscious didn't want you to inhale the smoke in the first place, so it is generally delighted to hear the news that you don't want to do that any longer, and keen to adjust anything to make that change easy for you.

If you look at it from the Subconscious mind's point of view - quite apart from all the health issues involved - shutting down the smoking habit means one less thing to bother with every day. It is actually easier for the Subconscious not to send the signals than it is to send them, so we are in fact saving it a task.

Interlude: Case Mysteries No.5

Why should this all be about smoking? Let's go wild and talk about something else for a little while. Of all the issues I deal with in hypnotherapy, getting rid of phobias is one of my favourites and right back when I started doing therapy, my second ever client I think it was, had a fear of water that had blighted her life for 35 years. She was unable even to splash water on her face, or put her head under a shower. She certainly couldn't swim, and it spoiled every seaside holiday for her. We got rid of it completely in three sessions, which is not bad for a beginner.

Nowadays I can usually wipe out specific phobias in a single session and I particularly like doing flying phobia sessions - partly because I used to be a bit uncomfortable about flying myself. I think a lot of people are, they just don't find it disturbing to the extent that it shows. I certainly didn't have a full-blown phobia but I felt pretty edgy about the whole thing and didn't look forward to getting on a plane. I looked forward to getting off, in fact.

Now I find the whole thing thrilling. I've never had any therapy myself to correct it, it's just that I've conducted so many flying phobia sessions that it has rubbed off on me, as suggestion will, and now I am not remotely bothered and really enjoy flying. Of course I still have that tiny thought, as I board the plane: "Will it be okay, or are we all about to die?" but I think that is just natural curiosity. I certainly do not feel afraid. I love the take off. I even quite enjoy the landing, which was the part I especially didn't like before - that bumping and screeching bit, followed by the unconvincing application of braking systems that seemed to hardly slow the plane at all at first... it was all a bit too real for me. But now I just relish the madness, and assume that somebody, somewhere knows what they're doing.

Incidentally that is not a suggestion I would use in therapy.

CASE MYSTERIES 5: THE WOMAN WHO CAME FOR AN ARGUMENT

These interludes, these "Case Mysteries" are really all about what happens in a session that does not result in immediate success, and I'm sure this will be the briefest and most obvious example of what *not* to do when you pop along to see the hypnotherapist. It is the case of:

<u>The Woman Who Just Came For An Argument, Apparently</u>

Now, despite the Pythonesque title, I wouldn't want you to think that there were any raised voices in this session. In fact it was all very proper and reasonable, so I had no reason to suspect, during the session itself, that there might be a problem, especially since flying phobias are one of my specialities. The woman in question - let's call her Coco, why the hell not? - seemed doubtful about all the things I was explaining to her, but there is nothing unusual about that. I do not explain things in order to convince people – only a successful result will do that. I explain things so that later they will have some idea what really took place, and also to help them to respond properly right away, though not all choose to do that.

You can lead a horse to water, as the old saying goes, but you cannot make it drink. Likewise you can explain to people how best to respond during the trance part of the session, but you cannot make them respond in that way. One of the things I make very clear to my clients is that later, when I talk to their Subconscious mind I will be putting forward lots of useful suggestions for consideration, and it will consider them. Then it will do what it bloody well likes but in deciding what that should be, one of the things the Subconscious will take into account is how the client apparently feels about those suggestions, how much enthusiasm there seems to be for the changes being suggested.

This is something the client can actually manipulate in their own favour. The hypnotherapist does not control that factor, but the client can, because we humans can adopt any attitude we like to what we are hearing. For example, we could choose to listen with indifference. We could choose to listen with amusement, or just about any other attitude we prefer. Here's the mood that works best: enthusiasm! So I invite the client to look forward - with natural enthusiasm - to being rid of the problem, and to welcome all suggestions along those lines with enthusiasm: "Great! That'll do for me, that's exactly what I came here for! That will suit me down to the ground!" That is the emotional attitude to adopt.

But of course if I didn't mention that, that is not what most people would do. A few might, because some people are just naturally enthusiastic people and that is how they approach everything. But most people are a bit more cautious than that and what they would probably do - if I didn't mention attitude at all - is sit on the fence emotionally, waiting to see if 'it' works before getting all excited about it. But that is not *responding*, that is *waiting*. And there is no 'it' - 'it' is the client. Nothing is changing while the client is *waiting* for something to come along and change them, and the Subconscious is less likely to act upon suggestions for which there is no apparent enthusiasm. Fence-sitting produces no successful change in any field, and hypnotherapy is no exception.

Since I explain this clearly to every client, you might think - since these people are paying good money for my advice and help, and since they apparently understand plain English - that they would then put that information to good use and so respond with enthusiasm. Because that would make a lot of sense, wouldn't it? "Welcome every suggestion with eager enthusiasm, right. I'll do that. Okay. Now I know how to respond perfectly to hypnotherapy... now the expert has filled me in with the necessary details, I'll just observe the expert advice..." Not difficult, is it?

So off we went into the trance part of the session, and not a flicker of doubt appeared on Coco's face, not a trace of discomfort in her posture throughout, as I delivered a particularly good performance, I thought, of the flying phobia removal therapy. At the end, as soon as Coco opened her eyes I said to her: "So! Did you find yourself in full agreement with everything I was saying?" expecting her to say "Yes, it all made perfect sense!" like people do after *accepting* suggestions. What she actually said was: "No, I was arguing with you every step of the way!"

Case Mysteries 5: The Woman Who Came for an Argument

You can lead a horse to water, but you cannot make it drink. You shouldn't hit it with a baseball bat either, although it might be sorely tempting. I was particularly disappointed, I remember, because I had just done such a cracking performance, and it was all a waste of breath. I remember thinking I wish I'd taped it. I was wondering if I would ever perform that part quite that well again.

Now please consider, reader: does the above scenario count as a failure? You might immediately assume it must; however I certainly didn't do anything different from what I had done in many other successful sessions, except that I considered it a particularly inspiring version on that occasion. Notice how that made absolutely no difference to the outcome, because she rejected every suggestion out of hand.

It matters not at all how relaxed she was, how deep in trance she might be – if that's how you feel about the suggestions, that's how you feel about the suggestions. I told her beforehand exactly how to respond, and then I put in a fine performance, which under normal circumstances (i.e. before a favourable client) would eliminate the problem. So there was nothing wrong with that aspect of the procedure.

Did Coco fail, then? Well, given that she *chose* to argue with me within her own mind, she clearly did not *intend* to change her emotional position on flying at that particular time. So she successfully resisted any attempts to get her to look at it differently. Who failed? Nobody. But she certainly did not do what I advised her to do: she did not accept all suggestions with enthusiasm. Or any of them, in fact.

However, it turned out she had another issue. She explained afterwards that she had come for therapy only because her family had pushed her into doing something about her phobia because it was spoiling family holidays. As well as the phobia, she had real resentment that she was not being understood by those closest to her. She was upset that her feelings were not being respected, just regarded as an inconvenience. She had told them all that she did not wish to go on the forthcoming holiday, and now she was being frog-marched into therapy (she felt) by a family that had just lost patience with her. She was afraid of flying, she was angry, she was upset, she was resentful – well, it is a bit difficult to suddenly become a fountain of eager enthusiasm when you're feeling like that, isn't it?

Could Hypnotherapy have helped this person further?

If Coco had revealed the emotional complications during the earlier, discussion phase of the session, I could have guided her through the maze of familial conflicts during the trance phase, but it only came to light afterwards. We could have addressed all this emotional baggage in a second session, but she did not want a second session. In fact she didn't even want the first one, which is why she was a bit tight-lipped about the complications to begin with.

In truth, Coco did not fail. In my opinion it was her family that failed: failed to understand, failed to be supportive and failed to respect her feelings. She was actually quite successful in resisting attempts to push her around but it wasn't a very positive situation, and it could have been a very different story with a little more respect and understanding. I don't think that is a failure, I think that's a shame.

It is also a shame that now - without any great insight into the way these things really work - she is also likely to associate hypnotherapy with these emotional conflicts, resentment, guilt and the illusion of failure, and - even though all of that could be eliminated through further and more accurately-targeted hypnotherapy - never consider it again.

Section Nine

The Stupidity of Nicotine Replacement Therapy

At the beginning of this book I welcomed skeptics, and if any are still reading at this stage, their skepticism should by now have shifted away from doubts about myself and the efficacy of hypnotherapy, and onto the nicotine addiction theory and especially NRT. Now comes the coup de grace: if anyone is still advocating NRT after reading this next section, they are either in blind denial or in the pay of the pharmaceutical companies. Since the vast majority of humans are neither, this marks the beginning of the end for the international poison factory that is Nicotine Replacement Therapy.

First, a little reframing. Here is a revolutionary observation:

The vast majority of the time, smokers don't smoke!

People who get through twenty or more cigarettes each day often have the impression that they 'always' seem to be smoking, and usually tell me that they smoke "heavily". But how long does it take to smoke a cigarette? Three minutes? A person smoking twenty, then, is only actively smoking for a total of one hour a day. Let us assume they are awake for the usual sixteen hours. Of course they don't smoke during the eight hours that they would normally be asleep. But in truth they do not smoke for fifteen out of the sixteen hours they are awake, either.

This means that a person smoking twenty cigarettes per day actually does not smoke at all for 23 out of the 24 hours of that day, or to put that another way, 4% of their time is spent smoking, and the other 96% of the time they normally abstain, which doesn't bother them a bit. Even a person who smokes sixty cigarettes per day only spends three of the sixteen hours they are awake smoking, or 12% of their time. For a full thirteen hours of the waking day they are already living in exactly the way they would if they were a non-smoker altogether. They are quite content to be without tobacco for all that time, which means that if you look at smoking as an habitual behaviour, which it is – instead of a drug addiction, which it isn't – then they are already 88% non-smoker, even before therapy begins.

People who smoke sixty a day are always astonished when I point this out to them. They thought they were smoking all the time. Far from it. By the way, I'm not suggesting for a moment that they don't have a serious health issue. Even passive smoking can kill people, so actively smoking any number of cigarettes is potentially lethal. I'm simply pointing out that they only smoke in response to a reminder signal, and the vast majority of the time *it isn't there*.

Also, have you noticed how many smokers are really just holding the cigarette most of the time? When I was still smoking I used to laugh at the way my brother, who lit up far more often than I did, didn't actually smoke most of it. He just sat there watching TV, holding it aloft like the Statue of Liberty. The cigarette smoked itself, the fumes just rose up and discoloured the ceiling. He was a thirty-a-day man whose lungs were remarkably clear, but he was ruining his ceiling. Or he would light up, stick the thing in the end of his guitar and play a song. By the end, the ash was tottering at an impossible angle, he would tilt the guitar to drop it into the ash tray, take a couple of puffs and put it out. If he ever dies from a smoking-related disease, they would have to create a new statistic category for him: a man who died mainly from passive smoking, yet only had himself to blame.

So given that smokers are spending most of their time without a cigarette in their hand at all, and even when they are holding one they only take a drag from time to time and so half of it just burns away by itself, why should any smoker need to wear a nicotine patch all day long? As I have pointed out above, smokers usually have zero nicotine input the vast majority of the time. As for the 24-hour patch, what kind of lunacy is that? It causes heart palpitations, nightmares and lost sleep. It raises further still the risk of strokes and heart attacks... and no-one smokes in the night anyway, for god's sake! Or hardly anyone.

The Stupidity of Nicotine Replacement Therapy

"I took it off to have a cigarette"

People wearing nicotine patches often find that they still feel an urge to light up anyway during the day, at certain times when they would usually smoke. Some people don't experience that – or not at first - but this is just a placebo effect that tends not to last, because there are so many social and emotional triggers involved in the operation of a smoking habit. Millions of people have now tried patches, gum or one of the other NRT products, so even if you have no personal experience of these products there is probably someone you know who could answer this question for you: "While you were using that, did you find that you still wanted to smoke?" The answer is nearly always "Yes". Or "Not at first, but after a while, yes". This clearly indicates that the urge to light a cigarette is not an urge to take nicotine, because they were taking nicotine already.

NRT = Newly-Reorganised Theory

Recently I noticed a new TV advert for NiQuitin lozenges, which was obviously trying to fudge the addiction issue now by shifting the emphasis a little away from being all about nicotine. It features a happy 'quitter' – who was clearly an actor, even if he *was* also an ex-smoker, his performance was way too confident for an ordinary person – declaring merrily: "NiQuitin takes care of my addiction, now all I have to deal with is my habit!"

Yeah, very clever. Notice how different that message is from the original way NRT was presented to the world. Let's remind ourselves how we got to this point, shall we? The theory that the urge to smoke was a 'need for nicotine' has been the simplistic message of NRT all along, and all previous adverts have stuck to that script. I remember particularly one TV campaign that showed a woman in her car with a bloke sitting in the passenger seat dressed as the devil. He was supposed to represent her temptation to smoke, and he was taunting her gleefully until she produced a pack of nicotine lozenges. Then he became terrified and begged her not to use one, and as soon as she pops the lozenge in her mouth he disappears in a puff of smoke, and she drives off happily, apparently without any problem whatsoever.

Pretty clear message, isn't it? The temptation to smoke is caused by your addiction to nicotine, so just take our nice, clean, clinically-approved nicotine instead and there will be no urge to smoke. And it is not surprising they were so confident about this simplistic message, because it had complete backing from the medical profession. Let me remind you that according to the British Medical Association, nicotine is:

"A drug in tobacco which acts as a stimulant and is responsible for dependence on tobacco."

Later in the same text, under the heading of "Withdrawal Syndrome", it states:

Withdrawal symptoms from *nicotine* develop gradually over 24-48 hours and include irritability, concentration problems, frustration, headaches and anxiety.

Notice how the BMA are unequivocal about attributing these feelings to the withdrawal of *nicotine specifically,* not just tobacco. No mention of habit here, is there? And there was no mention of habit in any earlier promotions of NRT because the emphasis was always on addiction, so it is interesting that they are beginning to change their tune. Now they are trying to have it both ways, by suggesting it is both addiction *and* habit, which covers them for the poor performance of the NRT product. If their marketing people are congratulating themselves over the genius of that new suggestion, I would point out that it still brings the smoker one step closer to the realisation that the method simply doesn't work, precisely because it's a habit.

The uncomfortable symptoms listed by the BMA may well be noticed by an habitual smoker who tries to force an end to the habit using willpower. The clear implication of the BMA's carefully-chosen words are that the withdrawal of nicotine is the cause of that. None of these symptoms are reported after the majority of hypnotherapy sessions I conduct with smokers. With all successful sessions there are no side-effects or withdrawal symptoms whatsoever. The BMA are wrong. If they were not, then all my smoking clients would be suffering those symptoms and I would get no messages of thanks or referrals.

Goalposts Back Where They Were, Please!

The Stupidity of Nicotine Replacement Therapy

The whole concept that is supposed to validate NRT has always been that the habitual smoker is smoking cigarettes because he is physically addicted to this 'drug' called nicotine, and that the craving - the urge to reach for cigarettes again - is a symptom of his body needing another 'dose' of nicotine. So to get out of this trap the people who manufacture NRT products suggest that smokers should take nicotine a different way in order to cease the more dangerous practice of smoking cigarettes, and then gradually wean themselves off the nicotine in a controlled, 'medical' sort of way. They also suggest they should take several *months* doing this, so they can sell you a lot of the poison gum, patches or whatever.

Well if you could wean yourself off the nicotine in gum, couldn't you just wean yourself off cigarettes? Ever tried that? Not many non-smokers created that way, are there? In fact just about every advisor in the field of smoking cessation - no matter what method they promote - will tell you that cutting down as a prelude to stopping does not work.

When is a Medicine Not a Medicine?

In any case, smokers contemplating the NRT approach just don't quite understand how it is supposed to benefit them to take their 'drug of addiction' a different way. And it's a fair point, isn't it? If they accept the suggestion that their problem is a physical dependence on nicotine then even if they have been on the patches for months, in their own eyes they have not achieved anything in terms of addiction, they have simply altered the delivery system. Many find they can't even succeed in doing that, and still want to smoke when they are wearing a patch. Some do smoke, thereby taking in even more dangerous concentrations of the poison nicotine. Some take the patch off, have a cigarette then put the patch back on... now they're *really* confused.

But if I announced to the world that I had developed a revolutionary new way of helping heroin addicts: "What you do, is get them to take their heroin a different way – to avoid the use of syringes, you see – then they can just wean themselves off heroin much more easily!" Does that sound plausible at all? Anyone want to invest in this? Let's get the Heroin Patch production line rolling, there's money to be made!

There are plenty of heroin users in the world and I'm sure they will be glad to be offered a reliable supply of good-quality heroin made by bona fide drug companies, rather than getting ripped off by dangerous gangsters all the time.

Actually let's not stop there, let's get rid of *all* our 'addictions' this way! We'll have a Nicotine Patch on one arm, some sort of Gambling Patch on the other, a Chocolate Lozenge nestling under the tongue, and we'll be getting a good night's sleep at last with the brand-new Booze 'n Snooze Vodka Patch stuck on our foreheads all night long. Patent pending, by the way.

What's that? You don't think that would work? You reckon heroin addicts wouldn't be cured that way? Because it makes no sense? Give that guy an honorary PhD!

Of course it is ridiculous. Giving a drug addict their drug of addiction simply continues their addiction. How have the drug companies got away with this all these years? NRT isn't therapy. It isn't a medicine. Even to people who believe in nicotine addiction, the idea is utter madness, and no-one would ever suggest it with a real drug addiction, except as a damage-reduction maintainance strategy. Maintainance and quitting are quite different things, as anyone working with opiate users will know very well. But at least with regard to the heroin problem, heroin really is at the centre of the issue. With tobacco, nicotine isn't even the real cause of the habitual behaviour in the first place, which means that NRT is madness with a silly hat on.

One smoker said to me, "You know, I can't understand it - I used to smoke strong cigarettes with quite a lot of nicotine in. I've changed brand five times, gradually reducing the nicotine content and now I'm on these with hardly any in at all – and I'm *still* smoking twenty a day!" He assumed that by reducing the nicotine levels he was weaning himself off nicotine and should then find it easy to quit later, being 'less of an addict' by then. Not a bit of it, he still had a compulsive habit of lighting cigarettes twenty times a day. Nothing had changed except the brand. Oh, and he was poisoning himself very slightly less.

Or possibly more, since the levels of other poisons such as carbon monoxide can actually be higher from the 'milder' cigarette.

By the way, aren't 'Mild' and 'Light' dangerously misleading terms where tobacco is concerned? Like having slightly harder or softer bullets, what difference does it really make? Marlboro Lights: what do they do? Give you a tumour that's not quite so heavy? A gentler heart attack?

The word 'mild' should never be displayed on tobacco packaging. Nor should 'Low Tar', unless they are also going to specifically mention all the toxins it is high in. These terms are finally being banned in some countries because they are dangerous suggestions, which help smokers to continue fooling themselves. All tobacco products should be marked:

Bloody Damaging
Even More Bloody Damaging
and:
Look, two hours in a comfy chair, mate, and this is history! You don't even have to do a thing, just look forward to being richer.

I'm not sure they could fit all that on a cigarette packet, though. Maybe that is why they don't list all the poisons, there is not enough room on the packet for the names of four hundred toxic chemicals, so they only specifically mention a couple. They assume you already know about the rest, you're breathing them in regularly every day. Your body knows them all intimately. Like knowing your killer.

Back to The Stupidity Of NRT, I wasn't finished with it

Have you ever heard of anyone lapsing into 'nicotine addiction' again via gum? Or lozenges? What I mean is, someone successfully stops smoking tobacco but *later on* starts chewing nicotine gum, or using the nicotine inhalator? Never hear of that, do you? If this genuinely was a drug addiction you certainly would hear of that, but no – it's *always* relapse into smoking tobacco. No ex-smoker ever sidled up to a work colleague and said: "Go on, give us a bit of that nicotine gum. I'm having a tough day!"

Actually - and this is a rather worrying development, since the last time I personally tasted nicotine gum - a client recently told me that current versions of the gum are becoming fairly pleasant because new flavours are available which are much more appealing than the original, which I recall being tough to chew, and rather hot and peppery. Why is this worrying? Because this stuff is marketed and licensed as a *medical treatment,* which you are not supposed to use for any longer than is absolutely necessary. Of course it doesn't have to be nasty but if they make it enjoyable, isn't that taking the whole thing in an inappropriate direction? No-one would approve of manufacturing steroids that tasted of chocolate, would they? And why should it be necessary to make the gum taste pleasant? Cigarettes taste foul, and it doesn't stop smokers buying those.

Yet however they taste, the drug companies are manufacturing products that nobody wants, not even people who believe they are addicted to nicotine. How do they sell so much product then? Simply through fear. Smokers have no desire to purchase NRT products - in fact they feel thoroughly unenthusiastic about using them, unlike the woman in the TV advertisement - but to some smokers the idea seems preferable to the consequences of smoking. Many smokers feel like they are under sentence of death. Many of them will indeed be killed by tobacco if they continue smoking long enough. Given that scenario you would expect NRT products to be hugely popular, far more popular than they actually are. When was the last time you heard someone singing the praises of nicotine products or recommending them to a friend?

"Requires willpower"

That's what it says on the NRT advertising and on every box of patches: "requires willpower". Well, *why* does it require willpower? If all you need is nicotine surely you just slap a patch on your arm and you're right as rain, just like the smokers in the TV ads. You've got your fix, you're sorted - what do you need willpower for? What are you fighting? If cravings really are 'your body needing nicotine' then all you would need is a supply of patches and you are smoke-free, why would you ever feel tempted to inhale acrid fumes again? Especially since you can wear a patch in any circumstances, it should be far more convenient these days than a smoking habit. NRT products have been around a long time now, most smokers have tried them. So why is there still such a huge smoking problem?

NRT = New Revenue and Taxes

This raises an important question: How serious is the government in effecting the most rapid change possible? There are many who suspect some deliberate foot-dragging here, and point to the massive revenues generated by tobacco taxes: £9,300,000,000 annual tax revenue as against £1,500,000,000 cost in extra healthcare due to smoking-related diseases. These are some of the estimated figures which put the U.K. Government's annual profit from the continuation of the smoking problem at around £7,800,000,000 annually. Purely in terms of income, it is not in the government's interests for smokers to become non-smokers overnight.

But it is also not in the government's interests to be seen to be doing nothing about the smoking problem. What better solution, a cynic might suggest, than a range of quit methods which do not really work for the majority, yet are viewed by the majority as a genuine offer of help? And if VAT can be raked in through the high-street sale of those products, so much the better, clawing back some of the expenditure in providing NHS Stop Smoking services, which in turn keeps more people in work, and out of the benefits system.

Lots of money moving around and around, involving lots of people employed producing lots of products and services, new smokers coming into the system all the time, partly replacing the relatively small numbers of people who do actually quit permanently. If the government suddenly replaced all that with a quit method like hypnotherapy that genuinely worked for the majority straight away, the only people who would benefit would be smokers, and those providing hypnotherapy services.

The government would rapidly lose massive amounts of regular revenue, as would the drug companies and all the people involved in the manufacture, packaging, transportation, wholesale, retail and marketing of both tobacco products and all the quit products like NRT, which would not be required any longer. Not just in the UK, either - as the success of hypnotherapy was proven beyond doubt by the results - but all around the world over the course of the next few decades. We are talking billions in lost profits here, for certain very powerful global players.

Now, what government is going to want to be pro-active in instigating that kind of global economic sea-change, just because it would save millions of smokers' lives? Especially since that would mean lots more people reaching pensionable age, when there are too many people doing that already.

Oh, I almost forgot – undertakers would lose out too. And florists. And the people who make inhalers, breathing equipment and oxygen bottles, that sort of thing. Wheelchair providers, artificial voice-box manufacturers - the cynic's list could go on and on, really, couldn't it?

The cynic might have a point. Whilst I am not really a conspiracy-theorist, nor a cynic either, I must confess to feeling some unease about the way the tobacco industry has been placed in the dock recently in the United States over smoking-related deaths. Especially since one of the main charges against them is that the executives of tobacco companies knew their products contained an addictive drug - nicotine – and sought to deny this to the public for as long as possible. As nicotine is not a drug at all, still less an addictive one and the whole thing is being misunderstood by all concerned, this charge is actually misconceived in the first place. It is perfectly possible that the tobacco executives secretly believed, erroneously, that nicotine was addictive and tried to conceal this erroneous belief, but it would be pretty ridiculous to charge them with that.

No, the part that really bothers me is that making the tobacco companies the official villians of the smoking story provides the perfect distraction from the drug companies, as they prepare to flood country after country with virtually useless NRT quit products, thereby maintaining the nicotine myth, slowing the inevitable demise of tobacco and squeezing yet more precious cash from the poor, much-abused and misled smoker, whilst giving them nothing in return but a poison.

Knowingly too, the cynic would say. Personally I'm not sure. From the perspective of a keen student of human behaviour, I am far more likely to lean towards the 'cock up' rather than the 'conspiracy' theory of how these things progress. Yet there are some suspect observations, when we look closely at how NRT is promoted and marketed: do the drug companies *know already* nicotine addiction is a myth?

Well, there is that very sneaky suggestion that quitting with NRT "requires willpower". If the manufacturers really believe cravings are nicotine withdrawal, then they should have every faith that their nicotine replacement device will eliminate cravings. Why would you then need willpower? What exactly are you fighting against? The warning that success will still require willpower is likely to result in the smoker blaming themselves if they don't actually quit with that method. Really the warning simply acknowledges that the product doesn't do what it is supposed to do. However, the inclusion of the phrase "Requires Willpower" might not be something the manufacturers chose to do anyway, it could be an advertising restriction, I'm not sure.

Then there is the fact that the drug companies recommend that you use the gum (for example) for three months before you even *start* to reduce it. Why? That's a lot of gum! Why not start reducing it after a month, or even a couple of weeks? The fact is, three months is considerably longer than most people's willpower will last anyway, which means that the smoker is likely to relapse into smoking behaviour *somewhere in the middle* of that extended programme. From discussing this with hundreds of smokers, I reckon the average is about three weeks. This again encourages the smoker to blame themselves, not the method, and possibly conclude later that if they had only stuck it out to the end, they might have been successful. This increases the possibility they might return to the product at some later date. Or maybe try the lozenge. Or that little inhalator thingy. Or the nicotine nasal spray.

Or the nicotine implant – will that be the next thing?

Or maybe the new promotional twist will be to *combine* nicotine with some other marketable product for which there is already a demand. How about a nicotine + sugar alternative you can put in your tea?

"New **Quit n Slim!**" Now you can quit smoking AND lose weight!"

Or a nicotine suncream?

"New **Quit n Tan!**" Now you can sport an unnatural skintone,

AND quit smoking!"

Or how about a nicotine/laxative combination:

"New **Quit n Shit**! Now you can..."

Endless possibilities, endless. Still the same old poison, though, isn't it? And may I just remind you once again at this point, dear reader, that there are many hypnotherapists up and down the country removing this problem in a single session with no willpower even being involved, no bad moods and no weight gain? So what is all this cost, effort, suffering and failure in aid of, Doc?

NRT = No Real Transformation

Why do the drug companies have to keep re-inventing NRT? Same reason there is always a new diet on the market. It's not solving the problem, so you have to keep slightly altering it and re-marketing it as if it is something new. So it is the combination of this slightly-altered package, with the marketing suggestion:

It's New!

...plus the eternal hope and desperation of the smoker that drives them to keep trying the latest version. As long as you can get the smokers to keep *blaming themselves* when it doesn't change anything – well, the dieting gurus have been getting away with this for decades, haven't they? And boy, is there a lot of money in that miserable game.

Still, at least dieting *works*... doesn't it? After all, we have more people reading diet books now, joining diet groups and buying diet products than ever before in UK history. No wonder the population is so slender and healthy!

Am I actually suggesting that NRT is no use, that it doesn't help anybody? How dare I? What about all the people who successfully quit that way? Well, some smokers manage to quit without using anything at all, so it follows that some are going to succeed in stopping themselves smoking even with a method that is not actively doing anything useful to help. It is called the placebo effect and is universally recognised as significant and real, even amongst the most skeptical of scientists. An example of a placebo would be something like a sugar pill which was presented in all seriousness as if it was a powerful medicine, and it is the extent of the patient's *belief* in the suggestion it is going to help that actually makes a difference. In other words it is a mild, simplistic form of hypnotherapy. (See Part Seven: The Placebo Effect, in Section Five *Why the Nicotine Addiction Theory is Wrong*.)

Also let us not forget that some smokers have quit by switching to Wrigley's Spearmint chewing gum or something like that, but this does not indicate that spearmint alleviates cravings or stimulates the 'nicotine receptors' in the brain. Just because a person changes their *response* to a craving, from lighting up a cigarette to eating fruit gums, doesn't mean the fruit gums had a real, active role in it or were an essential ingredient in the process.

So, even nicotine gum – the least effective of the NRT products – is bound to have a small percentage of successes. Mainly because it is gum (chewing is *something to do*), but also because of the smoker's assumption that nicotine is relevant so it should help. The rest of the effect is really just suggestion: advertising, marketing and the endorsement of medical authority and government. These are huge promotional advantages which hypnotherapy has never enjoyed, yet I am absolutely confident my methods are at least three times as effective as NRT, even without any of that kind of promotion. I am certain they would be proven to be so in any properly-conducted, extensive trial with a long-term follow-up. I'm sure the millions of smokers out there would be very interested in the results of such a trial.

So the fact that the drug companies can point to a small percentage of successes here and there does not validate their method. It is not remotely surprising that some people manage to quit even with the nicotine gum because in addition to all the above, smoking is going out of fashion very rapidly, at least in the developed world. All quitting methods can be expected to yeild more successes progressively under those circumstances, obviously, because the average smoker's motivation to get free is increasing all the time. The same is true of hypnotherapy, but it is the vast difference in the real success rates that is the point. Hypnotherapy beats every other method by far, especially when it is expertly done.

The Current Strategy is Costing Lives

There is no excuse for hesitation or delay in establishing the truth beyond doubt as quickly as possible, and then immediately acting upon it. There are many lives at stake, and any foot-dragging in governmental or medical circles would be nothing short of negligent because around 120,000 more smokers in the UK are killed by tobacco with every passing year. It is no good these people in authority trying to defend the status quo by saying "We've done this", or "we've spent that" because that is not the point. It is time for the powers that be, especially in the medical profession, to stop trying to pretend hypnotherapy and acupuncture do not exist or are unproven, and stop pretending that NRT genuinely was the best solution just because that official stance suits the drug companies. People are dying in vast numbers, the drug companies are making a killing at the taxpayers' expense, and it is time the killing stopped.

Lots of Cash but No Change

The Stupidity of Nicotine Replacement Therapy

It is true to say that in the U.K., the New Labour government has done more to tackle the smoking issue than any previous government – mainly because previous governments did virtually nothing to tackle it, and when you look at the vast amount of income raked in through tobacco taxes, it is easy to see why. The biggest single change in the U.K. - as in some other countries - is the banning of tobacco smoking in all enclosed public places. It is telling that the government actually didn't want that to happen, arguing instead for a partial ban. Fortunately Parliament won the day, so hooray for Parliament because smoking is just a habit. After a month or two everyone will have adjusted and no smoker with any sense will be bothered at all.

Banning advertising, banning smoking in public places, lots of scare campaigns and the endless hiking of prices - these will all have real effects and smoking will gradually decrease further. Amid all this, spending tens of millions on NRT products and quit services seems - at a glance - like money well spent, doesn't it?

<u>Might be a Good Idea to Look At It More Closely Then, Eh?</u>

The NHS Stop Smoking Services provide counselling and NRT products as well as the medication known as Zyban. £138 million was spent on these services from 2003 to 2006. A further £112 million was allocated for 2006-7.

In 2004 alone, two million prescriptions for NRT were dispensed "worth a total value of £44 million." According to the Department of Health:

"NRT or Zyban doubles the chances of a smoker successfully quitting and use has increased substantially year on year."

That sounds good on the face of it, doesn't it? Doubles the chances of a smoker quitting, eh? Bear that statement in mind, I shall be returning to it in due course.

How many people do you know personally who have tried NRT products at some time? Of all those attempts to quit using tobacco, how many succeeded that way permanently? The truth is, most of the smokers in the U.K. today, especially those who have been smoking for more than five years, will have tried at least one NRT product at some time. This is partly because the British Government decided to make them available on prescription from 2001. Vast amounts of taxpayers' money has rolled into the coffers of the drug companies since then. Yet it is very difficult, for some reason, to get any detailed statistics for the number of smokers currently in the UK, or sufficient statistics regarding the changing trend in the number of UK smokers since 2001, so that we could compare it with the falling trend in tobacco smoking in the previous five year period, from 1996 to 2001, before NRT was made available on prescription.

The Department of Health has previously reported that the number of smokers has fallen from 28% of the adult population to 25%, during the period from 1998 to 2004. That is a reduction of 1,200,000 smokers. But why are they not telling us how this breaks down, so that we can compare 1998-2001 with 2001-2004, and clearly see the actual impact of NRT being made available on prescription? There are huge amounts of money involved, where is the evidence it is not being wasted?

Some of the ongoing reduction in smoking is due to the fact that tobacco is becoming increasingly unfashionable - simply a continuation of the falling trend in tobacco use since 1948, when records began. According to a 2007 factsheet published by ASH:

After 1982, the rate of decline slowed, with prevalence falling by only about one percentage point every two years until 1990, since when it levelled out. However, an analysis of data taken from the Government's monthly Omnibus survey demonstrated that between 1999 and 2002 there was a decline in adult smoking of around 0.4% per annum. This rate of decline has continued.

This document is dated March 2007. It vaguely suggests that the rate of decline has remained at 0.4% since 1999, does it not? But that is not good, is it? Because it also says that between 1982 and 1990, the rate of decline was 1% every two years, which of course is 0.5% annually. This indicates that not only has the rate of decline slowed since the 1980s, but also that the 0.4% decline has not changed since 1999. This despite the British government making NRT available on prescription from March 2001, at massive cost to the UK taxpayer. Are we to conclude from these figures that Government sponsoring of NRT has made absolutely no difference to the general, oh-so-gradual reduction in smoking prevalence over the last six years? In the same ASH article, under the sub-heading *Cigarette smoking and age* there is a hint at this:

Between 2004 and 2005 the only age group to record a fall in smoking prevalence was the 35-49 age group.

This means that the two million NRT prescriptions dispensed during 2004, worth a total value of £44 million according to the DoH – *and* all the NRT products bought privately as well, from supermarkets, pharmacies, petrol stations and similar outlets in that year, at a cost to consumers of God only knows how much – made zero impact upon the number of smokers in the UK outside of the 35-49 age group. Perhaps the people who approved Nicotine Replacement as a medication in the first place would like to explain that. And all those who recommended that it should be made available on prescription at the taxpayers' expense. Perhaps the BMA would like to comment. Perhaps ASH would like to explain why they continue to recommend these products, given their own observations of its apparently total lack of effectiveness quoted above.

You see, we also have to bear in mind that some of the reduction in that group is due to the fact that smoking is becoming increasingly inconvenient, with more and more public places becoming no-smoking areas. Some of it can be attributed to the ruthless increase in tobacco taxes year on year. Some due to the horrifying media campaigns designed to shock the smoker into quitting. Some is due to the stark warning that SMOKING KILLS on every tobacco product. Another important change has been the recent banning of tobacco advertising, so that tobacco is no longer presented as if it were just another consumer product.

All of this must have had some effect, and of course public money was used to make all that come about too. So has the mass supply of nicotine products at the taxpayers' expense made any contribution at all? Well, let's look at some press releases from the Department of Health shall we? They should know.

Statistics published on the Department of Health website concerning NHS Stop Smoking Services for the period April to September 2003 state that nearly 80% of smokers using those services were given nicotine products. These services cost £14.9 million for that short period alone, a great deal of it, of course, going to the drug companies. The DoH press release states that 129,800 smokers set a "quit date" through this service, and that at the 4 week follow up, 68,600 had, and I quote:

"successfully quit (based on self-report), 53% of those setting a quit date".

This press release clearly implies that the success rate of these services, and therefore the products used is 53%. That's fantastic news! Maybe they *do* work for most people, the old patches. After all, isn't that exactly what you hear about NRT anecdotally: from your friends, your work colleagues, your family or your own experience? Most smokers have tried these things by now - isn't this the story you've consistently heard, over the years? Half the people who try NRT successfully stop smoking? No, it isn't. So why are we getting that impression from the Department of Health website?

53% Did What, Exactly?

First of all, how many smokers lie about how much they've been smoking? What is the real value of this "self report" statistic? Some people, doubtless, will have genuinely not smoked at all for four weeks. A proportion of those may never smoke again, but certainly not all of them. Probably not many of them actually, as we shall see. Then again, some would-be "quitters" will feel disinclined to admit the products and the services failed them, especially when talking to the very people who provide the service. Some may be of the opinion that *they themselves failed*, rather than the products, and feel more comfortable in front of their 'counsellor' pretending they didn't. Some people just tell the nice medical people what they want to hear. It simply isn't accurate, is it, this "self-report" business? I'm not disrespecting smokers, here, it's just human nature and it is not being acknowledged in this press release by the DoH, for obvious reasons.

In the same press release, it is noted that this figure of 68,600 "quitters" is 23% up on the number the previous year, which was 55,700. This sounds very positive, doesn't it? Until you take into account that nobody followed up those 55,700 beyond four weeks, and that any or all of them could have started smoking again – and even gone back the following year to try again! Are people allowed to try again and again? Of course they are. Which means that some of the 68,600 this time round were also heralded as successes last time round, when in fact they weren't long-term successes at all. How many smokers have been counted twice or more? Elsewhere the Department of Health do manage to acknowledge that long term success is a fraction of the 'success' at the four-week point, so we have to ask: Should those people be counted *again* as a success this time, just because they can manage not to smoke for four weeks again - if indeed that "self-report" is even true?

Also, is it not astonishing that no-one at the Department of Health should have paused to question just how any standard quitting method could suddenly become 23% more successful than it was the previous year. Yes, smoking is going out of fashion progressively, but not so dramatically from one year to the next that it could account for apparent changes in product performance to that degree in a sample the size of 129,800 smokers. Any sober scientific review of performance should have spotted that as evidence of a problem with the way success was being measured, because it is obviously contrary to logical expectations, but no – they were so busy hyping the services they didn't even notice that what they were suggesting about the success rates was in fact silly.

Oh yes, the Department of Health has been very careful not to claim, but merely imply a success rate of 53%, when the facts are vastly different from that. Let's face it, nicotine products have been around a long time now. If they really had that kind of success rate, there'd be hardly any smokers left by now and happy bands of ex-smokers would be singing the praises of nicotine patches and gum to the remaining handful of die-hards.

Why are NHS Stop Smoking Clinics encouraged by the Department of Health to count anyone who reports stopping smoking for four weeks as an official "success"? If the DoH were ever to do any decent research into hypnotherapy, I'd expect them to follow up results for a lot longer than four weeks. Never smoking again, that's what I call a success. Now obviously it is impossible to conduct an indefinite follow up, but honestly, how many smokers have never stopped for four weeks? That does not make them a non-smoker! When I was a smoker, I was always stopping and starting again. I could have been counted as seven or eight official successes all by myself.

Perhaps this particular method of manufacturing the illusion of success was modelled on the original example of the American Food and Drug Administration (FDA) when they decided to licence NRT based on its results at six weeks, totally ignoring the placebo factor and the much poorer results at one year. Now, who remembers the reported success rates for placebos in drug trials that I asked you to bear in mind at the end of Section Five, Part 7? That is correct, 35% success. Now I should like to quote the Department of Health once more, as they attempt to assure you that your tax money is not just being wasted. This was taken from their website on 28/03/06:

The Department of Health funded an evaluation of the NHS Stop Smoking Services programme, which was carried out by a team led by Glasgow University. The evaluation included an overview of the development and staffing of services, an analysis of characteristics associated with the more successful services, conclusions on the targeting of disadvantaged smokers, a summary of cost-effectiveness, and a pilot study of long-term effectiveness which looks at the extent to which smokers who successfully quit smoking after four weeks are still not smoking after a year.

Just to interject for a moment: this report is fairly recent, including information from data published in 2005 and 2006. The DoH do not mention exactly when this evaluation was carried out, but it is interesting that the investigation into the long-term effectiveness of these methods is described here as a "pilot study". They began providing these services in 2001, the cost has already gone into hundreds of millions... and they are only doing a pilot study into long-term effectiveness now, five whole years after they started? We could have had this information years ago. Oh well, let's see what they have to say anyway:

The main findings were that:

- The services can contribute to a (modest) reduction in health inequalities

- Long term quit rates for the services show about 15% of people remain quit at 52 weeks, which is comparable with earlier clinical trials

- The services are cost effective in helping smokers quit.

This means that a smoker who tries to quit with the NHS Stop Smoking Service and NRT/Zyban is up to four times as likely to succeed than by willpower alone.

Note that 15% figure attached to the phrase "Long term quit rates". Dramatically different from 53%, isn't it? Well if you think that is shocking, read on. It gets far worse.

"Four times more likely to succeed" is puzzling too, because this is the same report – in fact it is the same page – which earlier informed us that "NRT or Zyban doubles the chances of a smoker quitting", so the actual assistance that these millions of prescriptions provide is unclear – but at the end of the day it hardly matters because these results are shocking, appalling, terrible. They are scandalous. 53% has dropped to 15% already? To an experienced hypnotherapy professional like myself, smoking cessation results at that level amount to abysmal failure. Even a sober and cautious claim for quality hypnotherapy by any authority in the profession would expect success 400% higher than that from just a single session. Fifteen percent? No wonder they preferred to tell us about 'self-reports' at less than a month! Also, this evaluation should have been done years ago. The NHS is supposed to be in financial meltdown, why continue pouring hundreds of millions of pounds into methods that fail at least 85% of the people using them?

(It really does get worse, too. I'm not kidding.)

Just to remind you why this is truly scandalous, let us quickly refer back to the *Daily Telegraph*:

a) The placebo effect is a powerful medicinal tool: in an average drug trial, 35 per cent of patients receiving dummy pills show an improvement in their symptoms.

b) In a recent study at Imperial College, London, patients with chronic genital herpes that did not respond to medicine were taught to practice self-hypnosis three times a week for six weeks. "The recurrence rate of the condition halved, which is a phenomenal result in these severe cases," says John Gruzelier.

c) Irving Kirsch, professor of psychology at the University of Conneticut, claims that data from the original trial on Prozac submitted to the Food and Drug Administration shows that placebo is 80% as effective as the active drug.

These claims are not coming from any private practitioner like myself, or even from the hypnotherapy profession, so it certainly cannot be dismissed as hype. 50% success for hypnotherapy reported there, according to Imperial College, London. Improvements in 35% of cases recorded just for dummy pills - in other words, the effectiveness of suggestion - which in the case of Prozac was almost as effective as the drug itself! That drug has since been prescribed to many millions of people at enormous cost. It is the most basic of suggestions that is achieving that success: "Here, this will help!" What kind of success would be observed in such scientific trials if that suggestion were expanded upon, made more specific, repeated regularly? No wait, that would be hypnotherapy. No profit in that for drug companies, obviously.

Anyway, what all this means is that NRT/Zyban and the NHS Stop Smoking Services, according to the Department of Health's own report and the team led by Glasgow University, function very poorly even as a placebo when we see the actual results at one year.

Let me just run that one by you again, because it is the most important sentence in the entire book:

NRT/Zyban and the NHS Stop Smoking Services, according to the Department of Health's own report and the team led by Glasgow University, function very poorly even as a placebo when we see the actual results at one year.

And this is supposed to be cost-effective? Compared to what – jailing people for smoking? Compared to hypnotherapy it is abysmal, and hypnotherapy has the added advantage of being 100% safe because the outcome is controlled entirely by the client's own Subconscious mind.

So we can see from this that the government is certainly spending an awful lot of taxpayers' money. But it is no good throwing money at the problem if you're throwing most of it away.

How It Could All Have Been Avoided

The really infuriating thing to people in my profession, is that none of this was necessary because all these facts were in the public domain long before the government decided to become the answer to the drug companies' wildest dreams. It is a fact that, if you telephone the NHS Stop Smoking Services, or indeed any of the Quit 'charities' and ask about hypnotherapy or acupuncture, you will be told that there is "no scientific evidence for the efficacy of those methods". This is simply not true, and has actually not been true for decades, as I will now show by telling you all about:

New Scientist Magazine and The University of Iowa

As long ago as 1992 - that is nine years before NRT was made available on prescription - *New Scientist* magazine published a report which began with the words:

"Hypnosis is the most effective way of giving up smoking, according to the largest ever scientific comparison of ways of breaking the habit. Willpower, it turns out, counts for very little." *New Scientist* vol136 issue 1845 – 31 October 92, page 6

This is not a hypnotherapy magazine, you understand, but a widely-read and respected scientific journal. This is exactly the sort of scientific evidence the people who promote NRT keep telling the public is non-existent. The article goes on to describe a comprehensive study carried out at the University of Iowa:

"statistically combining the results of more then 600 studies covering almost 72,000 people from America, Scandinavia and elsewhere in Europe".

Hardly a small sample, I think you will agree. According to this study, smokers have only a 6% chance of quitting with willpower alone. So when the promoters of Nicorette tell you "You're twice as likely to stop smoking with Nicorette" what they actually mean is that you have about a 6% chance without it, which rises to a staggering 12% chance –or so they claim – if you chew their gum every day for months on end. How many people would buy Nicorette gum if they knew that? It is obviously nothing but a placebo, and a poor one at that.

In fact, the Iowa study found only 10% success for the gum, and a slightly better result for the patches if counselling was provided as well, but still rising to only 20%. This indicates that NRT is apparently performing more poorly now than it was in the late 1980s and early 1990s, if we compare that 20% figure reported in 1992 with the 15% figure the Department of Health is apparently stating now. What do you reckon: are smokers simply becoming less inclined to *believe* in NRT now than they were when it was first developed? Are we seeing that lack of faith playing itself out in the real long-term results? Or were the earlier follow-ups not so long-term anyway, and the actual failure rate even worse than the Iowa results suggested? Either way, it is grim, and makes you wonder how these products got approved in the first place.

Now, let's just take another look at how the Department of Health actually phrased the news that its tardy pilot study was turning up an 85% failure rate:

- o Long term quit rates for the services show about 15% of people remain quit at 52 weeks, which is comparable with earlier clinical trials

The Stupidity of Nicotine Replacement Therapy

"Which is comparable with earlier clinical trials"? Is it just me, or does that sound to you like they are trying to suggest that we shouldn't be appalled and dismayed that '53% success' at the four-week self-report stage has dwindled to a miserable 15% at one year, because earlier trials had found this as well! This is supposed to make it okay, is it? Actually it makes it a whole lot worse because what it really means is that this shocking failure rate was the basis upon which the massive NHS programme was approved in the first place, nine years after a respected scientific journal reported strong evidence that hypnotherapy – which is entirely safe – was far more effective than the poison patches and the poison gum.

Are we to believe that the U.K. Government decided in March 2001 to make NRT products available on the NHS at the taxpayers' expense on the basis of pathetic figures like these? Or were they told something else? Who recommended it? What studies were they looking at, and how come they didn't know what *New Scientist* and the University of Iowa knew? I knew it, and I am certainly not privy to the best scientific advice available to government. *New Scientist* is fairly widely read, how come the medical profession didn't know?

Nicotine is extremely poisonous. Why is the British Government encouraging the routine, unnecessary poisoning of thousands of smokers who wish to quit? Not only with NRT, but with Zyban too which has been suspected of contributing to the unexpected suicides of a number of people? On the basis of what "success", precisely, did the government decide to endorse and pay for NRT and Zyban with taxpayers' money? Was the evidence and advice put forward to the government *significantly different* to that found by the independent study cited above? If so – how different? If the real results for NRT turn out to be falling well within the normal range expected of placebos – and they do – surely *safer* placebos should have been backed instead. Nicotine can cause cancer, heart attacks and strokes, whereas placebo medications are traditionally harmless. Hypnotherapy cannot possibly harm the client, since all responses are considered and directed by the client's own mind.

Perhaps the government decided to back NRT without bothering to find out, independently, whether it actually did anything useful or if it was just a placebo in reality - with the unusual disadvantage, as placebos go, of also being highly poisonous? Either way, the NHS Stop Smoking Services have turned out to be the one element of New Labour's smoking initiative that has revealed itself to be a very expensive failure, and it should never have happened at all because that shocking failure rate of 85% was "comparable with earlier clinical trials". Oops.

(Not only that – it gets worse.)

When is Great News Not Great News?

When it is not telling you what you want to hear. Why did this very significant article about the study at the University of Iowa sink without a trace? Because it was in nobody's interests to publicise it more widely, which requires large amounts of money. Nobody's interests, that is, except millions of smokers and a few thousand hypnotherapists. In contrast, when the drug companies launched the nicotine lozenge its arrival was announced in the national press with tremendous fanfare:

"NEW MIRACLE SMOKING CURE"

was one headline, taking up the whole front page of the Daily Express, if I remember correctly. It didn't prove to *be* a miracle smoking cure, did it? Not surprising really, since it was just the same old poison again. So who decided to describe it in that way, and why? Who paid for that? How did they make that happen, it's fantastic promotion! Did the *New Scientist* report of 1992 spark similar great excitement in national newspapers about hypnotherapy? Did it even get a *mention?* Even if it did, it probably wouldn't have been any editor's idea of a front page story. But why not, since it offers potentially life-saving hope to all of their smoking readers? Why the massive promotion of one alleged smoking solution, and complete disinterest in the other?

Scientific evidence for the success of hypnotherapy does exist, in fact according to the Health Education Authority: "Research shows that there is more scientific evidence for hypnotherapy than any other complimentary therapy." So if you were ever told by some wind-up toy of a quit counsellor that NRT-promotional mantra: "There is no scientific evidence for the efficacy of hypnotherapy", either they didn't know what they were talking about - which is bad – or they knew they were lying. Which of course is much worse, as the outcome of that conversation could have a real bearing upon your health and survival.

The University of Iowa study also reported a 24% success rate for acupuncture, which makes it at least twice as effective as the nicotine gum, and a 29% success rate for exercise and breathing therapy, no medications involved. Sounds a lot cheaper than £44 million spent on poison prescriptions just in 2004 alone, doesn't it? That was the year smoking rates did not reduce at all, except amongst 35-49 year olds, according to ASH. If the NHS had just opted for exercise and breathing therapy and left nicotine and the drug companies out of it entirely, they could have had 29% success across the board, according the to massive Iowa study. And doesn't that sound like the sort of thing HEALTH services ought to be doing, not dishing out millions of prescriptions for poisons masquerading as medicines?

Hypnotherapy came out best in the Iowa study, but what was really interesting about that success is that the quality of hypnotherapy they were reporting upon was very basic and poor, compared to expert modern hypnotherapy. The approach was simple direct suggestion, or "just listening to cassette tapes"! These approaches are bound to reduce potential success considerably, because the idea that someone will stop smoking simply because you tell them to while they are in a trance is a moronic interpretation of the art of hypnotherapy. And cassette recordings are no substitute for live, one to one sessions with an expert therapist – yet it still beat all other methods.

Yes, as long ago as 1992, this major scientific statistical review established that even in that very basic form, hypnotherapy topped the list at 30% - three times more effective than the nicotine gum that is still being prescribed today. At *your* expense, taxpayer. And you are being told this is "cost effective" while the drug companies are having to have the floors of their accounts departments reinforced because of the weight of all that cash they are raking in from the NHS. At the same time, nursing staff on the wards complain of basic things like dressings often being unavailable or in short supply. Once wasted resources like this are identified it is criminal to allow it to continue.

What Hypnotherapists Call Success

A hypnotherapy expert interviewed within the *New Scientist* report of October 1992 did comment that modern hypnotherapy techniques could be expected to double that 30% success found in the Iowa studies even with a single session alone. Christopher Pattinson, Academic Chairman of the British Society of Medical and Dental Hypnosis said that the latest techniques:

"... achieve success rates of up to 60 per cent from a single session."

I would add that it would be higher still with a back-up session available if needed. His assertion is consistent with my own findings as a therapist, taking into account my further comments on that subject in the later section *Success Rates* (Section 14 Volume II).

One particularly annoying quote in the 1992 article comes from the director of the anti-smoking group ASH, David Pollock. We are told Pollock commented that he was:

"surprised by the success of hypnosis, which anecdotal evidence had suggested was not very effective."

Anecdotal evidence? You want to try looking at the real evidence Pollock, you clown. Oh wait, I forgot – there isn't any, is there? Just like it still says on the ASH website today (at time of writing):

"Hypnosis, acupuncture or other treatments may help some people but there isn't much formal evidence supporting their effectiveness. Our advice is to use with caution..."

Oh, neat little negative suggestion there, ASH! Caution, eh? Hypnosis sounds a bit scary then, better avoid that maybe. No let's be honest, Pollock & Co: your *advice* is to use NRT or Zyban, and anecdotal evidence suggests that ASH is really just a shop window for the drug companies' quit products, posing as an independent medical anti-smoking advice service.

This is what you will find, folks, if you go surfing through the websites of ASH, Quit, NHS services and various other 'medical' sites, they are all pushing the NRT products with great confidence and enthusiasm, and sometimes Zyban, at the same time virtually dismissing all other quitting methods like hypnotherapy and acupuncture as if they are highly unlikely to work, or might even be risky. People have killed themselves whilst taking Zyban, and nicotine replacement products all increase risks of heart attacks and strokes. It's just that in the weird world of medical science, deaths below a certain percentage of the total treated allow the medication to be officially endorsed as "safe". Hypnotherapy and acupuncture have never killed anyone, and never will. That's as safe as you can get.

So we shouldn't be surprised to find that the largest pharmaceutical company in the UK, GlaxoSmithKline, sponsors the Quit website, and also supported the ASH conference in Cardiff in 2002 – how independent are these Quit organisations really? By the way: Zyban, Nicorette, NicodermCQ and NiQuitinCQ are all manufactured by GlaxoSmithKline. No wonder ASH are very keen to make sure we are all thinking in terms of nicotine, nicotine, nicotine!

Listen up Mr Pollock, You Might Learn Something

The London-based hypnotherapist Valerie Austin, in her book *Stop Smoking in One Hour*, first published in 2000 – a full year before the decision to provide NRT and Zyban on the NHS – reported the Iowa findings again and added references to three other significant scientific studies finding very exciting results for hypnotherapy to stop smoking, which actually date back several decades:

67-68% Success for hypnotherapy in published research findings by Watkins, Sanders, Crasilneck and Hall.

88% Success with hypnotherapy based on one year follow up: M. Kline, (1970) International Journal of Clinical and Experimental Hypnosis.

94% That is 94% of 1000 people stop smoking with hypnotherapy, after 18 month follow up: T. Von Dedenroth, (1968) American Journal of Clinical Hypnosis.

These are the sort of studies that supposedly did not exist, when actually some have been around since before man set foot on the moon. A long while before actually, since hypnotherapy has been wilfully ignored by medical institutions for over 150 years, as I explain later in Volume II.

Valerie Austin also claims that she can beat all of the studies she mentions with a success rate of 95%, using "The Austin Technique". This can be done in one hour, apparently. Instead of commenting specifically on that, I would refer the reader to my detailed comments on that subject in *Success Rates* (Section 14, Volume II). Suffice to say that we, as expert hypnotherapists specialising in the field of smoking cessation, are in a completely different league from NRT and Zyban. We have real success rates indicating real success, not tiny success rates proving massive failure.

Numbers Games

Now, one of the objections I have anticipated from the NRT brigade is that the numbers they can treat with medications is far higher than could be treated by hypnotherapists, since there is currently a limited number of hypnotherapists who are expert in this field. To which I would reply:

a) That is a lousy excuse for prolonging failure. If the medical profession had not been pretending hypnotherapy was of little use – despite officially recognising its efficacy in 1955 – it could have been successfully developed as a normal aspect of NHS services for over fifty years, in which case NRT would never have existed and neither would a lot of other medications.

b) If the government had done their homework properly and discovered that the most effective method was in fact hypnotherapy, many more hypnotherapists could have been trained and set to work over the last five years, not just to help with smoking but many other health issues too. So the sooner we get started the better, obviously. Acupuncture is also more effective than NRT/Zyban, so that method could be brought on board to help with demand too, with none of the health risks currently posed by NRT/Zyban.

c) Even if the NHS had done nothing else for the last five years but hand out cassette tapes of hypnotherapy, and organised some breathing and exercise therapy which would have improved their patients' general health as well, according to the Iowa findings they could have doubled their long term success, with no prescription costs and without poisoning anybody. It would have avoided a lot of litter from pharmacies too.

When is a Mistake Not a Mistake?

When it is *known* and yet not corrected. On March 18th 2005, *The Times* Health Editor Nigel Hawkes reported upon a warning voice being sounded from fairly high up within the NHS. Under the headline:

NHS 'missing target on smoking'

the newspaper reports that the Deputy Medical Director of Northumberland Tyne and Wear Strategic Health Authority, Eugene Milne, had warned in the *British Medical Journal* that the targets set by the Government to cut the number of smokers through the NHS Stop Smoking Services were not going to be met, according to his assessment of the situation.

The report as it appears in *The Times* is bad enough, but it also raises another question about the real NHS success rates which was left unclear in the report by Glasgow University. *The Times* reported:

"In 2003-04, 20,103 people used the service, of whom 9,910 were not smoking when checked after a month. Dr Milne estimated that 35-40% of them would still be non-smokers at the end of a year – that is 3500 to 4000 people.

Now, that does not mean that NRT/Zyban has a success rate of 35-40%. It means that 35-40% of the 9,910 people listed as 'successes' at four weeks would be actual long-term successes, which would work out at 18-20% of the total 20,103 using the service. We now know this is likely to be an over-estimation of long-term success thanks to the pilot study reported by the Department of Health, which makes the rest of Dr Milne's warning even more serious. But it also raises a worrying uncertainty in the Department of Health's summary of the findings of the pilot study by Glasgow University:

- Long term quit rates for the services show about 15% of people remain quit at 52 weeks, which is comparable with earlier clinical trials.

This is what I meant when I said it gets worse. That statement is not what it appears to be. 15% of people *remain* quit? Does this mean 15% of the total treated in the first place, or only 15% of the self-reported "quitters" at four weeks? Because if it was the latter - and it certainly sounds like that because of the word "remain" - that would amount to a long-term quit rate of just seven or eight per cent of the total treated! Since that is about the same as willpower according to the Iowa study, that would lead us to the horrifying conclusion that the NHS Stop Smoking Services are virtually a complete waste of money.

Even using his overestimated figures for long-term outcomes, Dr Milne concludes that:

"...the best cessation services can do is to reduce smoking by somewhere in a range between 0.1 and 0.3 per cent a year. The Government has set a target of reducing smoking from 26 per cent of people to 21 per cent by 2010. Dr Milne predicts that the stop smoking services are unlikely to achieve even half this figure, and may produce less than a fifth of it."

In other words, a one per cent reduction instead of a five per cent reduction - and that warning is based upon estimates for long-term results that we now know are over-optimistic, suggesting that the ongoing 0.4% year on year suggested by ASH is about the best we could expect. Now, allow me to refer back to a point I made much earlier in this section, which may at first have seemed far-fetched to some readers. I remarked that:

> Purely in terms of income, it is not in the government's interests for smokers to become non-smokers overnight. But it is also not in the government's interests to be seen to be doing nothing about the smoking problem. What better solution, a cynic might suggest, than a range of quit methods which do not really work for the majority, yet are viewed by the majority as a genuine offer of help?

I must confess that until I really started looking into this, I had always assumed that the NHS programme and the NRT/Zyban approach was simply a genuine governmental mistake: bad judgement, poor advice, heavy lobbying by the drug companies for market share and so on. But the more closely you look at it, the more it starts to look as if this is not simply a mistake. This is looking more and more like a policy which does exactly what it is supposed to do. In fact, if someone were to deliberately set out to create a stop-smoking service that appeared to be very proactive on the face of it, but actually changed virtually nothing, they could feel very pleased with themselves if they came up with exactly what we have now in the NHS Stop Smoking Services.

We are all paying for it financially. But who is going to have to pay a much heavier price? How many thousands of people are going to have to lose their mum, their grandad, their sister, their best friend or their son over the coming years, as this hugely expensive policy makes very little difference to the overall numbers of smokers? This is a scandal which stinks to high heaven, and 120,000 people in the U.K. alone are paying with their lives every single year. If it is simply incompetence, that is bad enough and heads should certainly roll. But if it is not even a mistake...

Let's call a Spade a Spade

'Nicotine Replacement Therapy' is not a therapy, it is a multi-million dollar industry based on a myth. It should not even exist. Nobody is addicted to a drug called nicotine. There is no *drug* called nicotine. Nicotine is a deadly poison. All of its effects are uncomfortable, useless, dangerous, damaging and therefore *simply toxic*. Smokers are not smoking for the effects of nicotine, they do not even know what it does. Nobody needs nicotine 'replacing', in fact it's the last thing they need. Nicotine in any form can directly cause heart attacks, strokes, damage to circulation and thrombosis. It can also cause cancer.

Habitual smokers do not really smoke because of nicotine at all, even if they are convinced they do. They do smoke because of cravings, but cravings are nothing to do with nicotine or anything else in the smoke. It is true that cravings disappear when the smoker lights up, but that is because a craving is really a mental prompt to repeat the habitual behaviour, triggered by the brain but experienced as a physical compulsive urge that seems to the smoker like a real bodily need.

The nicotine theory has always been wrong. That theory is not supported by the real results of NRT because the patches and gum are an enormous failure in reality. And even in the cases of the small number of people have found NRT helpful, that tiny proportion of all the smokers who have tried those products is entirely accounted for by the placebo effect. Since the Subconscious *produces* these craving signals, it is not remotely surprising they can be *altered* by the placebo effect. What is surprising, perhaps, is how few people report feeling that benefit when compared to better results reported for other placebos in the treatment of unrelated conditions, as detailed in *The Telegraph* report. And unlike all other placebos, nicotine is not safe. As for Zyban, that has certainly been a factor in unexpected deaths amongst ordinary people who were simply trying to quit smoking for the sake of their health.

'Cravings' are very familiar to all of us, not just smokers. We get lots of cravings, they are not all about tobacco. I can prove what they really are by demonstrating how easily hypnotherapy can shut them down - whether they be urges to smoke, or to chew fingernails, eat chocolate, buy things you don't need, gamble or drink excessively... to mention only a few issues we routinely resolve with the hypnotherapy method.

You see the real irony is, the tobacco companies were right when they denied tobacco smoking was addiction, whether they believed they were lying or not! It is not addiction. It's not nicotine. It's a wrong guess. It's a big mistake. It's the biggest medical mistake of the twentieth century, that's what it really is. And it has paved the way for a deadly poison to be marketed worldwide as if it was a medication, when the actual results show it to be no help at all because it scores no higher than willpower in long-term effect.

NRT = Not Really Treatment

Here is the most stunning piece of evidence yet, to indicate the absolute stupidity of NRT/Zyban and the NHS Stop Smoking Services. Again it comes from *The Times* article and it concerns one of the methods Dr. Milne used to try to predict future results:

> "An alternative way of looking at the issue is to use established figures for how many people need to be treated with anti-smoking aids such as nicotine patches or the drug bupropion [Zyban] in order to achieve one long-term quitter – what doctors call the "numbers needed to treat". Evidence indicates that for nicotine patches or gum, the figure is 17, and for bupropion it is 8."

Now I'm no mathematician so you might want to get out your pocket calculators and check this out for yourselves, but I reckon that translates into a 'success' rate of 12.5% for Zyban and 6% for NRT. Zyban cannot be prescribed without unpredictable risk that has already caused grave concern in dozens of cases. Many of my clients told me that they stopped using it because they were alarmed by the way it made them feel. And its success rate is *half* that of acupuncture, which has never harmed anybody.

The 6% quit rate for NRT reported here clearly shows that the Glasgow University review did indeed mean 15% *remain* quit, but without clarifying that as only about 7% of the total treated, for the obvious reason that they did not want to draw attention to a failure rate of 93%. Since 6% success is exactly the figure the Iowa study found for willpower alone, that more or less amounts to ZERO improvement with NRT - and in this instance the information is coming from the Deputy Medical Director of a Health Authority.

Of course they are missing their target, their method is useless and yet they are wasting millions on it annually. And this performance is comparable with earlier medical trials? What numbskull authorised the national implementation of that policy? Or perhaps we should ask "what Machiavellian political genius", depending upon what they actually intended to achieve. So - what do you think, taxpayer? Ever get the feeling you've been had?

OK - but So What, Hypnotist?

There may be some of you out there thinking: "So NRT has a very low success rate, so what? Tell us something we *don't* know! At least a few people are helped, surely that's something, isn't it?"

But just consider this: if the government had been laying on sessions of acupuncture, or homeopathy through the NHS for vast numbers of smokers - spending hundreds of millions of pounds of taxpayers' money on that since 2001 instead of NRT, and it became established that 94% of that was a complete waste of money and willpower would have achieved the same results anyway - would you expect the government to continue with that policy once they knew the results were as poor as that? How could they possibly justify it?

Yet this is exactly what has happened with NRT. And they know! These are government statistics from the Department of Health, and every month I seem to stumble upon more research turning up the same figures, some of it going back years. Like this for example, quoted in a book published in 2002:

<blockquote>
Schneider *et al* showed that mere dispensing of nicotine gum actually resulted in a lower quit rate with active gum than with placebo treatment (**8%** nicotine gum, **13%** placebo gum)... Of course most patients simply buy and apply the patches like sticking plaster. Without any behavioural help, **we can therefore expect very low quit rates with the nicotine patch** (according to Allen V. Prochazka in his article *New Developments in Smoking Cessation*, **in the order of <u>5 per cent</u>**).

From *Don't Stop Smoking Until You've Read This Book*,
Dr Harry Adler and Dr Karl Morris, How to Books 2002
</blockquote>

Now just let me remind you once again about that press release from the Department of Health for April to September 2003, which informed the public that 68,600 people using NRT during that period had:

"successfully quit (based on self-report), 53% of those setting a quit date".

The difference between 53% and 5% is so enormous that this amounts to seriously misleading the public about the effectiveness of these services.

Taxpayers' money is taxpayers' money, it doesn't belong to the government. The government cannot just give it away or throw it away on projects that obviously don't work without having to account for it. And whatever mistakes may have been honestly made at the start, to continue with nicotine-based products now that the abysmal results are an established fact is impossible to justify and would simply amount to corruption. It has to be scrapped without delay.

GlaxoSmithKline are not going to like it, but they are just going to have to face the reality. Game over, boys.

Marketing, Slander and Excuses: How Everyone was Hoodwinked

i). The Promotion of a Poison

Take It As Read: The subtle use of suggestion in 'objective' analysis

There are many groups and organisations with an active interest in the maintainance and promotion of the nicotine myth, and first I want to offer just one typical example of how they do this, whilst appearing to be rigorously objective in their assessment of the smoking problem. Again, whether you suspect this actual lack of objectivity is entirely deliberate, or just lazy and careless will depend upon your personal attitude towards these groups but the *effect* of their misrepresentation of the true situation is just as bad either way. It is very misleading to the public.

Most leaflets and fliers promoting NRT, whether they originate from the NHS or some other organisation, will simply recommend nicotine products as if nicotine addiction were already a fact beyond question. However, some medical websites and those of the various 'quit' charities promoting NRT and Zyban will skim over the addiction debate for a page or two, just so that the medications they are recommending appear to be validated. As I showed earlier, the Royal College of Physicians' website untypically goes into considerable detail – giving me an opportunity to challenge some of the actual 'evidence' – but most sites do not risk that, or else they cannot be bothered to get into the details at all. Instead, they give a cursory nod towards the real debate, which they then *suggest* has already been satisfactorily concluded in such a way that nicotine addiction has become the only scientifically-approved interpretation of the smoking problem.

A typical case in point is the anti-smoking group ASH (Action on Smoking and Health). ASH describes itself as a "campaigning public health charity", but is really the creation of some elements of the medical profession who "were frustrated by the slow rate of progress in tackling tobacco by successive governments" ...or so we are told by ASH, at any rate. Most of the website is given over to promoting quit strategies that have NRT/Zyban as their key factor, whilst damning all other approaches with faint praise or worse. But just before ASH really get into the swing of that, they summarise the debate by briefly mentioning that some voices have questioned the idea that nicotine is addictive, although they do manage to suggest that the only people who have ever questioned this are the tobacco companies themselves, so the implication is that "they would say that though, wouldn't they?"

Having raised the question though, they then have to answer it *as if objectively*. What I want to demonstrate here is that their answer is not really objective at all, but heavily weighted with suggestion which aims to manufacture a sense of certainty about the nicotine theory in the very way the phrases are constructed. What follows is just a tiny part of the text, because I don't want to bore you with long lists of examples, but this is absolutely typical of the way suggestion can be woven in, without the ordinary reader noticing it at all. Unfortunately for them, being a Grandmaster of Suggestion – a veritable Wizard, indeed – I noticed it straight away. In a section which purports to objectively analyse the 'evidence' for addiction, ASH lists on the website the following symptoms which they present under the heading:

Nicotine Withdrawal Symptoms:

Another marker for addiction is the occurence of withdrawal symptoms following the cessation of drug use. For smokers, typical physical symptoms following cessation or reduction of nicotine intake include craving for nicotine, irritability, anxiety, difficulty concentrating, restlessness, sleep disturbances, decreased heart rate, and increased appetite or weight gain.

Now at first glance, that might seem acceptable enough. But look how insistently the writer of that paragraph uses the word *nicotine,* when that particular detail is supposed to be in question. The writer has no doubt, apparently, that everything he is describing is not only an observable symptom, but is surely caused by, or directly linked to nicotine specifically. Look how the sentences are constructed:

1. The writer chooses to describe the experiences of the smoker deprived of tobacco under the heading "Nicotine Withdrawal Symptoms", not Tobacco Withdrawal Symptoms.

2. The expression *withdrawal symptoms* is used twice, as if it were already certain that this is what those experiences actually are - as if that were already proven, when in fact this is only what they may appear to be, and no such thing has been proven at all, it is merely being assumed. As I have already shown, this is in fact wrong.

3. The writer also talks of the "cessation of *drug* use" (not tobacco use)

4. refers to "symptoms following the cessation or reduction of *nicotine* intake", not tobacco consumption...

5. ...the first of which symptoms he lists as "craving for *nicotine*", rather than an urge to smoke again or a craving for tobacco.

Now I am not just splitting hairs here, because the writer goes on to assert:

"The fact that these symptoms can be attributed to nicotine, rather than behavioural aspects of tobacco use is shown by the finding that withdrawal symptoms are relieved by nicotine replacement therapy (gum, patches etc.) but not by a placebo (ie. products that do not contain nicotine)."

Then without giving any actual details whatsoever to support that assertion, and without the slightest pause, the ASH website continues: "For further information about using nicotine as an aid to stopping smoking see Fact Sheet No.11 What Happens When You Stop Smoking."

Now, hang on a minute! That was a very quick transition from *describing symptoms* to promoting nicotine-based aids to stopping smoking! Surely ASH is supposed to be an independent charity giving advice on tobacco and health, not a shop window for NRT products! But this is exactly what we find all over the place, if we go surfing through the websites of ASH, Quit or the NHS services, and many medical or quasi-medical sites, they are all pushing the NRT products with great confidence and enthusiasm – and with almost identical messages, so it is all suspiciously co-ordinated - and often Zyban too, whilst at the same time virtually dismissing all other quitting methods like hypnotherapy and acupuncture as if they are inferior or dubious approaches.

Since I have already dealt with the issue of the 'NRT versus placebo' trial in Section Five there is no need for me to reprise that here, but just contrast the way suggestion is operating in the ASH text quoted above, and these following statements from the same sources regarding alternative or complementary approaches to stopping smoking, as we consider:

ii). Peddling Doubt

Take It From Us: Unsubtle suggestions to rubbish non-drug alternatives

The government-approved quit organisations and 'charities' promoting NRT/Zyban and also various medical authorities and pharmacy outlets would all have you believe their approach is the only way, or the only tested and approved way to stop smoking. Actually it performs so poorly in reality it is barely superior to willpower but they do not want smokers to know this. They certainly don't want smokers to take other approaches seriously and they mainly seek to avoid this possibility by not mentioning other methods at all on most of their promotional literature.

This is at least only marginally dishonest as it doesn't attack other methods, it simply suggests by omission that smokers have no alternative to NRT except willpower, or continuing to risk their life by smoking.

However, when these people do decide to mention alternatives, what they have to say is usually brief, dismissive, misleading, poorly-researched or not researched at all, cautionary or mildly alarmist, or just untrue. Here are some examples from printed leaflets and websites I have happened upon over recent months:

From the ASH website:

Acupuncture and Hypnosis: A review of alternative stop smoking aids found little evidence to support the effectiveness of either acupuncture or hypnosis as a means of stopping smoking but such methods may suit some smokers.

"A review?" This is so vague and unsubstantiated it has no more validity than gossip. "May suit some" clearly suggests "won't suit most", which is certainly not true of hypnotherapy in my experience.

From the NHS Stop Smoking Pack sent out to telephone enquirers:

Other aids to giving up: Hypnosis, acupuncture: Some claim very high success rates. Be careful – there is no magic cure and none of these methods have been scientifically proven. If in doubt, call us.

If in doubt call the NHS? If you have questions about hypnosis or acupuncture for God's sake don't call the NHS, that would be like asking me about hip joints. If you are looking for real scientific evidence about hypnosis, you could ask the University of Iowa about the 48 hypnotherapy studies they looked at, involving 6000 smokers, which led them to conclude it was the best quitting method of all. And of course the other studies mentioned elsewhere in this book.

From ASH director David Pollock, quoted in New Scientist magazine as being:

"surprised by the success of hypnosis, which anecdotal evidence had suggested was not very effective."

From registered charity 'Pharmacy Healthcare Scheme', in their *No Smoking Day & Your Pharmacist* leaflet. First, NRT and Zyban are promoted under the heading: *Proven Drug Therapies,* after which it says this, under the heading *Alternative Therapies:*

> Many therapists (hypnotists, acupuncturists etc.) advertise services for smokers who want to stop. While some people find them helpful, they are not tested in the same way as drug therapies like NRT and Bupropion [Zyban]. Some therapies can help boost your confidence or help you relax when quitting, but they are not magic cures. Reputable therapists will explain how their treatments will help – however you'll still need to deal with the nicotine addiction and habit aspects of smoking in the usual way. You usually have to pay for these therapies.

Notice how this writer also uses the expression "some people find them helpful" to appear objective whilst actually suggesting by implication that most people will not. The vast majority of people trying NRT/Zyban will certainly not be helped, but this well-known fact is not mentioned by this registered 'charity' trying to sell NRT here, in order to ensure complete unfairness. Notice also how "not tested in the same way" is used to suggest "not tested".

To hypnotherapists, the most offensive part of the above quote is the suggestion that all we have to offer the public is a bit of relaxation and a boost to your confidence, which is not advice at all but the peddling of total ignorance and inaccuracy. The suggestion that such therapies are not magic cures is patronising to the public - they *know* that! It is interesting that this "no magic cure" phrase also cropped up in the NHS Stop Smoking Pack. The real purpose of that expression is to destroy your hope that acupuncture or hypnosis will make a significant difference, and then the dagger of disappointment is driven home in the pharmacy leaflet with the assertion that:

> you'll still need to deal with the nicotine addiction and habit aspects of smoking in the usual way.

Liars! Fools! I cannot speak for the acupuncturists, who may wish to make their own comments about that statement, but speaking for the hypnotherapy profession I cannot let this outright lie go unchallenged. Hypnotherapy normally removes cravings and eliminates the habit entirely when it is conducted properly and readily accepted. In my practice, as in many others, this is the normal outcome of a smoking session. This fact in itself proves there is no such thing as nicotine addiction and leaves the new non-smoker with *nothing* to deal with, except their astonishment that all those doctors, scientists and pharmacists were just proved 100% wrong.

You usually have to pay for these therapies.

Pathetic. This implies that theirs is a superior method *just because* you may not have to pay for it! Actually you will anyway, even if you get these things on prescription, unless you qualify for free prescriptions. If you are a taxpayer, you are actually the person who is paying for all the NHS quit services in the UK, including the enormous costs of NRT and Zyban, whether you smoke or not. In stark contrast, the existence of all the hypnotherapists and acupuncturists in the country costs you nothing, unless of course you decide to ignore the stupid, misleading 'advice' above and opt to judge for yourselves by giving non-drug options a try.

Reputable therapists will explain how their treatments will help – however you'll still need to deal with...

In other words your therapist is only "reputable" if he tells you that his therapy won't help much because you will "still need to deal with the nicotine addiction and habit aspects of smoking in the usual way"! Boy, is that Catch 22 - that implies that if your therapist talks of easy success, he must be a liar! This is a subtle and cynical manipulation of the smoker's usual low expectations of success. Notice also how the pharmacists' leaflet uses this statement to *imply* the professional superiority of his own traditional reputation: your friendly, local pharmacist in his trusty white coat, almost like a doctor in fact, with the patient's best interests at heart. If that was true, why so keen to suggest that alternative therapies won't help the patient? Why not just be positive and encourage people to explore all avenues?

Well, it could be because this organisation genuinely doesn't know how successful hypnotherapy can be in helping smokers. If so, they should not be offering any advice about it at all. Or it could be because the pharmacist is actually just running a business, selling stuff, and that is the real aim of this leaflet. It presents itself as if it is medical advice, but it is really just an advert for stock items carried by the store. Why is this group a *registered charity?* The real aim is not helping the smoker get free, that comes secondary to selling him stuff. For months on end, preferably, as the drug companies 'advise'. None of these people want him discovering hypnotherapy and actually getting rid of the problem, especially since that might get him thinking about other ailments he might be able to get rid of in the same way, instead of going to the pharmacist and buying products made by the drug companies.

Time for a couple more? Well, there's the one from the ASH website I mentioned previously. Notice how similar it is to the NHS quote, and that both of them are phrased like warnings:

"Hypnosis, acupuncture or other treatments may help some people but there isn't much formal evidence supporting their effectiveness. Our advice is to use with caution..."

Then there is this, taken from TobaccoFree.org on 30.12.2005. This is the website of The Foundation For a Smokefree America, which is an organisation created by Patrick Reynolds, grandson of tobacco company founder RJ Reynolds. After recommending NRT and Zyban, which are claimed on this site to have success rates after one year of 15% and 30% respectively - more than double their success as reported by the UK Department of Health – the site goes on to suggest:

Alternative Therapies:

Alternative therapies such as hypnosis, acupuncture and herbs have been shown to be far less effective than the above methods. Several controlled studies found they were ineffective.

Notice how vague that is, very similar to the ASH quote in fact, and clearly just intended to be discouraging, without troubling the reader with any facts or details whatsoever. The suspicious word there is "controlled", which is meant to imply 'rigorously scientific' through the use of a control group, but also reminds us that if you exercise enough control in the way you assess any alternative therapy, you can make it seem ineffective. Interestingly though, the American site also reports good success rates for other non-drug approaches, including "the venerable Mayo Clinic", which is highly regarded by well-schooled hypnotherapists too, who will be aware of the Mayo brothers' impressive success in using hypnotherapy as an aid to anaesthesia in surgery over several decades.

It is also interesting that the above quote about alternative therapies has, at the time of writing, apparently now been removed from the site, and replaced by much more detailed text about the Subconscious mind, and although most of that content is not very accurate, they are at least working with the right tools now, so fair play to them! Unfortunately the same cannot be said for the Royal College of Physicans, who dispose of such treatment approaches thus:

Hypnosis and Acupuncture

Hypnosis and acupuncture hold a special place among a range of existing treatments for smokers. While most other treatments are practised only on a very limited scale, the number of commercial advertisements for acupuncture and hypnosis suggests that these two approaches are popular with smokers. The Cochrane group has reviewed nine studies of hypnosis and 16 trials of acupuncture, and concluded that evidence of specific efficacy is lacking. Some people can of course be helped by numerous different unproven procedures, via non-specific and placebo effects.

Source: www.rcplondon.ac.uk 30/12/2005

Why does it not occur to the RCP to wonder why hypnosis and acupuncture are so popular with smokers, even though they have to pay privately for them, if they are no specific help as this dismissal suggests? Also, who are the Cochrane group? What was their aim? What studies did they look at, and who did those studies anyway? How were those studies conducted in the first place? Who analysed the results, and to whom were they reporting their findings?

Nine studies of hypnosis were reviewed, it says. Obviously none of these included the studies mentioned by Valerie Austin, in her book *Stop Smoking in One Hour*, first published in 2000, a full year before the U.K. Government's decision to provide NRT and Zyban on the NHS. Just to remind you, some of these date back quite some time:

67-68% Success for hypnotherapy in published research findings by Watkins, Sanders, Crasilneck and Hall

88% Success with hypnotherapy based on one year follow up: M. Kline, (1970) International Journal of Clinical and Experimental Hypnosis

94% That is 94% of 1000 people stop smoking with hypnotherapy, 18 month follow up: T. Von Dedenroth, (1968) American Journal of Clinical Hypnosis

Evidence of specific efficacy is hardly lacking here, why did the Cochrane group choose to ignore these studies? Also, a review of nine trials is a rather minor project compared to the study at the University of Iowa, where the analysis of hypnosis alone included:

48 studies covering over 6000 smokers, [which] gave an average success rate of 30 per cent for this method.

This study, which was first reported in the *Journal of Applied Psychology* in the Autumn of 1992 and then picked up by *New Scientist* and reported again in October 1992, showed that out of all the quitting methods reviewed in 600 scientific studies:

...for most smokers the most effective technique was hypnosis, in which smokers go into a deep state of relaxation and listen to suggestive tapes.

Right, that's 600 scientific studies in all, 48 of which were classed as hypnotherapy but were actually just deep relaxation combined with listening to recorded tapes, which is the poorest method of doing hypnotherapy, so it only reached an average of 30% success. But this still beat willpower, nicotine gum, patches, and aversion therapy. So what sort of success rate does hypnotherapy get when it is done properly, Doc? Maybe this accounts for its popularity with smokers, eh? It simply works, and smokers have been discovering for themselves that this is indeed the case, despite the best efforts of medical authorities and drug companies to mislead smokers about that and steer them back to the poison patches and the poison gum, and that scary Zyban, which has been implicated in fatalities.

Smokers talk to each other, you know. And although NRT adverts are splashed all over the windows of every pharmacy, on billboards and the TV, smokers do not recommend those products to each other, which is why after all these years the drug companies still have to spend so much money every year promoting them. And although, as the RCP observe:

...the number of commercial advertisements for acupuncture and hypnosis suggests that these two approaches are popular with smokers...

...these adverts are almost exclusively confined to the local classified business directory, and the web. You hardly ever see hypnosis or acupuncture advertised in newspapers, you never hear adverts for it on the radio, on TV, or see it on a billboard. Yet these methods are very popular with smokers, as the Royal College of Physicians remarks. Put the pieces together, Sherlock: massive year on year promotion of NRT by drug companies, yet the products are hardly ever recommended smoker to smoker. Miniscule promotion by hypnotherapists and acupuncturists by contrast, because most of our turnover is from exactly that form of promotion - personal recommendation, one smoker to another.

There's nobody subsidising us. We private therapists cost the taxpayer nothing. No medical authority recommends us, in fact they often do the opposite, as I have shown. Governments ignore us. Exciting scientific studies showing success for hypnotherapy are totally ignored by all these people, except where they decide to call it psychoneuroimmunology, so they can take it over for themselves as if it is a medical procedure, which it isn't, and pretend it isn't hypnotherapy, which it is. Indications of tiny success rates in scientific trials for NRT and Zyban are hailed as significant, and "proof" of efficacy, even though they actually perform poorly even within the normal placebo range. At the same time, any results for hypnotherapy and acupuncture are dismissed by such comments as:

Some people can of course be helped by numerous different unproven procedures, via non-specific and placebo effects.

...as if that did not apply equally to NRT and Zyban! So far, the drug companies and the medical authorities have had it all their own way, but as the recent amendment to the Reynolds site indicates, the times they are a-changin', and smokers will not be fooled forever by misinformation. Lie all you want, they will find you out. Smokers talk to each other, you see. When people contact my office seeking hypnotherapy, it is not unusual for them to say "You've been recommended to me..." Nobody ever walked into a pharmacy and said:

"Everyone's going crazy about your nicotine gum, please say you still have some supplies available...!"

And that is not surprising because the success rates are so low they cannot seriously be regarded as success rates at all. The real reason the NRT advocates keep telling smokers there is "no magic cure" is to try to convince them that failure is the norm, to be expected, so that they can continue the pretence that NRT actually has a 'success' rate, be it ever so low. But the people at the sharp end of handing out these therapies, especially the doctors, are struggling to maintain any enthusiasm at all for these "Proven Therapies", which in reality have proven not to work for 94% of smokers. Yet the medical authorities remain determined to stick with the poison patches and the poison gum. Just listen to the desperation in this astonishing case made by the Royal College of Physicians, in which they try to argue that a success rate of 6% is still good, as we marvel at:

iii). Beggaring Belief

Take Heart, Doc: Mony a mickle maks a muckle!

Some of you may not know that phrase, so I'll explain. It is a Scottish expression which suggests that we should not be scornful of tiny quantities because if there are enough of them, it amounts to a lot. This seems to be the principle underpinning the following passage, in which the Royal College of Physicians (Setting Higher Medical Standards, don't forget!) explain that although doctors, especially GPs, feel very disheartened about giving medical advice regarding smoking, due to the abysmal results of NRT, they really shouldn't be, because:

The barriers to action amongst GPs include lack of time, perceived lack of skills, and the perception that success rates are low. The last of these may be particularly important in engaging the interest of GPs. Appreciating the difference between success rates and the numbers reached may help: intensive treatments that achieve high cessation rates but reach limited numbers will usually produce fewer ex-smokers than less intensive approaches which reach many smokers.

"Intensive treatments that achieve high cessation rates"? This is the first time we have heard from a *medical* source that there might be such a thing. Are they referring to hypnotherapy and acupuncture, or are there other approaches that also get better results than current medical services? Either way it doesn't matter, apparently, because according to this argument it is better to treat all smokers with a lousy treatment than some of them with a good one. This is pure sophistry. Notice also how they imply that these are the only two options that could possibly be considered, when in reality various changes of a non-treatment nature - like banning smoking in public places for example - can bring down the overall numbers too, so that superior treatments can be focused on the remainder.

Changing public perceptions would also be a very useful way of hastening the demise of tobacco. It would be easy and cost-effective, for example, to make a series of interesting television programmes that would demonstrate to smokers that they are not, in fact, smoking for pleasure even if they thought they were, and that tobacco does not alleviate stress, yet explain where the misunderstanding has come from. That is just one simple example of a range of new measures that could change smokers' attitudes radically in a short space of time, if the government really wanted to get serious about it. Look how much money and effort they are happy to invest in their election campaigns, all the major political parties. Is the health and survival of British citizens not worth that kind of investment? Sure, they run scare campaigns sometimes, but instead of just trying to frighten smokers, a campaign to raise general awareness of the utter pointlessness of smoking would probably get a much more positive response. That sort of message would increase the number of people genuinely motivated to quit and improve their chances too, by eliminating the mental attitudes that make smokers imagine that tobacco has a use.

In fact the combination of many factors, including the best treatments available whatever they prove to be, is the formula that would be the most effective in reality. But just look how the rest of this RCP passage actually tries to make a success rate of only 6% sound worthwhile:

Thus, brief advice from GPs (defined as up to three minutes) may encourage 'only' about 2% more smokers to stop compared with normal care control, but this apparently low figure applied nationally to all GPs would be enormously worthwhile and cost effective. With an average of about 9,000 patients and 2,600 smokers (29%) in a five-partner practice, brief advice could help more than 50 (2% of 2,600) additional smokers each year in that practice to stop. Nationally, this would produce about 300,000 additional ex-smokers. With NRT added to usual care the result would be about 156 (6% of 2,600) extra ex-smokers per practice, or almost one million nationally. *Downloaded from www.rcplondon.ac.uk 30.12.2005*

First of all, these figures are exaggerated! In order to get one million ex-smokers at a 6% success rate, you would have to treat 16,666,666 smokers, and there are nowhere near that many smokers in the UK. According to ASH there are about 12 million smokers in the UK, which is 28% of men and 24% of women. That statistic is dated January 2005, so unless the RCP is reporting that the number of smokers in the UK has suddenly leapt by 4.6 million in a year or so, I think we can safely conclude that the writer of this piece is trying to make NRT's 6% hit rate sound more potentially useful by exaggerating the total theoretical numbers involved by almost 40%. Oooh, perhaps that's what they meant by Setting *Higher* Medical Standards...

Quite apart from the phenomenal cost to the taxpayer of providing several months-worth of NRT prescriptions for 16,666,666 people, and the cost of 833,333 hours and twenty minutes of GP's time used up by spending three minutes talking to each of them – God knows what that amounts to - what is an hour of a GP's time worth these days? - the fact that it will not help 94% of them at all means that only the Mad Hatter and the March Hare could possibly describe that as "enormously worthwhile and cost-effective". Even the dormouse could probably spot the problem with that, and he's asleep.

In fact if we follow the RCP's 'reasoning' to its logical conclusion, the ideal scenario would be to get lots more people smoking year on year, so we can treat millions more yet, and get the overall effect of this miserable 6% apparently higher still! When is a lousy treatment not a lousy treatment? When you use it on millions of people. We really are in Wonderland now, aren't we folks?

So, let's get this straight. Here we have the Royal College of Physicians admitting that advice from GPs makes about 2% difference, but if you add NRT at the taxpayer's expense, that rises to a staggering 6%. Come on guys, that is a failure rate of 94% whichever way you look at it, no wonder the poor old GP doesn't want to precious time or energy on this! Meanwhile, these same medical authorities will advise smokers that hypnotherapy and acupuncture are 'unproven' methods. How dare they, when by their own admission their method is almost completely useless!

In fact, this figure of 6% is even worse than the shockingly poor results for NRT reported by the University of Iowa as long ago as 1992. Listen to what their findings were, as presented by *New Scientist* magazine fourteen years ago:

The least successful method turned out to be advice from GPs, which appears to convince virtually no-one to give up. Sheer willpower proved little better, with a success rate of only 6%. Self-help, in the form of books or mail-order advice, achieved modest success – around 9%, whilst nicotine gum was a little better at 10%.

So NRT was getting slightly better results fourteen years ago than it is now. Now it is down to 6%, exactly the same as willpower in fact, probably because doctors and smokers alike have virtually no faith in it at all these days, cancelling the slight traces of a placebo effect completely. No wonder the drug companies advise the poor hapless purchaser of the NRT product that it "Requires Willpower". In fact they might just as well sell you an empty box which just says "requires willpower" on it. It would get exactly the same success but without the poison.

Frank Schmidt, one of the researchers conducting the Iowa study, remarked:

We found that involvement of physicians did not have as big an impact as we expected... We speculate that the reason is that it is the content of the treatment that matters, not the status of the person giving it.

The RCP don't think the dismal failure of the treatment is a problem though because they conclude thus, following their surprisingly frank admission of a 94% failure rate for NRT:

These apparently low absolute figures are worthwhile and extremely cost-effective compared to many other things doctors do, and this message needs to be conveyed clearly to health professionals.

"Compared to many other things doctors do"? Surely the RCP are not suggesting that a failure rate of 94% can be seriously regarded as worthwhile and extremely cost-effective *because* many other things doctors do are even more of a failure than that?

<u>The Naked Truth</u>

OK I've really got to stop now, I'm beginning to feel too sorry for the general practitioners to continue with this. Let's just wheel on the little boy, here: the Emperor has got no fucking clothes on, I think we can all agree on that now, can we? The drug companies are the tailors and there *is no medicine,* it's just an empty box with WILLPOWER written on one side, and GOTCHA! in invisible ink on the other.

And if anybody reading this is thinking: "No, you're wrong, my husband stopped with the patches!", then all I have to say to that is: "Well done to him, and tell him to read the bit about placebos, I think he'll find it very interesting."

Section Ten

The Compulsive Habit Structure

Let's not make this complicated, I hate it when people do that. Whatever school of thinking you may represent - layman, counsellor, psychologist, hypnotherapist, psychoanalyst, whatever – just beware of the people who want to make everything sound highly technical and complex, they are usually just thrilled with the idea they are cleverer than other people. They need therapy, that's all. They have issues. They need to stop being so impressed with difficulty, it doesn't help.

For example, I could dream up a way to divide Compulsive Habits into eleven types, but I won't because it is totally unnecessary. I could use complicated terminology to define the differences. When I was an academic I spent many boring years doing postgraduate studies in contemporary critical theory, I could easily make all this sound dauntingly difficult in a way that would win me a significant identity in academia, and leave everyone else confused and unclear. Let's not.

In the interests of simply being *useful*, I propose a distinction between two types of Compulsive Habit:

1. The Simple Compulsive Habit, which has no beliefs attached to it, and

2. The Complex Compulsive Habit, supported by ideas and beliefs.

I shall be returning to these shortly.

Behaviour Habitual and Compulsive

The idea that there is such a thing as 'involuntary behaviour' is quite wrong. All behaviour is voluntary, but some of it is directed by the conscious mind, and some by the Subconscious. If there is a conflict, caused by oppositional aims between the Subconscious and the conscious mind, usually one will overrule the other in the end. Where habits are concerned, it is the conscious mind which is more likely to be overruled ordinarily. The conscious mind may then choose to regard the behaviour as involuntary just because *it* didn't aim to continue it. The Subconscious simply does not know this and ultimately succeeds in carrying out its aim, unaware that this may be causing a problem elsewhere.

New decisions, and the behaviour resulting from them are conscious-directed and generally regarded as 'voluntary'. Where there is no conflict with the Subconscious, that is easy enough. It is repetition and regularity that turns it into habit. For convenience sake, and so that we don't need to waste lots of time thinking consciously about the same old daily tasks or actions, the Subconscious takes them over as soon as they become predictable and repeats them 'on autopilot', on the basis of the pattern we have developed as the norm over weeks or months. Usually the conscious mind retains the perception that it is still directing the behaviour.

This shift to Subconscious control can happen surprisingly quickly, a new habit can be formed in a matter of days. Remember starting back at school in September, in a new classroom, with a new desk or seating-position in that room? How long before that has become 'your' desk? Even after three or four repetitions it would seem 'wrong' to sit anywhere else, wouldn't it? This is how quickly the Subconscious latches on to patterns that repeat. You feel gently compelled to sit there, you do that automatically, and if someone else sits there, you object: "Hey! Get out of my seat!"

Of course this is a simple functional habit. There is a compulsion to do it, but there is little tension or anxiety about things like that usually, you don't feel imprisoned within it. You are aware that you could sit somewhere else. There might be some feelings of tension and anxiety in 'obsessive compulsive' cases, and of course people on the autistic spectrum, but for most people there are no fears or false beliefs reinforcing that behaviour, so you can still regard it as if it were simply a free choice, or a preference. There is no conflict either, because there is no danger or risk in continuing to sit in the same seat, whereas there is a risk in continuing to smoke, for example.

So the smoker's habit can be seen to be more complex. As well as routinely lighting up, the smoker may also believe that he is addicted, and so be afraid of the daunting prospect of 'withdrawal', and also perhaps believe smoking is helping him deal with everyday stress, and so perceive an advantage in continuing to smoke. On top of that he may be conflicted because of the cost, or fears about his health and so on. Either way, these behaviours *and some of the beliefs* have passed to Subconscious control in reality, no matter what the conscious mind chooses to think or decide about the smoking later.

Most habits are behaviour patterns that roughly follow the clock, or our routine, and the sequence itself is often habitual so that one habit follows another in the same typical order it usually does, as is convenient. We feel comfortable when functioning like this, hence the unwelcomeness of any criticism of our habits. But none of this is set in stone, and we could make the effort to vary it if we have a good reason to, but it is an effort, and it is much easier to return to the previous pattern later than to maintain the effort. This is because whilst we are functioning on autopilot the conscious mind has no work to do, so there is no mental stress or tiredness generated. In short, the mind is being highly efficient, re-running established programmes so that we don't have to analyse.

Whilst we are operating under Subconscious direction, the conscious mind is free either to idly observe the usual behaviour, or more likely amuse itself with thoughts of other things, which is more entertaining. Or more negatively, the conscious mind might be stressing about the habit itself, if the person has chosen to beat themselves up about it: "I wish I could stop doing this/why can't I stop doing this/I'm such a weak person" etc. This is totally unnecessary. It is just frustration caused by the conscious mind still believing it controls all our behaviour, or ought to be able to do so. This has never been true, but the idea that the behaviour is therefore 'outside' that person's control is also not true. It is being successfully carried out by the Subconscious, which could change or stop it anytime, but is unaware the conscious mind is opposed to it – or any of the reasons for that.

Some habits however do not *simply* follow the clock or our routine, there may be more complexity in the programme than that. For example, the smoking habit can be quite complex in terms of detail compared to the singularly pointless habit of twisting your hair around with your finger until individual hairs snap. Not everyone does this – not everyone can - but it is a common enough phenomenon and an excellent example of a Simple Compulsive Habit. Clearly, it has no beliefs attached to it that are supporting the habit. It may occasionally be flirtatious, it may be just idle fiddling or it may be triggered by stress in some cases, but no-one in their right mind would regard it as a successful stress-relief strategy, or useful in any other way. It cannot possibly be pleasurable. It is obvious to anyone, even the person doing it that it is usually just meaningless and destructive, although not dangerous. Smoking as a behaviour is rarely admired either, yet there may be a tacit acceptance, by the onlooker, of the idea that it is actually relieving the smoker's stress – an impression common enough even amongst non-smokers, as that notion is universally familiar even though it is completely untrue.

People who compulsively eat chocolate are an interesting case, because that is almost in the Simple category, but not quite. Many 'chocoholics' will fall into strong compulsive patterns, but there are hardly any beliefs involved. Most will regard it as simply an unhealthy and indulgent habit – and therefore a 'bad' habit - yet there are sometimes one or two ideas or notions supporting the habit too. The 'chocoholic' may believe they can't stop, or even that they are in some way physically addicted. They probably believe they eat it for pleasure or comfort, and that it isn't doing them any good in terms of health, but apart from that there is no psychological complication. Also, there are a limited number of triggers that produce urges to eat chocolate, it isn't usually going to happen twenty or thirty times a day like the smoking pattern often does. For example, a typical trigger might be a certain regular event such as a work-break, or the start of a favourite TV show. Products containing chocolate are often advertised on TV before or during popular soaps, or else the manufacturer may sponsor them exclusively. The UK's top TV soap *Coronation Street* was sponsored by a leading chocolate manufacturer for years, ensuring the suggestion of eating chocolate is regularly repeated in association with another pleasurable indulgence (watching their favourite show), with the maximum number of viewers on the receiving end of that suggestion. The ultimate aim is to fuse the two brands, hopefully to the benefit of both. The original products were of course literally soaps, perhaps the ultimate domestic product as its use is virtually universal. Some products lend themselves to this form of advertising better than others, naturally: it has to be something many people buy, and generally regard as a 'good' thing, otherwise the intensive repetition would become annoying or upsetting. Pimple cream no, chocolate yes.

Other triggers might be seeing someone else eating chocolate, or noticing a shop that sells chocolate. Billboards of course are the direct suggestion. "Have a break...*have a KitKat*" or the less-successful slogan "Thank Crunchie it's Friday", which didn't last for obvious reasons. Clearly these direct suggestions are not just presenting the product but trying to link it to a regular routine event, aiming to generate long-term habitual patterns of behaviour that end up being hard to break with willpower alone.

The *compulsive* element is the key to understanding all troublesome habitual behaviours, including some aspects of genuine addictions like heroin, which will inevitably have a strong Compulsive Habit element to them - as well as any real physical dependence - because of the repetitive daily patterns that have built up around the dependence. Whatever we call this compulsive factor – an urge, a need, a desire, a craving, a compulsion – it is always the same thing: a signal from the Subconscious mind to the conscious mind, aiming to prompt us to do something. These physical sensations and mental compulsions will vary from person to person in terms of strength and frequency, depending on a number of factors, but they are entirely generated by the human mind and are nothing to do with the contents of the chocolate bar, or chemicals like nicotine, as I have already shown. Real withdrawal symptoms can now be truly identified as those which can never be removed by hypnotherapy in any case, as the Subconscious is not creating the experience in the first place so it cannot shut it off.

Got the **urge**? Get to **Burger** King!

Advertisers have learned - through decades of experience of what works and what doesn't - the mechanics of compulsive behaviour, especially when it comes to eating and drinking. The slogan above – and the old one for *Impulse*, a female body spray: "Men just can't help acting on Impulse!" - playfully attempt to link compulsive urges with a particular brand, and it is the impulse or urge *prompting* us to do something which is at the centre of those suggestions, the advertisers are directly referring to it. They are not telling us what the perfume is like, or explaining the special offers on at Burger King – no, they are going right for the Red Button that prompts you to *act*. It is highly effective, but it is not sophisticated because on this level our behaviour is not sophisticated. Which is precisely why none of this needs to be made out to be any more difficult than it is, and also we can enjoy the playfulness within it. This is all about feelings, sensations and the satisfaction of desires. Sometimes we misread that as *need* just because it can feel like a need, but actually there is rarely any real need involved, even if the person experiencing the urge honestly believes there is.

It is just a Signal

Signals from the Subconscious mind can occasionally become pretty insistent, especially if a matter is genuinely becoming urgent (such as a raging thirst), but usually they are just little reminders for our convenience and they are sent out automatically most of the time. We feel them in the body, like a pang, and they are otherwise rather indefinable should we try to describe or locate them precisely, but of course we know what they mean. Hunger is one, as is thirst. The urge to light a cigarette, bite into a Mars bar or buy a scratchcard are generated by exactly the same system, but unlike hunger or thirst there is clearly no physical gain as far as the body is concerned. On the contrary, there may even be disadvantage or damage resulting, which the conscious mind might have been informed about previously. But did anyone warn the Subconscious? No, probably not. Most people don't know they *have* a Subconscious mind, they certainly don't realise it needs detailed information if it is going to get everything right. They understand that about the conscious mind of course, which is why we have education. It is just as true of the Subconscious, or else it will make honest mistakes.

Doctors don't seem to recognise that their patients have a Subconscious mind either, or that most of their behaviour is controlled by that. So they don't talk to the Subconscious mind at all. Instead they lecture the patient's conscious mind about habitual behaviour controlled by their Subconscious, implying that they ought to be able to change that behaviour with a conscious decision which the Subconscious knows nothing about, and a conscious effort they cannot sustain for long. Even if they do that, they are vainly attempting to resist Subconscious directions that only become more insistent if you choose not to respond at first. Then the doctor lectures them again. And again... sometimes implying by this stage that the patient is being stupid, when in fact it is the medical profession who are being stupid, continuing to wilfully ignore the straightforward solution to all this as if it doesn't exist: hypnotherapy. Or in other words, the wholly practical matter of supplying useful information to the whole of the mind, not just a tiny part of it.

Since the Subconscious may not have the right information, then it is no surprise that there may be a negative result to the compulsive action, but there is certainly a positive intention – or at the very least, it is less taxing for the mind to continue the established behaviour if the Subconscious repeats it automatically, because thinking is then no longer necessary. Often though the compulsive behaviour is actually supposed to be helpful - carrying out the action is supposed to make us feel better, or succeed in some aim. In reality it might not, but that was usually the idea behind it, the trigger that prompted the behaviour. The key to understanding this is suggestion, and we will be looking at the particular beliefs and suggestions that support the smoking habit in the second volume. But it is now time to define the thing I have been talking about. Forget addiction, here is the reality about gambling, drinking, nailbiting, smoking, shoplifting, snacking and a hundred other common enough behaviours that might become a bit of a nuisance:

The Compulsive Habit Structure

<u>Stage one:</u> Voluntary behaviour becomes regular through repetition.

<u>Stage two:</u> The Subconscious recognises the now-predictable pattern, and takes over responsibility for the repetition of that behaviour under the usual circumstances. This will include the provision of impulses that prompt the behaviour at a suitable moment but are unlikely to trouble that person in other situations where that behaviour did not usually occur.

It is crucial to understand that the Subconscious mind, once it has taken over the running of the behaviour, will be totally unaware of any later conscious decision to alter or cease the behaviour. This is precisely why New Year resolutions rarely make the slightest difference in the medium to long-term. In hypnotherapy, one of the main things we do – which no other therapy really does – is explain directly to the Subconscious that the behaviour it now controls is under review, instigated by the conscious mind. Of course, the Subconscious may not necessarily feel inclined to change the behaviour just because of that, so it is important to also explain the reasons for the review. But as long as the Subconscious doesn't even know there is a problem, or a new decision, it is unlikely to reconsider the behaviour spontaneously unless the usual circumstances change significantly, because the Subconscious is not analytical in the same critical sense that the conscious mind is. It simply repeats the established pattern, and the conscious mind has limited power to oppose that. The power it does have – willpower – usually cannot be sustained for long anyway.

There are ocasionally exceptions to this: particular circumstances when the Subconscious might suddenly choose to change the behaviour without any therapeutic intervention, such as women suddenly finding it easier to quit smoking when they become pregnant for example. In that case there is an obvious change of priorities, but there can also be cases of a spontaneous reduction in Subconscious impetus to continue the smoking habit. It simply becomes less motivated to drive the repetition, allowing conscious resolutions to win out because there is less conflict over it. Usually though, repeating the established pattern for years on end is the familiar experience.

Stage three: Following the shift from conscious to Subconscious control, the conscious mind either:

- does not notice that this change happened at all and continues to believe the action remains a matter of conscious choice, or

- notices, but never becomes concerned about the change, or

- notices and becomes concerned.

Stage four: If the conscious mind does become concerned about this change, then there may follow attempts, using periodic temporary conscious efforts (willpower) to *resist* the compulsive urge which aims to prompt the behaviour, and override the Subconscious-directed action with deliberate inaction, or some other action. It is crucial to understand that this strategy is doubly flawed (see *The Willpower Myth*, Section 12 Volume II). These disadvantages make permanent cessation generally unlikely. (This is actually just the norm, but is usually regarded by the self or others as 'failure', causing all kinds of unnecessary emotional complications which often slow the course of therapeutic change. Limiting beliefs such as "I'm just a terrible person", "I'm such a failure" or "I've let everybody down" can so consume a person's thoughts that positive responses become difficult to generate at all, especially at first.)

Stage five: If these conscious efforts to resist compulsive urges fail - as they usually will, hence the expression 'Old habits die hard' - there may be attempts by the conscious mind to *cover up*. This is done either by rationalising – coming up with 'reasons' to explain the behaviour away and make it seem a free conscious choice after all, or by hiding the behaviour itself: doing some or all of it in secret.

Acting as if/Pretending/Believing the behaviour is still a matter of conscious choice – still a deliberate act of conscious freewill, as it once was – is of course *denial,* and hiding the behaviour is a part of that too. There are two aspects to denial: denial to others, and denial to self. How much the conscious mind is self-aware regarding the extent of denial strategies can vary, not just from person to person, but in the same person at different stages of the habit's development, from not aware at all, to complete recognition. Whether that sort of recognition is 'confessed' to others or not, mere conscious recognition probably won't alter the Subconscious-driven behaviour at all. But any degree of self-awareness regarding the loss of conscious control - if it is not properly understood (as is usually the case) as behaviour that is now under the control of the Subconcious - can cause *conscious distress,* leading to any one of the following reactions:

A). Resignation of self to habit – giving up on the idea of conscious choice - either happily, or unhappily.

B). Breakdown – an emotional crisis usually followed by:

i): Religious conversion: Give up autonomy to church/God

ii): Support Network conversion: Give up autonomy to the structured approach of a Twelve Step programme such as A.A., and so accepting the explanation of the 'addictive personality' proffered by people who know virtually nothing about the Subconscious mind. They mean well though.

iii): Spontaneous Total Aversion: Give up the behaviour itself permanently without help, and without any particular beliefs. This is usually mistaken for an impressive display of willpower, which it is not. It is simply the instinct for self-preservation, yanking us back from the precipice. This is a stronger instinct in some than in others.

C) The Search for Useful Therapy:

i): Straight to a good hypnotherapist. A couple of sessions should nail it in most cases. Three or four at the outside, if there's a conflict.

ii): Long fruitless quest, trying various self-help approaches and inappropriate therapies that don't work for that problem, or therapists that are low on talent. This can reinforce the notion that it is terribly difficult to change the behaviour, when really these are just the wrong methods.

iii): Go into 'analysis' for months or years (really, <u>don't!</u>)

D) Run away: Dramatic change of scenery like going to Australia, Thailand, Bolivia or canoeing down the Congo (often doesn't work, also might get kidnapped or killed is additional drawback).

E) Self-destruction (Does *work*, in one sense, but not necessary: see C.i)

The Simple Compulsive Habit

Actually, most of our behaviour is habitual. Quite a lot of it has a compulsive element to it too, and most of it is useful. The doorbell rings, you head for the door. You just feel compelled to do that, you don't think about it usually. The phone rings, you pick it up. You get up in the morning, you put the kettle on. Why? Did you think that through beforehand, did you analyse it? No. There is no need. Morning means kitchen, kitchen means tea or coffee, kettle is inevitable.

Of course there will be a few people reading this who say very smugly to themselves: "As a matter of fact you are wrong, I don't answer the door. When people telephone me, I just let it ring, I am no slave to the telephone, I don't care about the needs of the person trying to contact me. And I hate the kitchen, I never go there. So you are wrong, don't lump me in with all your helpless compulsive folk, I think for myself!"

Don't you hate people like that, people who just feel they have to disagree with everyone, for no good reason? Actually they are just doing it compulsively! They can't help it, it is another compulsive habit. There are lots of them. These people don't even realise they are doing it. They haven't analysed it, and if you tell them they are just compulsively disagreeing with everything you say, they will immediately deny that, and say: "No I'm not, I am just expressing my true opinion as a matter of fact!" They really believe this too, they are in total denial. In fact they are stuck in total denial concerning everything and there is usually no hope for any of them. The ones who are reading this will not be alarmed about that though, because they will not recognise themselves from that description and don't believe that I am right about any of this anyway. In fact they won't be reading this, they only read websites - the younger ones, that is. The older ones are more likely to be watching television programmes about consumers' rights, or writing letters of complaint to the council, or the local health authority.

Maybe you know someone like this. You can have some fun with them, believe it or not. Challenge them, by saying: "Okay, you claim you are not just disagreeing compulsively. Prove it by agreeing with me just *once*. Just agree with me once, can you do that?" And they will immediately claim that they can, of course they can. Make it easy for them too: state something that no normal person would feel the need to disagree with, like "Democracy is preferable to dictatorship." Then you can enjoy watching them struggle. Watch the inner conflict written all over their face, as the rational part of their mind that knows the generalisation is basically true battles it out with the compulsive (Subconscious) part, which can use the infinite resourses of the creative Imagination to dream up a plausible objection or two, and in the end they will say: "Actually, I don't want to be awkward, but there are one or two potential problems with that statement, it isn't *necessarily* true." And you will say: "See? I told you you are unable to agree with anything!" and they will say "Ah, no – actually it is your fault, for making a statement that is in fact more problematic than it first appears", and at that point you have to resist an overwhelming compulsive urge to bury a fire-axe in their skull, which you suddenly feel would be more gratifying than continuing to converse with them.

We all have moments like this, I think it is healthy to talk about them.

Where was I? Oh yes, simple compulsive habits. Now sudden *impulses*, like the urge to bury a fire-axe in a certain person's skull - whether those impulses are just mild, or overwhelming - these are nothing to do with compulsive *habits*, obviously, for the vast majority. If you happen to be a serial axe-murderer, you may have been about to raise a question there, but I think it is appropriate to regard that kind of compulsive habit as Well Out of the Ordinary, and I'm sure there are lots of other books written about things like that. Please don't come to me, if that is the sort of issue you have. Although someone once did actually, but that is another story. And they had already been through the penal system over that one, so it wasn't a police matter anymore... how did I get onto this? Oh yes, nailbiting, that's what I was about to point out. Nailbiting is another Simple Compulsive Habit, with no beliefs supporting the behaviour.

Okay - I know you're probably a bit curious about the other thing there, but try to get back on track now - a person who bites their nails knows that they have a bad habit of biting their nails. That's it. They don't imagine they are doing it for pleasure, or that it helps them with the stress in their life. They might notice that at times of stress they do it more, but they recognise that as an *anxiety reaction,* which is exactly what it is. Smokers may have that response too. As stress levels increase, they might reach for the cigarettes and smoke more of them. But the smoker may be under the impression that they are doing that on purpose because it helps - and that is a potentially deadly mistake. Stress causes blood pressure to rise, and so does nicotine. The combination can be fatal, and in fact thousands of smokers die each year precisely that way.

Easy Peasy Lemon Squeezy

As far as the brain is concerned, the operation of a compulsive smoking habit and the operation of a nail-biting habit are almost identical, they are both compulsive hand-to-mouth habits. Setting ideas and beliefs aside, and also any consideration of possible consequences, the behaviour itself is the easiest thing in the world for the brain to operate. The Subconscious orchestrates automatic driving behaviour for God's sake, it can direct the chewing of nails or the smoking of a cigarette as easily as it can blink. And of course, the Subconscious can shut the behaviour and the signals down too. The prompting signal is just a part of that operation, it has nothing to do with the chemical composition of either the tobacco smoke or the fingernails.

To eliminate the habit of nailbiting with hypnotherapy we just bring the matter to the attention of the Subconscious, which was simply repeating it on autopilot because it then requires no thinking, no input from the conscious mind at all. We explain that the activity is damaging and that it looks bad, and then ask nicely for the Subconscious to cancel that behavioural programme, since it serves no purpose and the client will be happier without it. I'm summarising of course, I spend quite some time doing that in a real session. Then the Subconscious shuts it down – not because the therapist says so, but because there is no earthly reason to object. The Subconscious isn't stupid, it just has the job of repeating predictable behaviour as part of its normal and extensive repertoire. It doesn't ordinarily analyse or review that sort of thing by itself, but it is certainly happy to change it, if that will help.

The Complex Compulsive Habit

Complexity does not mean difficulty, let's get that straight right away. The human mind is fantastically complex, but that does not make it difficult to work with unless there are significant factors you do not understand. Not understanding how to work with the Subconscious mind makes it very difficult to get rapid changes in human behaviour or outlook, especially if you are dealing with habitual or emotional matters.

So a complex compulsive habit – which is only *potentially* complex, it isn't necessarily so – is really just a simple compulsive habit with a few snags. These are the beliefs and ideas that may be associated with the behaviour both at a conscious and Subconscious level. Now, all you new and would-be hypnotherapists out there, take note: removing these beliefs and ideas at a Subconscious level is essential if you wish to prevent relapse into smoking. A lot of you will know that, but here's the thing: removing them at a conscious level is also important. Don't forget, it was the conscious mind that made a decision to try smoking in the first place. It doesn't control compulsive habits but it did instigate the behaviour initially, so don't leave it out. Both mental departments have their own beliefs and ideas, and they all need addressing if we are going to do a thorough job.

All too often, you see, therapists neglect one side of the mind or the other. NHS quit counsellors will spend ages talking to your conscious mind, and not realise the Subconscious is oblivious to all that. With any habit, like smoking, that will result in very few successes. Some hypnotherapists will roll their eyes at that sort of ignorance, then go ahead and repeat the same mistake in reverse, by hardly talking to the conscious mind at all. How do I know? Because people tell me. I always ask the client if they have used hypnotherapy for anything before, and if they have, then I ask them all about that experience. Most hypnotherapists do the job properly, but some scarcely bother addressing the conscious mind in any detail at all.

Now I know why this is so. It is partly because no-one ever told them it is important, and you can get reasonable enough success rates even if you don't bother. It certainly is quicker not to bother, and time is money after all. Partly it is because they cannot be bothered explaining the same detailed matters hundreds of times a year. But beneath all that is an assumption: since we are not expecting the conscious mind to fix the problem, why bother talking to the conscious mind about it?

Precisely because it was the conscious mind that started it all in the first place, and we don't want it to do that again somewhere later on down the line. If we wish to prevent relapse later, getting rid of the supporting beliefs and suggestions at both conscious and Subconscious levels is essential. Let's do the thing properly, then we won't have to do it all over again later.

Another Little Complication

As well as the 'simple' and the 'complex', there is also the 'emotional' compulsive habit - although these are less common - where the behaviour has a powerful emotional component, such as anger, grief or guilt. Really this is more of a complication than another subgroup, so it can be regarded as part of a complex habit for some people, but it needs flagging up because the effective removal of that factor is absolutely essential or the behaviour will not change permanently. For example, a woman whose drinking habit developed following the death of her child is not going to respond to attempts merely to address her drinking habit as if it was a straight health issue. We have to know what we are *really* dealing with, and get the priorities in line with the particular Subconscious priorities of that individual. Otherwise we can expect our positive suggestions for change to be ignored by that person's Subconscious.

Having said that, a hypnotherapist has to tread carefully with matters like that, because the client may not have intended dealing with that emotional issue when they sought help over their drinking, and may not wish to deal with it either. They may not even be ready to acknowledge its relevance. The best way we can handle it is to explain the situation, make sure they understand and then let them decide how they want to proceed, if they wish to proceed at all. I always remind them that they can also consult a different therapist if they would like a second opinion, and make sure they have all the options clear in their mind. Drinking habits are often easy to change with hypnotherapy if there are no emotional complications, but if there are, we need to address them. It is helpful for therapists to bear in mind that if a person is very reluctant to deal with the emotional component, they probably weren't truly ready to stop drinking anytime soon anyway - even if their conscious mind proclaims that intention. So we weren't likely to get lasting change by any approach as long as that was the case, and nobody likes wasting their time. If the client in that kind of case baulks at addressing deeper issues that are closely connected with their drinking or drug-taking in the therapist's estimation, that's okay, that tells us all we need to know. I then just wish them luck and let them walk, you cannot drag people through a process of positive change.

The Variable Cultural Components

Compulsive habits can also be made more complex by prevailing cultural attitudes towards that particular behaviour, which not only varies from culture to culture, but also varies *within the culture*, over time. To give examples roughly relating to UK culture at this, the start of the 21st Century, compulsive habits may be regarded as:

Socially Permissable: In other words, there is no 'shame' in it. It may not be an admirable tendency, but other people find it easy enough to live with: chocoholics, nail-biting, hair-pulling, cleaning, collecting, hoarding, list-making, performing, attention-seeking, acceptable risk-taking such as skydiving or bungee jumping etc. Tobacco smoking is still just about within this category, but is teetering on the edge of:

Socially Frowned-Upon: In other words, 'shame' and 'blame' more likely: Rocking, and other emotional rituals; the so-called 'obsessive compulsive disorders', gambling, habitual drinking, drug abuse, sexual promiscuity or 'perversions', unacceptable risk-taking such as drink-driving or dangerous driving, lawlessness, theft, fighting, bullying, general anti-social or criminal activity which has become regular, opportunistic, spontaneous or compulsive ("I don't know why I did it really, but that's just me, I'm a *bad* lad" - this self-perception being one of the beliefs that supports the habitual problem behaviour.)

Socially Beyond the Pale: These are impulses and tendencies that are disapproved of even by the people in the previous category. Includes:

Serial murderers, paedophiles, cannibals, psychopaths, international heroin traffickers and mafia bosses etc. Precisely how the heirarchy works within this category is debatable. Is a paedophile worse than a cannibal, or is it the other way around? What we all agree on, though, is that feeling compelled to touch the light-switch thirty times before you can leave the room might be a little intense, but it is just not in the same league as having a severed head in your fridge.

These *really* extreme behaviours can become compulsive habits by the same process that any behaviour can, but these individuals are most unlikely to present themselves for hypnotherapy. We hypnotherapists are most unlikely to regret that fact. If however a serial murderer and sometime cannibal were to go through a deep and meaningful transformation – genuinely - and then become a hypnotherapist themselves, they might become quite good at helping other maniacs to turn away from mayhem and horror, and learn to be piano tuners instead. Or care for the elderly, or something. I'm idly speculating here of course, I'm not suggesting we should put any valuable resources into finding out. Let's not throw open the gates of Broadmoor Prison Hospital on a whim! Oh, you weren't going to. Yeah, fair enough.

By this stage in the book, some of you may have recognised so-called 'attention deficit' tendencies in my mental processing. Before this officially became a disorder it was generally regarded as creativity, or simply having a good imagination. Thank God we now understand that this is wrong, and that new medication can help dreamy people to be less creative, and pay more attention to analytical people who would otherwise bore them rigid. If I'd had the benefit of that sort of medication when I was at school, I might not have been hated quite so much by Mr Whittaker, the mathematics teacher who seemed determined to convince me that I was stupid, when in fact I was just so painfully bored I used to self-harm with a pencil-sharpener blade during his lessons.

Not depressed, not crazy, not even unhappy – just *fucking* bored.

Back to the real explanations

So, we have the behaviour as it operates: the mechanism, including the *impulse* - the signal that prompts the behaviour. Then we have the reaction or attitude of the conscious mind - how it interprets what is going on, and how it has chosen to respond to that so far. Then we may also have to take into account how that kind of issue is perceived - by the operator, and also by the culture. Complexity here means that complications can arise from these various perceptions, as many of them are *misunderstandings* that may involve: unhelpful criticism and proscription, shame, blame, fear, secrecy, denial and damage to self-esteem – all of which need to be taken care of in the ordinary therpeutic process in order to eliminate the problem completely.

I am aware that all this might seem daunting to a person who doesn't normally handle this sort of thing, but to a good hypnotherapist this is all in an ordinary day's work. We do this sort of thing all the time.

Yet another little complication: Secondary Gain

The Compulsive Habit Structure

Some compulsive habitual behaviours may seem simply negative on the face of it, and yet have an 'advantage' to the client that is not immediately obvious to the therapist... or even to the client. For example, a person who has got into the habit of making themselves sick to avoid gaining weight – if they sometimes try to hide this by pretending to be physically ill - may find that they get more attention when they are 'ill' than they normally do, and without realising it consciously, they develop a secondary Subconscious motivation to become 'ill' again, whenever they are feeling a bit neglected. This does not mean, I hasten to add, that people who habitually make themselves sick are 'only doing it for attention', that would be an incorrect interpretation of what I just stated. But if it is a factor in a particular client, and the therapist does not pick it up at first, we can expect a resistance to change from the beginning. On a conscious level, the client may be genuinely unaware of this factor, until in therapy when their Subconscious brings to the table the subject of how little attention they *normally* get, then the penny drops.

In more anti-social behaviour such as the habitual criminal may be repeating, like robbery or drug-dealing, it is not always simply the immediate and obvious gain that is driving the behaviour. For instance, if a gang-member believes, deep down inside, that he would probably be a complete 'loser' in the game of life if he did not have a criminal career, then returning to crime is entirely predictable regardless of what punishments are meted out. Crime not only seems to offer this person far greater financial gain than they expect they could earn legitimately, but criminality and the 'code' of that sub-culture also becomes their identity and belief structure. The world of the lawful then becomes 'another world' which they feel free to plunder because it is a world to which they do not feel they belong, they feel rejected by it. Trying to address the criminal behaviour itself, without helping that person to construct an acceptable alternative identity for themselves is likely to achieve little – unless of course they happen to have reached a point of personal disillusionment with the criminal subculture anyway. Even then, the secondary gain of local status and reputation - and that thing criminals are always whining on about, "respect" - can prove formidable barriers to permanent change. It's all about self-esteem at the end of the day.

It may even be that local status, reputation and respect are actually the primary gain - for some criminals at least - and profit the secondary gain or bonus. Money matters more to some than to others, but everyone would prefer to be highly regarded by their peers. Am I suggesting hypnotherapy could help people turn away from crime more easily? Absolutely, but only if that was their real aim. Targeted at criminals generally across the board hypnotherapy would be a waste of everyone's time, but offered to certain hopeful individuals it could prevent the kind of opportunistic recidivism that is caused simply by 'involuntary' habitual compulsion, by getting Subconscious responses in line with new conscious resolutions. In terms of legal and penal costs it would save far, far more than it would cost to do, and would transform some of those individuals' lives. Just a thought.

To sum up:

The idea that some of our behaviour is outside our control is an illusion caused by the over-estimation of the conscious mind's field of influence, and a lack of understanding of the Subconscious, both of which are pretty universal. This has led to the myth of addiction in tobacco habits, and also gambling, drinking, chocolate-eating and other common repetitive behaviours. Tobacco smoking is not really drug use at all as I have shown, any more than chewing gum is eating. Looks a bit like it, but it's not.

Even where the habitual behaviour does involve drug use – such as alcohol, cannabis, ecstasy, amphetamines and cocaine – the compulsion to repeat the behaviour is not truly withdrawal, as withdrawal is observed in the opiates like heroin and morphine. It is a mental compulsion not a bodily need - even though that compulsion can often be felt as a bodily *experience,* which is obviously the main factor which has caused all the confusion. Just as the overwhelming urge to eat a whole packet of biscuits is not a true bodily need but may feel like hunger, the overwhelming urge to take some more cocaine is also a Subconscious habitual drive. Addiction would be a misunderstanding in either case.

It has often been said that crack cocaine – the freebase, smokable form of the drug – is the most addictive drug there is. Certainly the drug causes enormous trouble socially, in terms of drug *related* crime and violence, not least because the instant high it produces is so intense that the immediate urge to recapture the high can become obsessive. To understand the behaviour properly, though – which is essential if we are going to find real solutions that help the individual to return to a productive, stable lifestyle – it is important to separate the issue of *the harm done in the long run* from the mechanics of *the habitual behaviour as it operates on a daily basis,* otherwise the activity ends up being defined largely in terms of the negative consequences, which is no way to make sense of it. Negative consequences may be no great surprise as an outcome in drug use, just as falling off a motorbike periodically may be no great surprise as a result of riding those machines regularly. But if you try to understand the behaviour of a keen biker through focussing upon the harm that results from the inevitable spills and crashes, you will draw a blank.

In considering illicit drug use, the traditional assumption from a medical point of view is that the extent of the harm that results from this obsessive, repetitious behaviour, coupled with the lack of regard *at the time of using* for the likely consequences, must mean that the drug has "unreasonably come to control behaviour" as the Royal College of Physicians put it when defining addiction/dependence. This is typical of the myopia of the conscious, rational mind - a patronising assumption based upon a dispassionate logical assessment of cause and effect which completely fails to take emotional drives into account and simply comes up with a wrong answer. Where compulsive habitual behaviour is concerned "reason" has nothing to do with it. Every person working in a medical field who also has a smoking habit should know this, because the contradiction involved in that is obviously "unreasonable". Yet the suggestion that *tobacco* must therefore be controlling *their smoking behaviour* is as ridiculous as suggesting that the gambler at the racetrack is controlled by the horses, or that the obsessive-compulsive mentioned above is controlled by the light-switch.

The same compulsive obsession observable in smoking crack, which in that case has been regarded as an effect of the drug, can also be seen at the blackjack table or the roulette wheel, with exactly the same disregard - at the time - for the likely consequences. Later, we may see the same confusion, despair and even suicide in both gambling and drug cases, proving beyond doubt that the apparent lack of concern was only a temporary condition, and since the gambler is not taking a drug anyway, clearly this kind of momentarily reckless, obsessive compulsive behaviour has far more to do with the way the human mind works than the activities it is obsessing about. Drugs might complicate things to some degree, but to simply blame the drug is both dumb and wrong, like blaming the dice for the gambler's ruin. When the gambler blames the dice, the non-gambler knows he is deluded. When the police chief blames the 'evil' nature of crack cocaine, how many people realise that his assumption is precisely the same error?

I have recently been working with a client who had been regularly using cocaine for fourteen years, including smoking crack in large quantities over the last decade. Now, it is important to make clear that I am not making wild claims here, because this case is ongoing, relapses have already occured (of course, just as I would expect in most cases of this sort) and the long-term outcome is still uncertain - but what is very interesting is how this case proves that addiction in cases like this is a misunderstanding, a medical assumption based upon the harm resulting from the behaviour, fear of the problem becoming rife and the general prejudice against illicit drug use which naturally stems from that. And also, of course, the fact that the user keeps returning to the drug despite the problems it causes.

What is most telling about this particular case is that this man would typically behave quite differently in differing circumstances – which on the face of it might make the drug use seem wilful, a deliberate act which he simply 'chose' to do sometimes, but not at other times. The drug habits stemmed from his upbringing in a fairly deprived area where drug use was rife. Habitual drug use was the normality of the

The Compulsive Habit Structure

family he grew up in, which makes some level of involvement almost unavoidable. However, as a young adult he developed a strong ambition to rise above all that, even though that ambition was not shared by the loved ones to whom he was nevertheless very close. A dilemma developed out of this: does he turn his back on his nearest and dearest so that he can stay clear of the drugs and build a new life, or risk getting dragged back into it by staying in touch?

Let's call him Solomon – why not, it's an impressive name. And it may surprise you to know that I like this man, and I really hope he has long-term success. His case is quite complicated, so it is by no means predictable what the outcome may be, but I never write anyone off early in the therapeutic process because experience has taught me that such prejudice can turn out to be quite wrong, which proves it nothing more than prejudice in any case. If you met Solomon socially, you would have no idea he had ever taken drugs. He looks youthful, healthy, very strong, good-looking and is very sociable when the drugs are out of the system. Even though he has been using these substances for years – taking large amounts during binges with other users that can go on for days – in his own case, he has to stop at certain regular intervals because his work is important to him.

Solomon makes very good money in the straight world, and because of that he doesn't have to work all the time. His work is honest and legitimate and he is very successful at what he does. He has a partner with children, and the family home is nowhere near the problem area he grew up in. Yet he remains very close to certain members of his own family, and it is usually when returning to visit them – they never come to his new area to visit him, they never venture off their home turf – that the compulsive urge to smoke crack returns, although it does not always overwhelm him. Sometimes he just visits, and leaves.

When he is working, he is completely away from the scene and uses nothing. This is not self-control: there is simply no way to safely conceal drug use because of the demanding nature of his work, so all cravings (prompts to repeat the behaviour) shut down. He has never found this very difficult, in fact he says it is rather a relief. Obviously if he had any kind of physical dependence upon the drug this would not be so. It is usually shortly after returning home that he typically becomes plagued with obsessive thoughts about cocaine. This is entirely because the urge to recapture the high is once again being generated by the Subconscious, but only because using is no longer ruled out by the greater emotional commitment to professional success and earning-potential, the main source of his prowess and self-esteem. Nothing must be allowed to threaten that directly, Solomon has evidently decided. Also he may have done a deal with himself Subconsciously in the past: as long as he could always prevent it from affecting his work, then using was okay.

Once he is home again, then, there is a terrible conflict: the Subconscious starts prompting the drug use once more, especially in certain situations, whilst the conscious mind – puny by comparison – attempts to oppose that with efforts of will that cannot be sustained for long... we are back to *old habits die hard* again. Notice how this is all going on within his own mind? It has nothing to do with addiction or withdrawal, or else it would surely happen *when he went off to work,* not kick in much later when he came back, after weeks of no cocaine at all, and no conflict.

The first session we did was after a typical binge, when his partner was threatening to kick him out, and indeed she accompanied him to the first session, staying during our initial chat and then leaving us to it. We got on well right from the start, which was a pleasant surprise to them. I think both Solomon and his partner were expecting him to be defensive and guarded upon meeting me, probably because they expected me to be very straight and perhaps a bit nervous about meeting the 'wild crackhead'. I would probably have felt the same at first, if I were him.

Following the initial session, he went away working again and felt very happy, very positive. At the time, he felt certain he would never smoke crack again, and was deliriously happy about that - which is a typical initial reaction after a first session on chronic drug use, which we can confidently expect will be followed by a relapse at some point in virtually all cases. Ending long-term drug habits is usually a process

The Compulsive Habit Structure

involving a number of sessions, and I have yet to see one case in which there was no relapse at all after the first session, which again makes it obvious that drug use is very different from tobacco smoking. The only exception to this is cannabis, which can also commonly be wiped out in a single session where all the factors are favourable. The difference does not lie in the substance itself, but in the social and emotional complications which typically vary from one type of drug to another. These influences shift over time too, both socially and individually.

Relapse should never just be dismissed as 'reverting to type' because it is partly a facet of the very nature of illicit drug use: it is rebellious behaviour in the first place. These people are accustomed to living dangerously, often taking risks that would scare the shit out of straight people, hiding things, lying and breaking the law on a daily basis. They are the least compliant clients we ever work with, and they bullshit others so often they don't even know, after years of it, if they are being honest with the therapist or not. They cannot be sure they are being honest with themselves, and probably don't have any idea if the therapist honestly can help them. Honest is not a concept they can handle with any confidence at all. If they are trying, though, you've got to give them a chance to change. Several, actually. After all they have experienced, if you only give them one chance you're not being realistic. We only have to refer to the many thousands of former drug users who quit the habit, to realise that these people are not hopeless cases just because their problems are complex. Relapses will have been a normal part of all those recovery journeys too.

The only physical symptom Solomon noticed after that first session was heavy perspiration for the first two nights, which surprised him but he was not alarmed or distressed. He interpreted this as 'his body getting rid of the toxins', but his mood was upbeat, so that can hardly be termed 'withdrawal'. What is curious about the heavy perspiration is that it had never happened before. Typically, he never had much trouble with this switch from using to non-using when it came to working anyway, so it can be seen that the assumed 'disregard for the consequences of using' can be conditional, and is therefore not simply caused by the drug. In other words, if the drug was "unreasonably" controlling his behaviour, he would have lost his job ages ago.

I also learned later that he always stopped using for two clear days before returning to work, for reasons I will not specify here, but it does prove that the drug is not controlling him, it is the other way around. I must stress, however, that this is not conscious control (willpower), but a hierarchy of desires. We are seeing conflicting Subconscious emotional drives in play: the old desire to get high being, at key moments, headed off by the new desire for financial and professional success. He also has a desire to be a good family man, but that is sometimes overridden by the desire to get high again. The idea that a person can be a loving, family-oriented person whilst still having a drug habit is an imprint of his own upbringing, but is regularly challenged by his partner. These challenges may have become a cause of Subconscious resentment that sometimes drives him back to 'his own kind', partly to punish her for trying to restrain his excesses (control him), and also due to a periodic crisis of confidence in himself that he really can lead a straight life successfully. After using again, he then comes back to his original dissatisfaction with that, which drives him to seek clean domesticity again. The cycle had been going on for many years.

Just One More Time...

Ironically, it is precisely because this has been going on for years that creates the impression that 'just once more' won't make any difference. In truth, the user has already had that 'just one more' so many times previously that it amounts to hundreds or thousands, it's just that they wouldn't ordinarily notice the reality of that little illusion unless therapy makes it clear, preferably to both mental departments. De Nile is not just a river in Egypt.

Notice, too, that if you remove the whole subject of *consequences* from all this, each drive reveals itself as essentially a *positive intent:* getting high (or in other words, feeling great), being successful and making lots of money, having the security of a loving wife and kids, a nice home in a pleasant area of town, and regularly visiting those members of his family who looked out for him the most when he was little, before they pop their clogs. Now it becomes obvious that the Subconscious is just swapping one aim for another according to the circumstances, and the only difficulty arises out of other peoples' reactions and objections, and his own conscious efforts to sometimes oppose the user-aim of the Subconscious, which creates a mental conflict. Really all this struggle and tension has no more to do with the actual effects of cocaine than the gambler's struggles with himself have to do with the development or outcome of a poker game.

Initial Disappointments

Like many substance abusers, Solomon overreacted to his first relapse after therapy began, mainly out of embarrassment and disappointment with himself. He assumed I would feel the same disappointment and be unimpressed, as if he had let me down or failed in some way. He began missing sessions or cancelling with spurious excuses. Then he turned his back on therapy for weeks, but I was able to keep tabs on the situation through his partner, who kept in touch and also came back later herself to quit smoking. This she successfully achieved in a single session despite her doubts – she had tried to quit by herself many times before – and despite the ongoing uncertainties over her domestic situation, a factor that can sometimes stall success. She is still smoke-free and very happy about that, singing the praises of hypnotherapy to all and sundry... who just look at her like she's raving.

Solomon returned to therapy recently, and we just picked up where we left off. Each relapse only reminds the user of the reasons they wanted to quit in the first place, and subsequent sessions can use these experiences to reinforce the resolve. But if you don't work with the Subconscious, you are reduced to working only with a part of the mind that is not driving the behaviour anyway, and has precious little power to oppose the part that does - which of course creates the illusion that the drug controls the user, and that the user is 'helpless'. It is a very convincing illusion, especially to the outsider. The gambler, by contrast, has no chemical substance to blame, and is just left completely confused about why he keeps 'making the same mistake' again and again, until his wife, kids and business have all disappeared and he is left desolate and alone, with self-esteem several hundred points below zero.

The most significant aspect of Solomon's experience is that when he is not using – which can be for weeks at a time – he is obviously perfectly normal. Indeed he is a strong and successful individual with drive and ambition – and not just the kind of grandiose fantasy that drug-users often ramble about either, because he turns his ambition into real success. Nor is he seeking escape from work 'pressure' when he relapses, he enjoys work. Rather it seems a case of wanting to have his crack and smoke it too.

The 'Getting Away With It' Factor

One more thing which seems almost universal amongst long-term users in these drug-binge relapses – and I suspect this is true in many cases of gambling, criminal activities and serial unfaithfulness too – is the buzz of breaking the rules and getting away with it. Each time the miscreant is forgiven, or the misdemeanor is not even detected, seems to confirm the notion that these behaviours can be consequence-free. Or that the miscreant is so lovable, feared, charming or needed that they will always be forgiven, or be able to talk their way out of it with promises of change. At the same time, there is often a conflicting fear attached to this: that their luck or the patience of others will run out. Then it becomes a tantalising guessing game, over whether all the remaining luck was already used up last time, or whether there might be enough left for Just One More Time...? So real change can be repeatedly deferred until luck really does run out.

Though obviously normal whilst drug-free, when he is using Solomon displays all the typical self-centred user behaviour and crack-head problems, and since most of his fellow users don't have any reason to keep stopping and starting, they just go on like that all the time, which is why everyone assumes they are 'addicted to the most addictive drug in the world, crack cocaine'. It certainly looks like that, especially if you know nothing about the Subconscious mind. In truth, the Subconscious is controlling it all very precisely, just as in the case of the compulsive gambler – but in both cases, completely unaware of the better intentions and rational concerns of the conscious mind with regard to the dangers of continuing.

The conscious mind is analytical, it can easily work out in advance that the further we go down this road, the nearer to disaster we get. But the Subconscious is simply not looking that far ahead, it is just impulsively responding to the situation and the circumstances. And yet, if a stronger Subconscious desire conflicts directly, that may override the impulse with relative ease, but the conscious mind played no part in that, even if it thinks it did. Either way, the Subconscious gets what it desires most of all at the time.

It is important to understand that this repetition of risky behaviour is not stupidity, nor is it self-destructiveness. It is just that these two separate mental departments view the thing differently, and without insight regarding the other part of the mind's standpoint. The Subconscious could easily change the behaviour... but it doesn't do what it's told, it does what it likes, so it might need persuasion. It is not analytical so it does not figure out the full nature and extent of the problem by itself. The conscious mind is analytical, so if it is not hiding its head in the sandy banks of De Nile it is able to work out the problem and the obvious solution, but it doesn't control the behaviour and only has willpower to throw at the problem if no competent therapist is talking to the Subconscious about it. This situation is usually misunderstood as a 'lack of control', when it is really a conflict of aims and a lack of insight, coupled with a tendency to defer change – a tendency which is generally based upon pleasure principles.

So we can clearly see from this that the compulsive urge to 'do it again' is not dependency or addiction, it is simply wrong to regard it that way. Put a compulsive gambler on a desert island by himself, and all thoughts of gambling will vanish for the duration. Put the smoker in hospital for a couple of weeks and they won't find abstinence difficult during that time, because there simply is no opportunity - just like the 'clean' situation when Solomon is working. These observations give the lie to the popular notion that crack cocaine is highly addictive, or that nicotine is more addictive than heroin. Put a heroin addict in any of those situations with no supply of heroin and they will inevitably be ill for a while before they begin to recover. That's addiction - and just to make matters a little more complex, it is a compulsive habit too.

Don't forget the beliefs!

Solomon's stop-start habit is not the usual pattern, it just proves that physical dependence is a misunderstanding, an assumption which is common even amongst users themselves. Do you think they are in a position to have insight? It's not impossible, but denial is far more commonplace, as is the natural impulse to shift the blame away from themselves. Any active Subconscious beliefs such as: *Cocaine makes me feel good* and *If I don't get some cocaine I'm going to have a rotten night* can also be supporting that habitual drive in users, as can the limiting belief *I am a coke-head and I cannot live without it*. Also the Subconscious fear that *If I stop partying I'm going to have to face the fact that my life has fallen apart* can sometimes be playing a part in all of this, as can the Thing you are really running away from in the first place – if indeed there is such a Thing.

Solomon has conflicting impulses: to run away (from the drugs everyone around him was using, the poverty and crime) and also return (to the family members he loves – as well as the drugs), followed inevitably by the impulse to return to his partner, tail between his legs, making promises again. Just because people have drug habits doesn't make them horrible people, you know. It might make them more unhealthy or even make them ill, but it doesn't mean they are evil. How many people in this country drink? When the HM Customs find cocaine by the ton heading into Britain, and warn us it's just the tip of the iceberg, who is all this cocaine for? And the heroin? And the vast amounts of cannabis being grown here in the UK these days, the millions of tablets of ecstasy? Who is it all for? If there are millions of pounds-worth of drugs coming into the UK every year, which certainly wasn't the case when I was born, doesn't it stand to reason there are millions more people regularly using illicit drugs than there was a generation ago? Is that why no-one really gave a toss in the end about Kate Moss snorting coke, even though the tabloids tried to ruin her with the usual hysterical hypocrisy? Have we reached the point where most of the readers just thought: "So?" Isn't it time we updated our stupid old misunderstandings of concepts like "drug user" and "addiction"?

All the typical complications I mentioned above – the user's beliefs - may add up to a significant problem for the individual with the habit, and they may need some expert assistance to overcome it, but the idea that the organic system of their physical being needs more cocaine is as ridiculous as the idea it needs a whole packet of biscuits.

Now, don't misunderstand the message of this book – accidentally or deliberately – by leaping to the conclusion that I am suggesting a session or two of hypnotherapy will magically turn every crack-head into a carefree, relaxed and healthy person, or that I could easily prevent someone from determinedly drinking himself to death by 'hypnotising' him. This kind of assumption has always been the cause of skepticism about hypnosis, and it irritates me so please don't be that intellectually lazy. Hypnosis isn't a treatment, it is an advanced means of communication that allows an opportunity for someone like myself to present a meaningful case for change to that person's Subconscious mind, because we need to win Subconscious approval for the Subconscious-driven behaviour to be changed.

The quality of the argument for change is most important, and it must address any complicating factors such as those explained above, because if we don't win Subconscious approval, we don't get change. A lame or poorly-presented case is far less convincing, so the real talent of a good hypnotherapist is rather like that of the skilled barrister: the ability to construct an appealing and sound argument and present it effectively. But here's the thing: once you win Subconscious approval, change becomes effortless, and is much more likely to be permanent.

It is precisely because these things are not usually being addressed in the conventional treatment of the above issues that change is notoriously slow, temporary or non-existent in the majority of people using other methods.

Relapse should not be regarded as disheartening either, but rather something to be expected as possible at any time. Relapse itself is nowhere near as significant as *how everybody reacts to it,* as I explain in Section 14, Volume II. Hypnotherapy, when it is properly conducted, gives us an opportunity to *work with* the Subconscious as well as the conscious mind - resolving conflicts and creating a much better opportunity for solving the problem and minimising the incidence of relapse, because you simply do not get that kind of opportunity if the Subconscious is not involved in the therapeutic process. Hence the popular belief these changes are 'difficult'.

Oh by the way, there's no such thing as an "addictive personality". This myth has been created by people who don't understand the Subconscious properly and do not work with it, because their training was not really in that area. The truth is, different people's minds have different normal operational modes, and this will be influenced by what they have learned previously *and* what they spend most of their time doing – as well as their innate faculties - so none of it is set in stone. How much their occupational role reflects their mental operational mode, and how much that mode is influenced by their occupation is a bit like the nature/nurture debate, but it is possible to develop the power and influence of any part of the mind, so the negative label of "addictive personality" is a lazy, pejorative misunderstanding.

Some people spend a lot of time with the analytical part of their mind in the driving seat, and consequently less of their behaviour will be driven by the Subconscious, hence less habitual and compulsive behaviour overall. These people will typically be less intuitive, less obsessive and also less imaginative, so they would lack talent in creative roles. They don't understand other people's behaviour if it is not just like theirs, so they do tend to criticise. These people also usually pride themselves on their 'self-control' and their 'common sense', when it would be just as accurate to say that their powerful Subconscious is being under-used. They get more mentally stressed too, and are likely to be a bit too serious or critical for their own good. They may typically excel in finance, legal roles, business and medical careers, but would be less likely to shine in the world of entertainment or in any of the arts. They would never invent anything unless it was a new kind of spreadsheet and they could never be much of a hypnotherapist – not that they would ever want to be.

Many people (including myself) spend half their lives in trance because it is much easier and we can do lots of things at the same time, worry less and be more creative. More of our behaviour will be repetitive and compulsive though, and we will be absent-minded and daydreamy more often. Rulebreaking is more likely in this category, as is impulsiveness, iconoclasm and habits others might regard as obsessive. The imagination plays a much more dominant role in our lives, which means we might be capable of sudden brilliance but are often too disorganised to capitalise on it long term, if left to ourselves, because we get swept away by other ideas too. The boldest examples of this mindset may just occasionally bring about a revolution in conventional thinking - in which case it looks like inspirational genius, but is really just the brilliance of the human imagination, the most powerful engine of creative change on the planet.

How noticable these attributes are in any one individual is all a matter of the degree to which they develop over time, but all these things are normal variations in human development, not disorders at all. And when activities of the conscious mind or the Subconscious are getting a bit out of hand – like in the so-called 'obsessive compulsive disorders' for example – we only need to redress the balance with some enlightening, expert hypnotherapy, because all that is really going on is that one part of the mind was working too hard, and didn't realise it was.

Interlude: Case Mysteries No. 6

What is the secret of great hypnotherapy? Well it isn't timing - that is the secret of great comedy, as is often said. I think the secret of great hypnotherapy is actually sincerity. So, as the old joke goes, if you can fake that, you can't lose. That's what my first hypnotherapy tutor gave me to understand, anyway. I think he was joking, I'm not entirely sure.

There are times, though, when timing can be important too, and although smokers routinely put off quitting attempts by claiming the time isn't right - "I'll quit after Christmas", "I'll quit before I'm 30", "I'll start cutting down after the holidays" - that is not what I'm talking about. To illustrate, I would like to present the case of:

The Otherwise Perfect Client

Some clients are difficult, it has to be said. Not necessarily because they are trying to be, although some apparently are, but often just because they belong to that category of clients I call the Hypnotherapeutically Disadvantaged. There are various types, and I won't list them all here but just give an example of one: the Totally Emotionless client. These people are rare, in fact they may even be a vanishing species. I certainly hope so. If they do vanish altogether, I doubt anyone will even notice, let alone care. Probably they are being quietly strangled one by one, by their nearest and dearest, and the authorities are not bothering to investigate.

I have never actually strangled one - not yet, anyway - but there have been times when I have only just managed to stop myself, by using advanced self-hypnosis techniques like digging my fingernails into the tender part of my wrist, and repeating in my head the suggestion: "I am a professional therapist, I have the patience of a saint, I am a professional therapist..."

The Totally Emotionless is probably the client hypnotherapists dread the most, because their motivation levels are about as close to nil as you can get without a medical crash team bursting in to resuscitate. The whole process of hypnotherapy runs on motivation, you see - aim, desire, hope, excitement, choice, optimism, determination – all fuelling the direction of the session. In short, you need to care, and the Totally Emotionless simply does not seem to care. At all. About anything.

Imagine these sentences muttered slowly in a dull monotone, with numerous unnecessary pauses: "I do want to stop smoking. That's why I've come. To see you. Yes. I've wanted to stop for a while now. My wife stopped. I stopped too. We both stopped. But only for a week. Then I started again. She didn't though. She's still stopped. But I started again. I do want to stop though, I don't want to carry on smoking. It's no good really, is it? I mean I know it's not doing me any good. I don't know why I started again. I suppose it was stupid really, when I don't want to smoke. I mean, obviously I do want to smoke, but I don't want to, if you see what I mean..."

Actually, looking at that now on the printed page the person seems quite talkative. But if you extend the above dialogue over about four minutes, you'll get a clearer impression of the way the Totally Emotionless 'communicates'. Now imagine spending a whole session with that person. My sessions are two *hours*. Now you're beginning to get it. And your fingers begin to twitch, and flex – and let's face it, no jury would convict, would they? Diminished responsibility, temporary insanity... not in the public interest even to go to trial, in fact. But I digress.

Tim – which actually may have been his real name, I don't know, but it certainly wasn't the name he gave me – was not like that. Tim was young and full of life, cheery and bright, and looking forward to being a non-smoker. From the moment he arrived, we were having a lively and intelligent conversation about this whole mad tobacco business, laughing about how sick we felt when we started smoking, how pointless it is and how stupid we must have looked when we were twelve, thinking we were all grown up and vomiting in the park.

Tim took in all the details and explanations with interest and enthusiasm, asking pertinent questions and seeming to be happy with the answers. In fact there was a point where I began to wonder if it was all going a bit too well.

Human communication is a funny thing. When it is stilted it can be awkward and embarrassing, and yet it can go too far in the other direction also, and start to run away with itself, so you feel like it is necessary to slow up a bit, and that's how I was feeling towards the end of that conversation. Hypnotherapy is ridiculously easy, compared to achieving the same results any other way, but even in hypnotherapy there can sometimes be a feeling things are going a bit too smoothly. Sometimes when I get that feeling during the pre-talk, there turns out to be some sort of hitch with the trance section, so I was half-prepared for that, but no - Tim took to the trance section just as happily and effortlessly as he took to everything else. It seemed as if he was indeed the perfect client, and I felt confident of success.

So did he. And so it was with genuine surprise that he found himself calling me up the very next day. I was surprised too, and I made no secret of the fact. He was still smoking, in fact there had been no response at all. This was the point which puzzled me the most, since it is quite rare for no response to happen at all, particularly when the session apparently went well. I was intrigued, and called him back in.

Now there was one thing I knew for sure. Something in particular was causing this. Of course there always is a cause, when there is an obstacle, but I knew this wasn't just one of the usual stumbling blocks that make a second session on smoking necessary in some cases. This, I felt sure, was something I had not seen before, or perhaps something I had been unaware of in the first session.

As it turned out, it was both. When Tim came back, we backtracked over everything we had previously covered and found no problem, just as I thought first time around. But when I asked him once again about his reasons for wanting to stop smoking at this point in his life, he gave me a different answer from the one he gave me in the first session. Originally he had listed all the health reasons for his decision to quit, as most people tend to do, in all probability just telling me what they assume I want to hear. But this time he also mentioned the financial aspect, and explained that money had been a major consideration when he first called me, because he had been forced to re-apply for his own job due to re-structuring at his place of work, and at the time we did the first session, he was not at all sure he was still going to be in work at all.

Nobody should have to re-apply for their own job. It is a horrible idea, the height of corporate ruthlessness. It's your job, you have already got it, it is difficult enough having to go through the process of winning the position in the first place. It is nothing short of cruelty to make you go through all that again just to remain as you are. Once you have got a job, you should be allowed to keep it provided you haven't done anything to make them regret giving it to you in the first place. It is bad enough when an organization decides to make people redundant, through re-structuring, downsizing or personnel-estranging, or whatever they decide next to call it when they fire people. But to make you re-apply for your own job makes it twice as bad, because if they then decide to get rid of you, that makes it seem like it is somehow your own fault!

Tim was a young man. He had a new mortgage, a baby girl and another kid on the way. He was the sole breadwinner. You would never have thought it from the way he carried himself through that first session, but he was worried sick. He didn't mention any of this to me first time around because he didn't think it was relevant. He had come to me to stop smoking, not to moan about his personal woes. He kept it all inside and conducted himself admirably, you never would have guessed there was anything wrong. But at the time of that first session, Tim had already been through the interviewing process and was waiting to find out if he still had a job. Two of his colleagues had already gone.

The Subconscious mind, folks, has an agenda. It consists of all the things that really matter to you, deep down inside, in your heart of hearts. At the top of the agenda are the things that matter most to you right now. Let's face it, for most people stopping smoking is not usually going to be at the top of the agenda, it would be ridiculous to expect it. Your children, the love of your life, your close relatives, your home, your self, your life's work, your best friends, your career, your passion (whatever that is), and as we move down the scale, your dog, your car, your football team, these are the sort of things that may also be significant to the emotional Subconscious. In addition there are new things you may be looking forward to: the trip of a lifetime, your daughter's wedding day, the birth of your first grandchild, your son's graduation. All the things that bring a lump to your throat and a tear to your eye, especially when you've had a couple of vodkas.

There was I, in that first session, enthusiastically encouraging Tim's Subconscious mind to look forward to a wonderful future as a non-smoker: feeling happier, healthier, wealthier and without a care in the world... and all the time he was deeply worried because his livelihood was hanging in the balance. Everything he had worked for - his home, his family and his self-esteem - all on a knife-edge, and no idea which way it was going to go. Until he knew what the future was actually going to be, he couldn't possibly relate to the future I was describing.

If the Subconscious isn't sure what to do, it does nothing. It plays safe, holding a steady course until it does know what to do. During the chat we had in the second session it dawned on me that with all of that awful and sickening uncertainty hanging over his head, there was no way Tim's Subconscious could get on board with me, happily accepting this rosy view of the future when stopping smoking was, comparatively, of precious little immediate significance on the Subconscious mind's list of pressing concerns.

The conscious mind thought it was important, yes - because the conscious mind is not emotional - ever the practical analyser, it had worked out logically that stopping smoking at that point in time would be a good idea whatever the job outcome, since money might be very tight if all income suddenly stopped. Smoking would be a particularly unjustifiable waste then, so why not get rid of it now?

Quite right, very reasonable. But that's not how hypnotherapy works! Fortunately this case had a happy ending, because Tim had secured his job shortly after the first session and so the emotional mood of the second session was far more conducive to optimism, freedom and positive change. He succeeded completely, and ever since then, thanks to Tim, I always remember to check that point - amongst many others - when searching for the cause of a delay in a client's response: "Is there anything important you are waiting to hear about, not sure which way it's going to turn out?" Every now and then, it turns out to be exactly the thing that needs to be addressed, for success to be unlocked.

Could the delayed success in this case have been avoided?

In my opinion, no. When major changes to the usual routines of life are looming, it is not unusual for the Subconscious to delay any response to suggestions to change something that is not an urgent priority. This is not inevitable, but it is no longer surprising to me when it happens. So if no other obvious cause for hesitation is detectable, it is well worth the therapist checking out this angle. Waiting for a house sale to go through, a medical operation coming up, a child seriously unwell, a prosecution pending... these are the sort of nail-biting issues which the Subconscious may regard as needing to be resolved before we can get on with changing something else, and I think this particularly applies to smoking.

What if Tim had lost his job? Well, I would have advised him to leave the issue for a short period to get over the immediate shock, and then once he had become accustomed to the idea that this had actually happened, and could get very practical about turning things around, the session would be more likely to succeed. Trying to do that immediately or during the first week would not be advisable, there would be too much emotional disorientation and if the Subconscious is not quite sure what it should do, it does nothing. However, in a healthy, normal, self-motivated individual it doesn't take long to recover.

NICOTINE: THE DRUG THAT NEVER WAS

A Pause for Breath

Well, that's it for Volume I. Why two volumes, you may wonder? Actually it is because I want people to be able to read my books on the bus, and a 750 page volume is not the kind of thing you can carry around. Also, I wanted to gather all the mild and uncontentious stuff into the first volume, all the things I could simply prove about nicotine through logical argument and the presentation of government figures and statistics, which all prove NRT is useless. It is like a shot across the bows for the people who should not have let that happen.

Volume II is a broadside.

"One day we will have a pill..."

So I woke up this morning, 31st May 2007, looking forward to putting the finishing touches to Volume I and getting it sent off to the lovely people who can magically turn it into a real book, and what do I hear on the radio? A new pill to stop people smoking, called Champix, will be available on the NHS within months. Studies show that half the people taking it successfully stop smoking, they said... a course of tablets over twelve weeks, or something like that. The cost to the NHS is only £160 per course, apparently.

I really hope these promising suggestions turn out to be true. But when Zyban was launched, similar hype was blaring from the newspapers, TV and the radio. The independent evidence I have quoted in this book now only gives it a 12.5% long-term success rate in reality. Since that is poor even within the placebo range, that is not a success rate. How much money was wasted on that? Are we about to get ripped off all over again?

I really hope this new pill turns out to be safer than Zyban and nicotine products. I really hope that the claim for 50% success is not superhyped, or based on short-term trials that do not take relapse rates into account, because that would be bogus marketing aimed at ripping off the taxpayer *again*. As I have shown in this volume, the difference between long-term and short-term quit rates can be as much as 53% to 6%, or in other words, a short-term influence that crumbles into complete and utter failure.

With a single session, good quality hypnotherapy has long-term success rates of 60% and up, for smoking cessation. (With a back-up session in the other 40% of cases, that overall success rate is higher still, but it's just not my style to boast about my real success rates – I refer the reader to my analysis of that matter in *Success Rates*, Section 14 Volume II, which looks at the problems of claiming actual rates for any kind of therapy.) Hypnotherapy is also totally safe, natural and the intelligent way, not only to get rid of old habits like smoking, but also: cannabis and cocaine use, alcohol habits, gambling habits, phobias and anxiety attacks, sometimes depression, confidence issues, sexual issues, emotional problems of all kinds, trauma recovery, stress and stress-related illnesses... well, the list goes on.

Can your new pill do all that, Doc? When is medical science going to stop playing with its chemistry set and grow up? The human being is a fantastically complex organism, not just a bag of chemicals that can be sorted out by chucking other chemicals into the mix. Still, the big drug companies want us to continue believing that chemistry is healthcare, and blindly trusting that doctor knows best, whilst meekly accepting that we lesser mortals should not presume to question this. But in reality the pharmacists and the doctors are so wrapped up in that chemical industry that they are even more dependent on it than the millions of customers popping the pills. Chemicals are not the solution for the human constitution, they are pollution... oh my God I'm turning into a rapper! Time for some self-hypnosis, I need to calm down.

Well, I hope you enjoyed this irreverent romp through the mad world of poison-pushing. I hope to renew the connection with many of you in Volume II, which actually starts out quite reasonable but then kind of goes on the warpath. I do hope it doesn't upset anyone, especially any of those really powerful people in authority. Mustn't upset the people who run the country... no, not the government, silly! I mean the BMA and the Royal Medical Colleges, those totally unaccountable people who scare governments to death. The ones my hypnotherapy instructor warned me never to upset, because they have the power - and certainly the temperament - to destroy the hypnotherapy profession. What he actually said was: "Whatever you do, don't upset the BMA!"

Now that was just a daft suggestion, wasn't it? Like showing me a Big Red Button and saying: "Whatever you do, don't push that!"

This is what I have to say to the BMA. This book is dedicated to those bright and intelligent men who were hounded out of the medical profession for pursuing their sound and promising investigations into mesmerism - which of course later became known as hypnosis - and particularly the brilliant Dr John Elliotson (1791-1868), who was President of the Royal Medical and Surgical Society and one of the Founders of University College Hospital, London, where he became its first Professor of Medicine. You will remember, in Section Five when we learned of recent exciting success for hypnosis in scientific trials from John Gruzelier, Professor of Psychology at Imperial College, London:

"The potential for mind-body medicine is enormous," says Professor Gruzelier, who is about to embark on trials of self-hypnosis for advanced breast cancer and early-stage HIV. "It's non-invasive, easy to teach and to do, and very cost-effective."

Non-invasive. Easy to teach and do. Very cost effective, and the potential enormous. John Elliotson knew that, *one hundred and seventy years ago,* when the Board of Trustees at University College Hospital demanded that he stop his public demonstrations of the medical applications of mesmerism. I tell the full story of what happened to these early heroes of mind-body medicine in Volume II, but the crunch came for Dr Elliotson when in 1838 the Council of the University passed a resolution forbidding the use of mesmerism in the hospital. Elliotson immediately resigned. The Dean of the University tried to persuade him to give up mesmerism so that he could retain his position in the hospital. Elliotson's reply will serve as the note that I hereby nail to the door of the headquarters of the British Medical Association. He declared that the University which he had co-founded:

"...was established for the discovery and dissemination of truth. All other considerations are secondary. We should lead the public, not the public us. The sole question is whether the matter is the truth or not."

Professor John Elliotson was right, and his critics were 100% wrong. Professor John Gruzelier knows it, and so does Dr Malcolm Kendrick and they are not alone. Throughout the medical profession there are thousands of honourable men and women who are genuinely dedicated to the health and wellbeing of the people in their care and are increasingly uneasy about the contradictions between natural, true health and long-term medication. My message to those people, who like myself would be full of admiration for Dr Elliotson's honourable and inspiring declaration, is this: If the overbearing power of an industry, and the prejudice and arrogance of authorities and institutions which refuse to admit they have made mistakes even when it is blindingly obvious - simply because they assume they are so powerful that they just don't have to - make you feel that you had better not say anything, better just keep your head down and keep your opinions to yourself... where is the honour, truth and decency in that? When poisons can pose as medicines, something is very rotten in the state of healthcare.

As I hurl this book straight at the Red Button that is going to set all kinds of alarms ringing at the the BMA - and the FDA, and NICE and all the rest of them - I am inviting all the honourable and decent people in the world of healthcare to reach out and push it too. Push hard, and keep pushing, because:

"The sole question is whether the matter is the truth or not."

John Elliotson, 1838